An Integrated Approach to Drug Discovery and Natural Products

An Integrated Approach to Drug Discovery and Natural Products

Editor: Scarlet Mount

AMERICAN
MEDICAL PUBLISHERS
www.americanmedicalpublishers.com

AMERICAN
MEDICAL PUBLISHERS
www.americanmedicalpublishers.com

Cataloging-in-Publication Data

An integrated approach to drug discovery and natural products / edited by Scarlet Mount.
p. cm.
Includes bibliographical references and index.
ISBN 978-1-63927-870-1
1. Drugs--Design. 2. Drug development. 3. Natural products. 4. Pharmacology.
5. Pharmaceutical chemistry. I. Mount, Scarlet.
RS420 .I58 2023
615.19--dc23

American Medical Publishers,
41 Flatbush Avenue,
1st Floor, New York,
NY 11217, USA

ISBN 978-1-63927-870-1 (Hardback)

Contents

Preface

Every book is a source of knowledge and this one is no exception. The idea that led to the conceptualization of this book was the fact that the world is advancing rapidly; which makes it crucial to document the progress in every field. I am aware that a lot of data is already available, yet, there is a lot more to learn. Hence, I accepted the responsibility of editing this book and contributing my knowledge to the community.

Natural products are an abundant source of various compounds for the discovery of new drugs. They are significant sources of novel drugs and good lead compounds for further modification in drug development process. The complex carbon skeletons and diverse structures of these products have resulted in an increased proportion of natural products that are being used in drug discovery. Natural products and their structural equivalents have made significant contributions to pharmacotherapy, particularly in the treatment of infectious diseases and cancer. Numerous therapeutic agents are derived from chemicals found in nature. Plant-derived medicines have been used to treat a wide range of pathological conditions. Anticancer drugs like vinblastine and taxol, and antimalarial drugs including artemisinin and quinine were discovered from natural products. This book provides comprehensive insights into drug discovery. It is compiled in such a manner, that it will provide in-depth knowledge about the role of natural products in drug discovery. This book will prove to be immensely beneficial to students and researchers in this field of research.

While editing this book, I had multiple visions for it. Then I finally narrowed down to make every chapter a sole standing text explaining a particular topic, so that they can be used independently. However, the umbrella subject sinews them into a common theme. This makes the book a unique platform of knowledge.

I would like to give the major credit of this book to the experts from every corner of the world, who took the time to share their expertise with us. Also, I owe the completion of this book to the never-ending support of my family, who supported me throughout the project.

Editor

1

BIOFACQUIM: A Mexican Compound Database of Natural Products

B. Angélica Pilón-Jiménez, Fernanda I. Saldívar-González, Bárbara I. Díaz-Eufracio and José L. Medina-Franco *

Department of Pharmacy, National Autonomous University of Mexico, Mexico City 04510, Mexico; angiepilon96@gmail.com (B.A.P.-J.); felilang12@gmail.com (F.I.S.-G.); debi_1223@hotmail.com (B.I.D.-E.)

* Correspondence: medinajl@unam.mx;

Abstract: Compound databases of natural products have a major impact on drug discovery projects and other areas of research. The number of databases in the public domain with compounds with natural origins is increasing. Several countries, Brazil, France, Panama and, recently, Vietnam, have initiatives in place to construct and maintain compound databases that are representative of their diversity. In this proof-of-concept study, we discuss the first version of BIOFACQUIM, a novel compound database with natural products isolated and characterized in Mexico. We discuss its construction, curation, and a complete chemoinformatic characterization of the content and coverage in chemical space. The profile of physicochemical properties, scaffold content, and diversity, as well as structural diversity based on molecular fingerprints is reported. BIOFACQUIM is available for free.

Keywords: chemical space; chemical data set; chemoinformatics; consensus diversity plot; drug discovery; molecular diversity; visualization

---

1. Introduction

The significance of compound databases in drug discovery projects is continuously increasing. In fact, compound databases and chemical data sets are a centerpiece in pharmaceutical companies and other academic and government research centers [1]. In addition to their role in compound databases, natural products have been a major resource in drug discovery [2,3]. As reviewed elsewhere, there are several drugs recently approved for clinical use that are natural products or synthetic analogues of hit compounds initially identified from natural sources. A notable example is the fungi metabolite migalastat (Galafold®), approved in 2018 for the treatment of the Fabry disease [4]. Not unsurprisingly, natural product-based drug discovery is being coupled with other major drug discovery strategies such as high-throughput screening and virtual screening. Natural products are again gaining attention in the scientific community to address novel and/or difficult molecular endpoints, for instance, epigenetic targets [5,6].

Several compound databases of natural products have been constructed, curated and often maintained by academic and other not-for-profit research groups. Notable examples are the Universal Natural Product Database (UNPD) [7] and the Traditional Chinese Medicine (TCM) Database@Taiwan [8]. Of note, UNPD is no longer available online but represents the efforts of an academic group to assemble a large natural product database. Reference [4] confirms that there are other compound databases that collect natural products from specific geographical areas and countries, such as NuBBE$_{DB}$ for natural products from Brazil [9] VIETHERB: A Database for Vietnamese Herbal Species was recently released to the public [10]. Other databases of natural products are discussed elsewhere [11–13]. Despite the fact that Mexico also has high levels of biodiversity, there are limited efforts to assemble a compound database of natural products. One example is UNIQUIM, recently reviewed by Medina-Franco [11].

The objective of this work is to introduce BIOFACQUIM as one of the first compound databases of natural products isolated and characterized in Mexico. In this proof-of-concept study, we discuss the assembly of the first version of this chemical data set along with a chemoinformatic characterization of molecular diversity, scaffold content and coverage in chemical space. The compound database is freely available via the web-interface BIOFACQUIM Explorer (https://biofacquim.herokuapp.com/), and is part of an initial effort towards building, updating and maintaining a compound database representative of the biodiversity of Mexico. Compounds in BIOFACQUIM are also available from ZINC15 at http://zinc15.docking.org/catalogs/biofacquimnp/

2. Materials and Methods

2.1. BIOFACQUIM Database

The database of natural products was assembled from a literature search. For the construction of the first version of BIOFACQUIM, the Scopus database (www.scopus.com) was searched using the keywords "natural products" and "School of Chemistry of the National Autonomous University of Mexico (FQ, UNAM)". This search led to a list of scientific papers and researchers that work with natural products. The eight journals that had contributed the most thus far were selected: *Journal of Ethnopharmacology*, *Natural Products Research*, *Journal of Agricultural and Food Chemistry*, *Journal of Natural Products*, *Planta Medica*, *Phytochemistry*, *Natural Product Letters*, and *Molecules*. As part of the search, three filters were used for the selection of the articles in each journal. The first filter was the search by institution (FQ, UNAM), the second was the search by publication year (2000–2018), and the last was the detailed analysis of the articles to identify if the procedure for the isolation, purification and characterization of the compounds from natural products was present. We want to emphasize that this is the first version of BIOFACQUIM; future versions will have natural products from more years, more peer-reviewed journals and more institutions, to achieve a database representative of the biodiversity of Mexico.

With the module 'Wash', from the molecular operating environment (MOE) program version 2018 [14], the database was curated. This was done to normalize and collect the most relevant information from the molecules. The data curation involved the elimination of salts, the adjustment of the protonation states, the optimization of the geometry by energy minimization and the elimination of the duplicated molecules. The default settings of the 'Wash' module were used.

2.2. Reference Data Sets

In order to characterize the diversity of BIOFACQUIM and to explore its coverage in chemical space, seven compound databases of broad interest in drug discovery were used as references. The structure files used in this work were taken from previous comparisons and chemoinformatic analyses of natural products [15]. The structures of the reference compounds were curated using the same procedure described to prepare BIOFACQUIM. Table 1 summarizes the reference databases and the number of compounds. Of note, the reference collections include seven data sets of natural products.

Table 1. Reference databases [15] compared for BIOFACQUIM.

Database	Size [a]
Approved drugs	1806
Cyanobacteria metabolites	473
Fungi metabolites	206
Marine	6253
MEGx	4103

Table 1. *Cont.*

Database	Size [a]
Semi-synthetics (NATx)	26,318
$NuBBE_{DB}$	2214

[a] Number unique compounds after data curation.

2.3. Molecular Properties of Pharmaceutical Relevance

The curated BIOFACQUIM database was characterized by calculating six physicochemical properties of therapeutic interest, namely: molecular weight (MW), octanol/water partition coefficient (SlogP), topological surface area (TPSA), number of rotatable bonds (RB), number of H-bond donor atoms (HBD) and number of H-bond acceptor atoms (HBA). The statistical analysis was done, with the program DataWarrior [16], by calculating the mean, median and standard deviation of the calculated properties. Based on these statistics BIOFACQUIM was further compared with other natural products databases ($NuBBE_{DB}$, cyanobacteria, fungi, marine, and MEGx), approved drugs, and semisynthetic compounds (NATx) (Table 1).

2.4. Scaffold Content

Scaffold content analysis enabled us to identify the most frequent scaffolds in compound data sets and, in this work, to compare the scaffolds containing approved drugs with those containing natural products. The scaffold content analyses also enabled us to identify potential novel scaffolds. The most frequent core molecular scaffolds of BIOFACQUIM were computed using the definition described by Bemis and Murcko [17], in which the core scaffold is obtained by systematically removing the side chains of the compounds. The most frequent scaffolds in BIOFACQUIM were compared with data from the literature (vide infra).

2.5. Visual Representation of Chemical Space

In order to generate a visual representation of the chemical space of BIOFACQUIM, two visualization methods were used: principal component analysis (PCA) and *t*-distributed stochastic neighbor embedding (*t*-SNE). PCA reduces data dimensions by geometrically projecting them onto lower dimensions called principal components (PCs). The first PC is chosen to minimize the total distance between the data and its projection on the PC and to maximize the variance of the projected points.

t-SNE is a nonlinear dimension reduction in which Gaussian probability distributions over high-dimensional space are constructed and used to optimize a Student *t*-distribution in low-dimensional space. The low-dimensional space maintains the pairwise similarity to the high-dimensional space, leading to a clustering on the embedding space without any significant loss of structural information. Further details of each visualization method of the chemical space are discussed elsewhere [18,19]. In this work, for *t*-SNE, subsets of compounds were retrieved from large reference data sets (Table 1), namely: 40 % of the Marine, MEGx, and $NuBBE_{DB}$ data sets (2501, 1641, and 886 compounds, respectively). For NATx and approved drugs, 1000 molecules were used. For cyanobacteria metabolites and fungi data sets the entire databases were employed (473 and 206 compounds, respectively).

2.6. Global Diversity: Consensus Diversity Analysis

Since the chemical diversity strongly depends on the structure representation, it is practical to consider multiple representations for a complete, global assessment. To this end, consensus diversity (CD) plots have been proposed as simple two-dimensional graphs that enable the comparison of the diversity of compound data sets using four sets of structural representations [20]; these are typically the molecular fingerprints, scaffolds, molecular properties, and number of compounds. CD plots have been used to compare the diversity of natural products and other compound data sets [21]. Briefly, in a typical CD plot the scaffold and fingerprint diversity are represented along the y- and x-axes, respectively. The diversity based on whole molecular properties of pharmaceutical interest is represented by a continuous color scale and the number of compounds is mapped into the plot using different size data points. Further details are provided elsewhere [20]. To generate the CD plot of this work, for the y-axis we used the area under the cyclic system recovery curve [22]. For the x-axis, we employed the median of the fingerprint-based diversity computed with MACCS keys (166-bits) and the Tanimoto coefficient. Both are established and are representative metrics of the scaffold and fingerprint-based diversity. Subsets of the compounds were retrieved from large reference data sets (Table 1), considering the size of the databases. For NATx, Marine, MEGx, NuBBE_{DB} and approved drugs, 2000, 1500, 1000, 800 and 700 molecules, respectively, were used. For cyanobacteria metabolites and fungi data sets, the entire databases were employed (473 and 206 compounds, respectively).

3. Results and Discussion

First, we present the results of the construction of the first proof-of-concept version of the BIOFACQUIM database followed by a first chemoinformatic characterization in terms of physicochemical properties, scaffold content, diversity and coverage in chemical space.

3.1. BIOFACQUIM Database

As described in the Materials and Methods section, after the first survey in Scopus with the researchers of the FQ, UNAM, three filters were applied to the eight selected journals. Each of the 92 scientific papers selected was analyzed individually to extract information about the natural products. Of note, in this manuscript we disclose the first version of BIOFACQUIM as a proof-of-concept collection in which current content may be biased by the type of compounds published by a research group (e.g., based on their expertise and/or the analytical techniques available to their groups) and the type of compounds and characteristics accepted for publication by a given journal (e.g., compounds with the biological activity of compounds with drug-like features). It is anticipated that these biases will be reduced as the content of BIOFACQUIM is updated in future releases, by increasing the number of research groups, number of journals and number of years covered (cf. the Conclusions section).

The current version of BIOFACQUIM contains the following information: identification number (ID), compound name, simplified molecular input line entry system (SMILES), reference (with the name of the journal, digital object identifier (DOI) number and publication year), kingdom (Plantae or Fungi), genus, species, and geographical location of the collection of the natural product. In addition, the biological activity, if it was reported in the publication, has been included. The current and first version of BIOFACQUIM has 423 compounds. It should be noted that 316 compounds were isolated from 49 different plant genera, 98 were isolated from 19 genera of fungi, and nine compounds were isolated from Mexican propolis (a sticky dark-colored hive product collected by bees from living plant sources). Figure 1 shows the distribution of compounds per year reported since the year 2000, as contained in the first version of the chemical data set. The compounds in the database that were published in 2018 are not included in Figure 1.

Figure 2 shows the chemical structures of representative compounds from the first version of BIOFACQUIM (discussed further below).

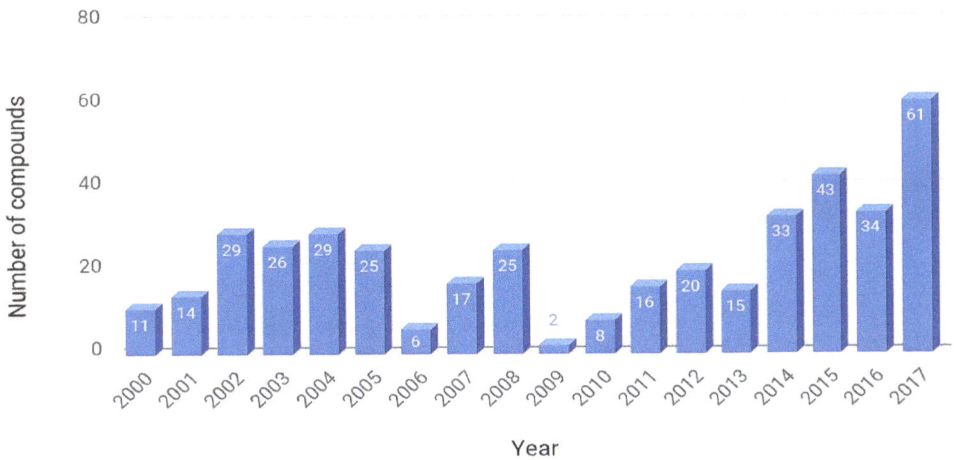

Figure 1. Distribution of compounds reported from 2000 to 2017, as contained in the first version of BIOFACQUIM. Compounds published in 2018 are not shown in this graph.

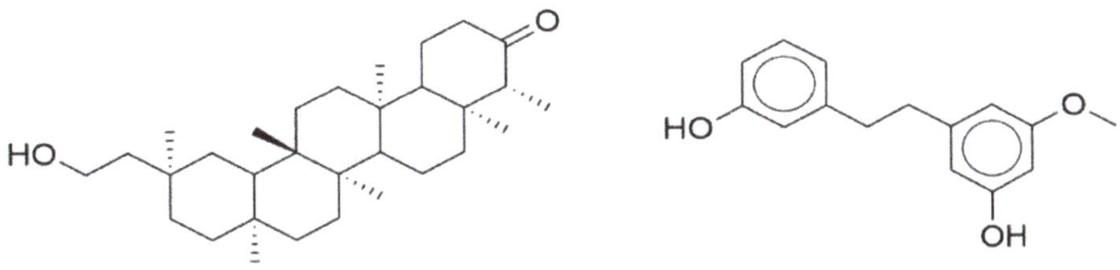

Figure 2. Select compounds contained in BIOFACQUIM.

3.2. Molecular Properties

Figure 3 shows box plots of the distribution of the six calculated physicochemical properties (vide supra) calculated for BIOFACQUIM. For comparative purposes, the box plots also include the distribution of the same properties of the seven reference data sets that were retrieved from the literature [15]. The corresponding violin plots are shown in the Supplementary Figure S3. The three main molecular properties, size, flexibility, and molecular polarity, are described by MW, RB, and SlogP, TPSA, HBA, and HBD, respectively. In these plots, the boxes enclose the data points with values within the first and third quartile; the line that divides the box denotes the median of the distributions. The lines above and below indicate the upper and lower adjacent values. The red asterisks indicate the data points with values beyond the upper and lower adjacent values. Summary statistics are presented at the bottom of the box plots. The figure also includes a table below each box plot with the maximum, median, mean, standard deviation and minimum values for each property and each data set.

According to Figure 3 (and the violin plots in the Supplementary Material), based on the mean of RB, BIOFACQUIM compounds have comparable flexibility to approved drugs. The figure also shows that, except for cyanobacteria metabolites, all databases have a median of up to five rotatable bonds (including approved drugs). The median and mean MW of BIOFACQUIM are 340.5 and 412 g/mol, respectively. Notably, BIOFACQUIM and $NuBBE_{DB}$ have the most similar MW profile compared to drugs. BIOFACQUIM has a median of 4 HBA, the same as that of the $NuBBE_{DB}$ and Marine data sets. Furthermore, BIOFACQUIM has a very similar profile of HBA compared to MEGx. Comparing HBD, BIOFACQUIM, $NuBBE_{DB}$, NATx, and cyanobacteria have the same median values, with similar profiles to approved drugs and higher standard deviations than approved drugs. Regarding TPSA, the compounds in BIOFACQUIM are those that share the closest values to the approved drugs. It should be noted that the cyanobacteria metabolite set has the largest distribution and the highest mean values of TPSA, being the double of the mean of the approved drugs. The distribution of the SlogP values indicates that, overall, natural products are slightly more hydrophobic than approved drugs.

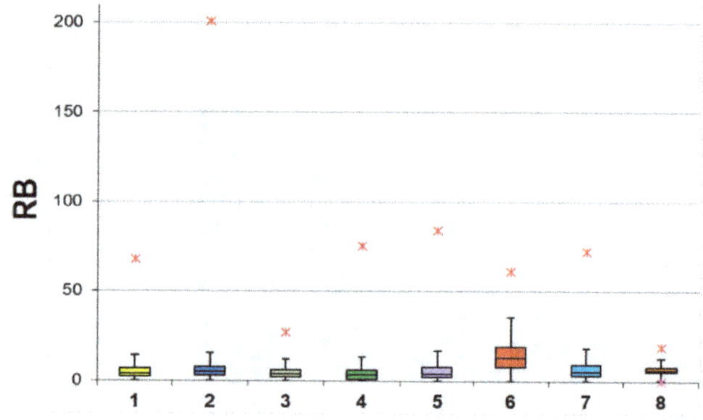

	BIOFQ	App	NuBBE	Fungi	Marine	Cyano	MEGx	NATx
Min	0	0	0	0	0	0	0	0
Median	4	5	4	3.5	4	13	5	6
Max	68	201	27	75	84	61	72	19
Mean	6.2	6.6	4.9	9.4	6.8	14.3	6.8	6.5
Std Dev	8.6	8.3	4.1	18.5	7.9	8.7	6.1	2.3

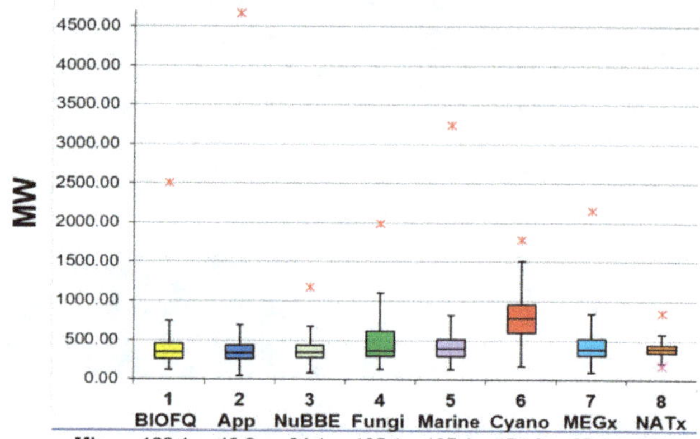

	BIOFQ	App	NuBBE	Fungi	Marine	Cyano	MEGx	NATx
Min	122.1	40.0	84.1	135.1	127.1	174.2	97.1	176.2
Median	340.5	334.3	344.4	364.4	390.4	785.7	388.3	395.4
Max	2501.1	4669.4	1171.0	1993.4	3236.0	1785.3	2151.3	849.0
Mean	412.0	384.6	358.6	528.6	445.2	771.6	451.9	395.4
Std Dev	293.7	255.0	133.1	431.3	238.3	288.4	243.6	65.7

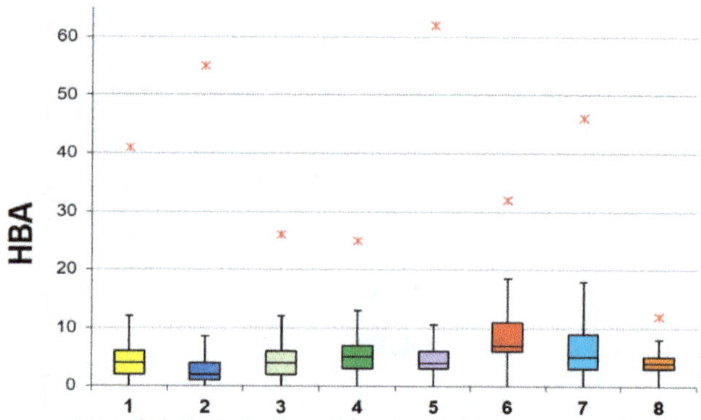

	BIOFQ	App	NuBBE	Fungi	Marine	Cyano	MEGx	NATx
Min	0	0	0	0	0	0	0	0
Median	4	2	4	5	4	7	5	4
Max	41	55	26	25	62	32	46	12
Mean	5.5	3.4	4.3	6.4	4.9	8.1	6.8	3.8
Std Dev	6.2	3.7	3.0	5.4	3.8	4.6	5.9	1.4

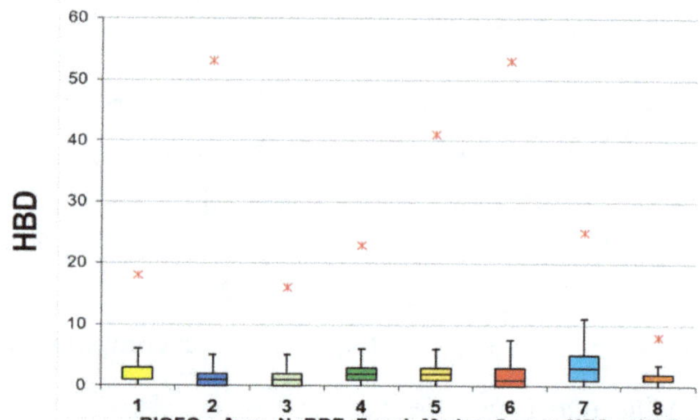

	BIOFQ	App	NuBBE	Fungi	Marine	Cyano	MEGx	NATx
Min	0	0	0	0	0	0	0	0
Median	1	1	1	2	2	1	3	1
Max	18	53	16	23	41	53	25	8
Mean	2.5	1.7	1.6	3.6	2.6	2.4	3.7	1.5
Std Dev	3.2	2.8	2.1	5.4	2.8	3.5	3.6	1.2

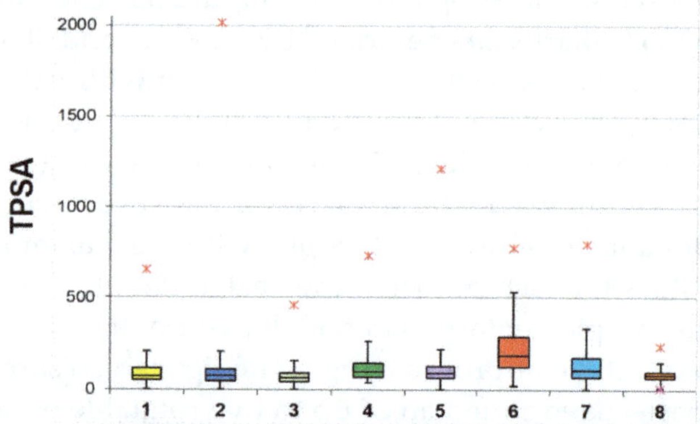

	BIOFQ	App	NuBBE	Fungi	Marine	Cyano	MEGx	NATx
Min	0	0	0	37.3	0	20.2	0	8.9
Median	71.1	75.1	64.6	99.3	88.5	185.6	104.6	79.4
Max	656.9	2014.5	459.4	734.2	1210.7	778.4	798.8	235.2
Mean	104.1	95.5	73.8	152.8	110.3	208.6	136.2	81.9
Std Dev	100.4	102.3	54.0	166.2	87.2	125.5	98.7	26.8

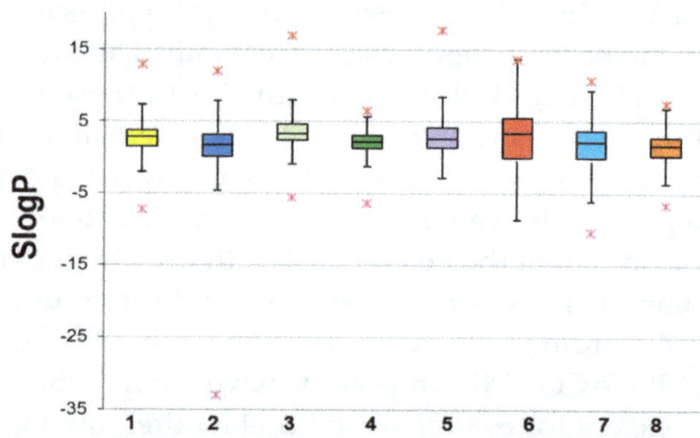

	BIOFQ	App	NuBBE	Fungi	Marine	Cyano	MEGx	NATx
Min	-7.3	-33.0	-5.6	-6.4	-31.0	-12.5	-10.4	-6.6
Median	2.8	1.8	3.4	2.1	2.7	3.0	1.6	1.8
Max	12.9	12.0	16.8	6.5	17.6	13.6	10.7	7.4
Mean	2.9	1.3	3.5	1.9	2.7	2.5	1.3	1.5
Std Dev	3.0	3.4	2.3	2.4	2.7	4.1	2.7	1.9

Figure 3. Box plots for the physicochemical properties of BIOFACQUIM (BIOFQ) and reference data sets (Table 1). The boxes enclose data points with values within the first and third quartile. The red asterisks indicate outliers. Summary statistics are included below each plot. RB: number of rotatable bonds; MW: molecular weight; HBA: number of H-bond acceptor atoms; HBD: number of H-bond donor atoms; TPSA: topological surface area; SlogP: octanol/water partition coefficient.

Taking together the results of the general profile of the properties, it can be concluded that the current version of BIOFACQUIM is, in general, most similar to the $NuBBE_{DB}$ and Fungi data sets. This outcome is in agreement with the findings that, while assembling BIOFACQUIM and analyzing the source papers in detail, the compounds were mostly isolated from plants and fungi.

3.3. Scaffold Content

Figure 4 shows the 27 most populated molecular scaffolds in BIOFACQUIM that included half (50.6 %) of the 423 compounds making up the database. Aside from benzene which is also frequent in several other compound databases [21], the second most frequent scaffold was a flavan-related scaffold (5 %), followed by 1,3-benzodioxole and dibenzyl core scaffolds (2.4 %). Interestingly, the last three frequent scaffolds in BIOFACQUIM are not the most frequent in other databases of natural products [15].

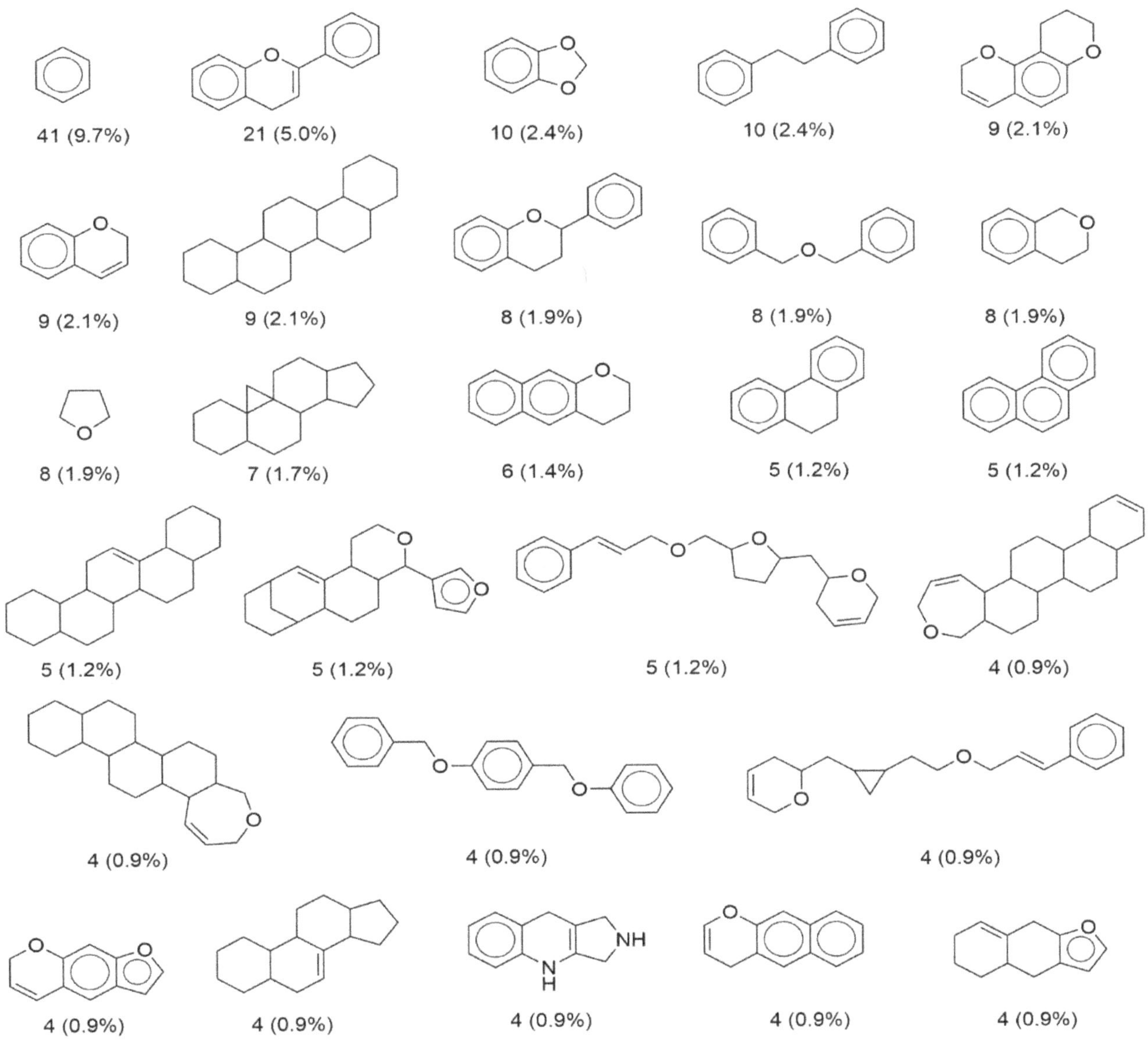

Figure 4. Most frequent scaffolds in BIOFACQUIM. The frequency and percentage are shown. The 27 scaffolds shown in the figure contain half of the total compounds in the database (50.6%).

3.4. Chemical Space

As explained in the Materials and Methods section, a visual analysis of the chemical space of BIOFACQUIM was done with two visualization methods, PCA and *t*-SNE. The visual representation with PCA was based on the physicochemical properties while the visualization with *t*-SNE was based on the molecular topological fingerprints.

3.4.1. Visual Representation Based on Properties

Using the program KNIME [23], we did a visual comparison of the chemical space of BIOFACQUIM and the reference databases. We used the "Normalizer" node in KNIME which gives a linear transformation of all values, the minimum and maximum of each database. Then, PCA was applied to reduce the dimensionality of the six calculated physicochemical properties and to compare BIOFACQUIM with the reference collections (vide supra, Table 1).

Figure 5 shows a visual representation of the property-based chemical space. Table S1 in the Supplementary Material summarizes the corresponding loadings and eigenvalues for the first three PCs. The first two PCs capture 84% of the variance while the first three recover 92% of the variance. Table S1 shows that for the first PC, the larger loadings corresponded to SlogP, followed by RB, whereas for the second PC the largest loading corresponded to HBD.

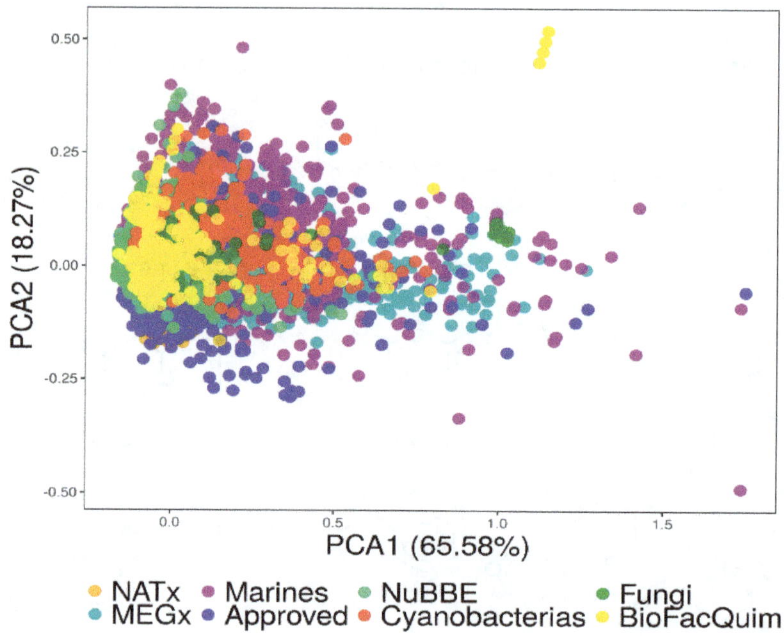

Figure 5. Visual representation of the chemical space based on the physicochemical properties of eight data sets. BIOFACQUIM (423 compounds, yellow); fungi metabolites (206 compounds, green); cyanobacteria metabolites (473 compounds, red); $NuBBE_{DB}$ (2214 compounds, light green); NATx (26318 compounds, orange); MEGx (4103 compounds, blue); marine metabolites (6253 compounds, lilac); US Food and Drug Administration (FDA)-approved drugs (1806 compounds, dark blue).

The visual representation of the chemical space in Figure 5 indicates that some of the natural product compounds occupy the same space as the already approved drugs. It also shows that there are molecules in BIOFACQUIM and the Marine set that cover neglected regions of the currently drug-like chemical space. Finally, Figure 5 suggests that BIOFACQUIM shares the chemical space of almost all Fungi and $NuBBE_{DB}$.

3.4.2. Visual Representation Based on Molecular Fingerprints

Figure 6 shows a visual representation of the chemical space of the current version of BIOFACQUIM based on topological fingerprints using *t*-SNE (see Materials and Methods). Figure 6a compares BIOFACQUIM with all other reference data sets. Figure 6b shows a comparison of BIOFACQUIM with approved drugs. Figure 6a shows three main groups or clusters in which all the databases have compounds. The clusters indicate that the visualization method and the fingerprints can distinguish three major core structures that would have detailed variations in the structure. Figure 6b indicates that there are compounds in BIOFACQUIM with high structural similarity to approved drugs. Notable examples are the compounds FQNP329 (chemical structure in Figure 2), similar to ethinylestradiol (App_75), and FQNP130, similar to choline (App_878). Other comparisons with *t*-SNE are shown in Figure S3 in the Supplementary Material.

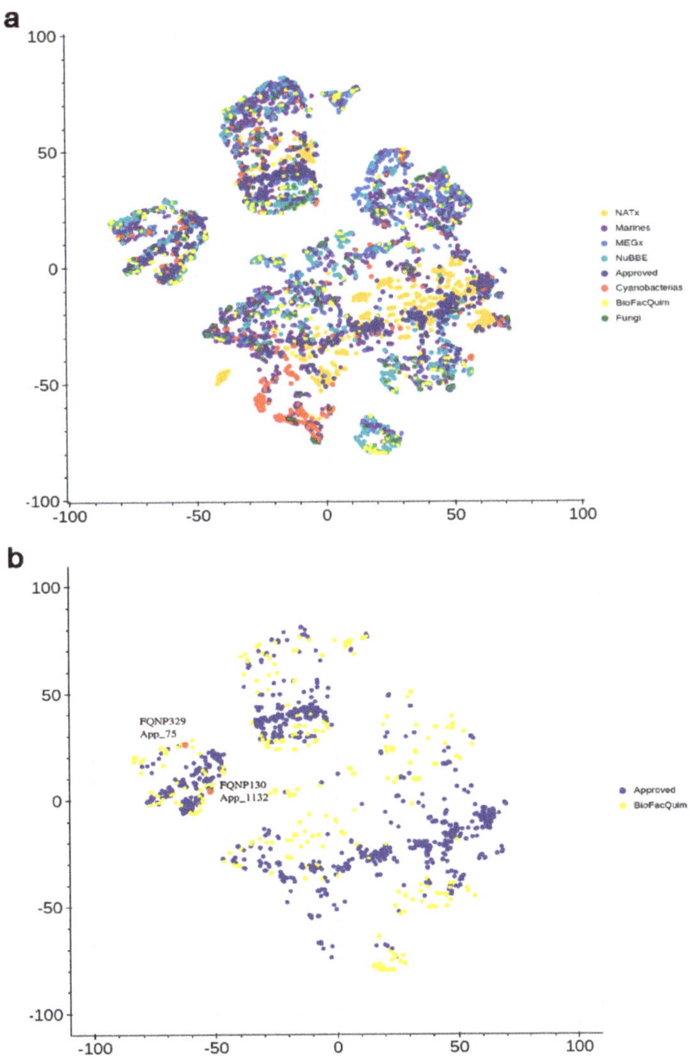

Figure 6. Visual representation of the chemical space of BIOFACQUIM compared with: (**a**) all reference data sets; and (**b**) approved drugs. The visualization was generated using *t*-distributed stochastic neighbor embedding (*t*-SNE) based on topological fingerprints. The red dots indicate the position of two representative compounds of BIOFACQUIM that are very similar to approved drugs.

Based on the assessment of the chemical space, in particular the position of BIOFACQUIM relative to other reference libraries in chemical space, it can be concluded that the compounds in BIOFACQUIM are very similar to drugs, based on their physicochemical properties (PCA) and structural fingerprints (*t*-SNE). Therefore, the chemical space analysis further supports the use of BIOFACQUIM in drug discovery projects.

3.5. Global Diversity: Consensus Diversity Analysis

As elaborated in the Materials and Methods section, a CD plot was used to compare the diversity of BIOFACQUIM with the diversity of the reference data sets, based on molecular fingerprints, scaffolds, and whole (physicochemical) properties. Figure 7 shows the CD plot, representing the

MACCS keys/Tanimoto similarity on the x-axis. Here, lower values indicate larger fingerprint-based diversity (further details of the fingerprint-based diversity assessment are presented in Figure S1 in the Supplementary Material). The y-axis of the CD plot represents the scaffold diversity where lower values (the area under the scaffold recovery curve—see Table S2 in the Supplementary Material) indicate higher scaffold diversity. The property-based diversity of BIOFACQUIM and each database was calculated as the Euclidean distance of the scaled properties. The values are represented on the color CD plot with data points on a continuous color scale. The darker color represents lower diversity while lighter colors represent higher diversity. Finally, the relative size of the databases is represented with different point sizes, where smaller data points indicate data sets with less number of molecules. The CD plot in Figure 7 shows that BIOFACQUIM and Cyanobacteria are found in the area representing low diversity of both scaffold and fingerprints. This may be attributed to the fact that this is the first version of the database. Regarding the diversity, based on physicochemical properties, the cyanobacteria metabolites were observed to have more diversity (e.g., lighter blue data point in Figure 7) than BIOFACQUIM. This is consistent with the analysis of the box plots discussed in Section 3.2. Figure 7 also indicates that approved drugs have high scaffold and fingerprint diversity that is consistent with previous reports [20,21].

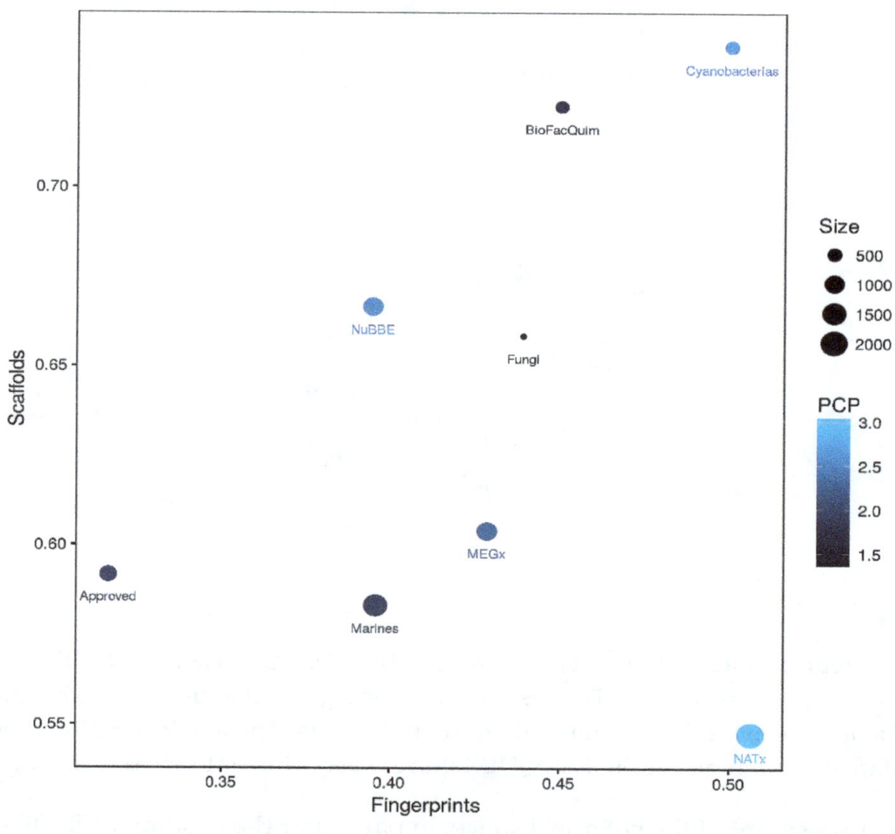

Figure 7. Consensus Diversity Plot comparing the global diversity of BIOFACQUIM with other natural product databases. The structural diversity (fingerprint diversity), calculated with the median Tanimoto coefficient of MACCS keys fingerprints, is plotted on the x-axis. The scaffold diversity of each database was defined as the area under the curve (AUC) of the respective scaffold recovery curves and is represented on the y-axis. The diversity, based on physicochemical properties (PCP), was calculated with the Euclidean distance of six scaled properties (SlogP, TPSA, MW, RB, HBD and HBA) and is shown on a color scale. The distance is represented with a continuous color scale from light blue (more diverse) to dark blue (less diverse). The relative size of the data set is represented with the size of the data point, smaller data points indicate compound data sets with fewer molecules.

4. Conclusions

BIOFACQUIM is a compound database of natural products from Mexico being constructed, curated and maintained by an academic group. The first and current version of BIOFACQUIM includes 423 compounds reported over the past 10 years at the School of Chemistry of the National Autonomous University of Mexico (UNAM). The compound database contains the chemical name, SMILES notation, reference (with name of the journal, year of publication and DOI number), kingdom (Plantae or Fungi), genus and species of the natural product, and geographical location of the collection. In addition, the biological activity, if it was reported in the publication, was included. The chemoinformatic characterization and analysis of the coverage and diversity of BIOFACQUIM in chemical space suggest broad coverage, overlapping with regions in the drug-like chemical space. The analysis also indicated that there are compounds in BIOFACQUIM with chemical structures very similar to drugs approved for clinical use that could, based on the similarity principle, be of pharmaceutical interest. Similar to other natural product databases, BIOFACQUIM can be used, via virtual screening, to identify potential lead compounds or starting points for additional optimization. The database is freely accessible through the website BIOFACQUIM Explorer, version 1.0 (https://biofacquim.herokuapp.com) and is part of the initiative D-TOOLS, described in detail elsewhere [24]. Compounds in BIOFACQUIM are also available from ZINC15 at http://zinc15.docking.org/catalogs/biofacquimnp/

One of the major objectives of this work, currently in progress, is to augment the size of BIOFACQUIM by expanding the search to other universities and research centers in Mexico, increasing the number of years and the number of scientific international peer-reviewed journals covered (with DOI number available). A second major objective of this work is to continue improving and maintaining the web-based interface BIOFACQUIM Explorer following general guidelines for the development and maintenance of public biological databases [25].

Author Contributions: Conceptualization, B.A.P.-J., F.I.S.-G., and J.L.M.-F.; methodology, B.A.P.-J., F.I.S.-G., and B.I.D.-E., formal analysis, B.A.P.-J. and B.I.D.-E.; writing and editing, B.A.P.-J. and J.L.M.-F.; funding acquisition, J.L.M.-F.

Acknowledgments: B.A.P.-J. is grateful for the support given by the subprogram 127 "Basic Training in Research" of the School of Chemistry, UNAM. F.I.S.-G. and B.I.D.-E. are thankful to Consejo Nacional de Ciencia y Tecnología, Mexico (CONACyT) for scholarships, numbers 629458 and 620289, respectively. Discussions with Oscar Palomino-Hernández to implement *t*-SNE are acknowledged. We also thank John Irwin and Khanh Tang for adding BIOFACQUIM in the database ZINC15.

References

1. Miller, M.A. Chemical database techniques in drug discovery. *Nat. Rev. Drug Discov.* **2002**, *1*, 220–227. [CrossRef] [PubMed]
2. Newman, D.J. From natural products to drugs. *Phys. Sci. Rev.* **2018**. [CrossRef]
3. Newman, D.J.; Cragg, G.M. Natural products as sources of new drugs from 1981 to 2014. *J. Nat. Prod.* **2016**, *79*, 629–661. [CrossRef] [PubMed]
4. Saldívar-González, F.I.; Pilón-Jiménez, B.A.; Medina-Franco, J.L. Chemical space of naturally occurring compounds. *Phys. Sci. Rev.* **2018**. [CrossRef]
5. Saldívar-González, F.I.; Gómez-García, A.; Chávez-Ponce de León, D.E.; Sánchez-Cruz, N.; Ruiz-Rios, J.; Pilón-Jiménez, B.A.; Medina-Franco, J.L. Inhibitors of DNA methyltransferases from natural sources: A computational perspective. *Front. Pharmacol.* **2018**, *9*, 1144. [CrossRef] [PubMed]
6. Thomford, N.; Senthebane, D.; Rowe, A.; Munro, D.; Seele, P.; Maroyi, A.; Dzobo, K. Natural products for drug discovery in the 21st century: Innovations for novel drug discovery. *Int. J. Mol. Sci.* **2018**, *19*, 1578. [CrossRef] [PubMed]
7. Gu, J.; Gui, Y.; Chen, L.; Yuan, G.; Lu, H.-Z.; Xu, X. Use of natural products as chemical library for drug discovery and network pharmacology. *PLoS ONE* **2013**, *8*, e62839. [CrossRef]
8. Chen, C.Y.-C. TCM database@Taiwan: The world's largest traditional chinese medicine database for drug screening in silico. *PLoS ONE* **2011**, *6*, e15939. [CrossRef]

9. Pilon, A.C.; Valli, M.; Dametto, A.C.; Pinto, M.E.F.; Freire, R.T.; Castro-Gamboa, I.; Andricopulo, A.D.; Bolzani, V.S. $NuBBE_{DB}$: An updated database to uncover chemical and biological information from brazilian biodiversity. *Sci Rep* **2017**, *7*, 7215. [CrossRef]
10. Nguyen-Vo, T.-H.; Le, T.Q.M.; Pham, D.T.; Nguyen, T.D.; Le, P.H.; Nguyen, A.D.T.; Nguyen, T.D.; Nguyen, T.-N.N.; Nguyen, V.A.; Do, H.T.; et al. VIETHERB: A database for vietnamese herbal species. *J. Chem. Inf. Model.* **2018**. [CrossRef]
11. Medina-Franco, J.L. Discovery and development of lead compounds from natural sources using computational approaches. In *Evidence-Based Validation of Herbal Medicine*; Mukherjee, P., Ed.; Elsevier: Amsterdam, The Netherlands, 2015; pp. 455–475.
12. Tung, C.-W. Public databases of plant natural products for computational drug discovery. *Curr. Comput. Aided Drug Des.* **2014**, *10*, 191–196. [CrossRef] [PubMed]
13. Chen, Y.; Garcia de Lomana, M.; Friedrich, N.-O.; Kirchmair, J. Characterization of the chemical space of known and readily obtainable natural products. *J. Chem. Inf. Model.* **2018**, *58*, 1518–1532. [CrossRef] [PubMed]
14. *Molecular Operating Environment (MOE)*, version 2018.08; Chemical Computing Group Inc.: Montreal, QC, Canada, 2018; Available online: http://www.chemcomp.com (accessed on 28 November 2018).
15. Saldívar-González, F.I.; Valli, M.; Andricopulo, A.D.; da Silva Bolzani, V.; Medina-Franco, J.L. Chemical diversity of NuBBE database: A chemoinformatic characterization. *J. Chem. Inf. Model.* **2019**. [CrossRef]
16. Sander, T.; Freyss, J.; von Korff, M.; Rufener, C. Datawarrior: An open-source program for chemistry aware data visualization and analysis. *J. Chem. Inf. Model.* **2015**, *55*, 460–473. [CrossRef] [PubMed]
17. Bemis, G.W.; Murcko, M.A. The properties of known drugs. 1. Molecular frameworks. *J. Med. Chem.* **1996**, *39*, 2887–2893. [CrossRef]
18. Van der Maaten, L.; Hinton, G. Visualizing data using t-SNE. *J. Mach. Learn Res.* **2008**, *9*, 2579–2605.
19. Osolodkin, D.I.; Radchenko, E.V.; Orlov, A.A.; Voronkov, A.E.; Palyulin, V.A.; Zefirov, N.S. Progress in visual representations of chemical space. *Exp. Opin. Drug Discov.* **2015**, *10*, 959–973. [CrossRef] [PubMed]
20. González-Medina, M.; Prieto-Martínez, F.D.; Medina-Franco, J.L. Consensus diversity plots: A global diversity analysis of chemical libraries. *J. Cheminf.* **2016**, *8*, 63. [CrossRef]
21. Naveja, J.; Rico-Hidalgo, M.; Medina-Franco, J. Analysis of a large food chemical database: Chemical space, diversity, and complexity. *F1000Research* **2018**, *7*, 993. [CrossRef]
22. Medina-Franco, J.L.; Martínez-Mayorga, K.; Bender, A.; Scior, T. Scaffold diversity analysis of compound data sets using an entropy-based measure. *QSAR Comb. Sci.* **2009**, *28*, 1551–1560. [CrossRef]
23. Berthold, M.R.; Cebron, N.; Dill, F.; Gabriel, T.R.; Kötter, T.; Meinl, T.; Ohl, P.; Sieb, C.; Thiel, K.; Wiswedel, B. Knime: The konstanz information miner. In *Data analysis, machine learning and applications: Proceedings of the 31st Annual Conference of the Gesellschaft für Klassifikation e.V., Albert-Ludwigs-Universität Freiburg, Freiburg im Breisgau, Germany, 7–9 March 2007*; Preisach, C., Burkhardt, H., Schmidt-Thieme, L., Decker, R., Eds.; Springer: Berlin/Heidelberg, Germany, 2008; pp. 319–326.
24. Naveja, J.J.; Oviedo-Osornio, C.I.; Trujillo-Minero, N.N.; Medina-Franco, J.L. Chemoinformatics: A perspective from an academic setting in Latin America. *Mol. Divers.* **2018**, *22*, 247–258. [CrossRef] [PubMed]
25. Helmy, M.; Crits-Christoph, A.; Bader, G.D. Ten simple rules for developing public biological databases. *PLoS Comput. Biol.* **2016**, *12*, e1005128. [CrossRef] [PubMed]

2

Eruca sativa Meal against Diabetic Neuropathic Pain: An H_2S-Mediated Effect of Glucoerucin

Elena Lucarini [1], Eleonora Pagnotta [2], Laura Micheli [1], Carmen Parisio [1], Lara Testai [3,4,5], Alma Martelli [3,4,5], Vincenzo Calderone [3,4,5], Roberto Matteo [2], Luca Lazzeri [2], Lorenzo Di Cesare Mannelli [1,*] and Carla Ghelardini [1]

1 Department of Neuroscience, Psychology, Drug Research and Child Health—NEUROFARBA—Pharmacology and Toxicology Section, University of Florence, 50139 Florence, Italy
2 CREA-Council for Agricultural Research and Economics, Research Centre for Cereal and Industrial Crops, 40128 Bologna, Italy
3 Department of Pharmacy, University of Pisa, 56126 Pisa, Italy
4 Interdepartmental Research Centre "Nutraceuticals and Food for Health (NUTRAFOOD)", University of Pisa, 56126 Pisa, Italy
5 Interdepartmental Research Centre of Ageing Biology and Pathology, University of Pisa, 56126 Pisa, Italy
* Correspondence: lorenzo.mannelli@unifi.it

Academic Editor: Pinarosa Avato

Abstract: The management of pain in patients affected by diabetic neuropathy still represents an unmet therapeutic need. Recent data highlighted the pain-relieving efficacy of glucosinolates deriving from Brassicaceae. The purpose of this study was to evaluate the anti-hyperalgesic efficacy of *Eruca sativa* defatted seed meal, along with its main glucosinolate, glucoerucin (GER), on diabetic neuropathic pain induced in mice by streptozotocin (STZ). The mechanism of action was also investigated. Hypersensitivity was assessed by paw pressure and cold plate tests after the acute administration of the compounds. Once bio-activated by myrosinase, both *E. sativa* defatted meal (1 g kg^{-1} p.o.) and GER (100 μmol kg^{-1} p.o., equimolar to meal content) showed a dose-dependent pain-relieving effect in STZ-diabetic mice, but the meal was more effective than the glucosinolate. The co-administration with H_2S scavengers abolished the pain relief mediated by both *E. sativa* meal and GER. Their effect was also prevented by selectively blocking Kv7 potassium channels. Repeated treatments with *E. sativa* meal did not induce tolerance to the anti-hypersensitive effect. In conclusion, *E. sativa* meal can be suggested as a new nutraceutical tool for pain relief in patients with diabetic neuropathy.

Keywords: diabetic neuropathy; neuropathic pain; glucosinolates; *Eruca sativa*; glucoerucin; H_2S; Kv7 potassium channels

---

1. Introduction

The development of neuropathy is a common long-term complication of uncontrolled hyperglycemia and the relief of neuropathic pain still represents a therapeutic challenge in patients affected by diabetes [1]. The management of diabetic neuropathic pain consists basically in improving glycaemic control as a prophylactic therapy and using medications to alleviate pain. Unfortunately, their use is limited by side effects and by the development of tolerance [2,3]. Recent evidence highlighted the beneficial effect of synthetic and naturally occurring H_2S donors in different types of persistent pain [4,5]. Among the natural compounds able to release H_2S there are isothiocyanates, which derive from glucosinolate (GSL) hydrolysis mediated by the enzyme myrosinase (β-thioglucoside glucohydrolase, thioglucosidase, EC3.2.1.147) or by the intestinal microflora [6–8]. These phytochemicals are contained in almost all the plants belonging to the Brassicaceae family and are responsible for many of their beneficial effects in animals, as well as in humans [6,8–10]. The GSL glucoraphanin (GRA) and the derived isothiocyanate sulforaphane (SFN), are the most widely studied due to their potent anti-inflammatory, antioxidant, anti-cancer, antibiotic, as well as neuroprotective effects [6,11–16]. SFN has also been tested in humans, demonstrating an improvement of glucose levels in patients with type 2 diabetes [17]. Nevertheless, its effect on the development of diabetic neuropathy was not studied. Recent findings highlighted the anti-hyperalgesic and protective effects of SFN in an animal model of chemotherapy-induced neuropathy [18] and its capacity to potentiate the antinociceptive effects of opioids in animals with inflammatory pain or diabetic neuropathy [19,20]. As in the case of other H_2S donors, SNF properties are closely related to the release of H_2S in vivo and the consequent activation of Kv7 potassium channels [4,7,18,21–23].

SFN represents a redox couple with erucin, another isothiocyanate which is derived from the metabolism of glucoerucin (GER), the most abundant GSL in *Eruca sativa* spp. oleifera Mill seeds [24–26]. Despite the limited studies on erucin, beneficial properties similar to SFN have recently been reported [27–29], as its ability to release H_2S in vitro and to mediate vasodilatation [30,31]. This also led to assume that the effects showed by SFN in vivo could actually be due to its rapid interconversion to erucin [32]. In 2015 Franco et al. developed a system to obtain a food-safe organic material starting from *E. sativa* (*Eruca sativa* Mill. Sel. NEMAT). This pressure defatted oilseed meal enriched of GSL, suitable to produce bakery products, aimed to realize a functional food [33]. The purpose of this study was to evaluate the antihyperalgesic properties (efficacy and tolerance) of *E. sativa* defatted seed meal (DSM), along with that of its active constituent GER, in a model of diabetic neuropathic pain induced by streptozotocin (STZ) in mice. The involvement of H_2S release and Kv7 modulation in the pain-relieving activity of *E. sativa* derived products were also investigated.

2. Results

2.1. *Eruca sativa* Defatted Seed Meal Characterization

Eruca sativa DSM was characterized in its main components: Proteins, % residual oil and its fatty acid profile, GSL content and profile, total free phenolic fraction, and myrosinase activity. Proteins were the main component of *E. sativa* DSM accounting for 36% *w*/*w* of dry matter. The mild oil extraction brought to a 20% residual oil component in DSM, which was characterized for fatty acid profile and resulted in particularly rich erucic, linolenic, oleic, and linoleic acids (37%; 16%; 15%; 12%, respectively). The GSL content accounted for total 138 μmol g^{-1}, with 98.6 % GER of the total GSLs, and the remaining GRA. Total free phenolic content was 8.9 ± 0.5 mg of gallic acid equivalents (Ge) g^{-1}, according to previous studies [34]. Residual myrosinase activity was 8 ± 2 U, with one enzyme unit (U) corresponding to 1 μmol/g DSM of sinigrin transformed in 1 min. The myrosinase activity was comparable to a previous study [28] and low in comparison to the myrosinase activity of cold extracted *E. sativa* DSM, which was about 24 U [28].

2.2. *Effect of Eruca sativa Defatted Seed Meal and Glucoerucin on Diabetes-Induced Neuropathic Pain*

Figures 1 and 2s how, respectively, the effect of acute oral administration of *E. sativa* DSM (0.1–1 g kg^{-1}) and GER (30–100 μmol kg^{-1}) in STZ-treated animals with and without myrosinase bioactivation. Four weeks after the STZ injection, mice showed a significantly decreased latency to pain-related behaviours induced by a noxious mechanical stimulus (Paw pressure test, Figures 1a and 2a) as well as by a thermal non-noxious stimulus (cold plate test, Figures 1b and 2b), compared with control mice treated with vehicle (Figures 1 and 2). *Eruca sativa* DSM was able to dose-dependently relieve pain in STZ-treated mice, increasing the paw withdrawal latency to the value of controls 30 min after the administration of both doses 0.3 and 1 g kg^{-1}. Furthermore, the higher dose (1 g kg^{-1}) of *E. sativa* DSM showed a long-lasting effect, since the animal's pain threshold was significantly increased up to 90 min after the injection (Figure 1a). The pain-relieving effect of *E. sativa* DSM was also observed in the cold plate test, though it is significant only at the higher dose (Figure 1b). GER, administered in an equivalent dose to that contained in the *E. sativa* DSM (100 μmol kg^{-1}) significantly reduced mechanical hyperalgesia in STZ-treated animals, though it was less effective than the meal. By contrast, the 3-fold lower dose of GER (30 μmol kg^{-1}) was completely ineffective (Figure 2a). The same trend was observed in the cold plate test (Figure 2b). It is worth noting that both the solutions of *E. sativa*, DSM and GER, lost their effect on pain without the myrosinase-mediated bioactivation (Figures 1 and 2).

Figure 3 shows the effect of the repeated treatment with *E. sativa* DSM on STZ-induced neuropathic pain in mice. The defatted seed meal was administered once daily for 8 consecutive days to evaluate the development of tolerance in these animals. The Figure shows the animal pain threshold 60 min after the treatments. The acute pain-relieving effect of *E. sativa* DSM (1 g kg^{-1}) remained constant over time, without the onset of tolerance. On the other hand, the repeated administration of *E. sativa* DSM did not influence the animal basal threshold, which was not different from that of STZ + vehicle-treated animals before the compound administration.

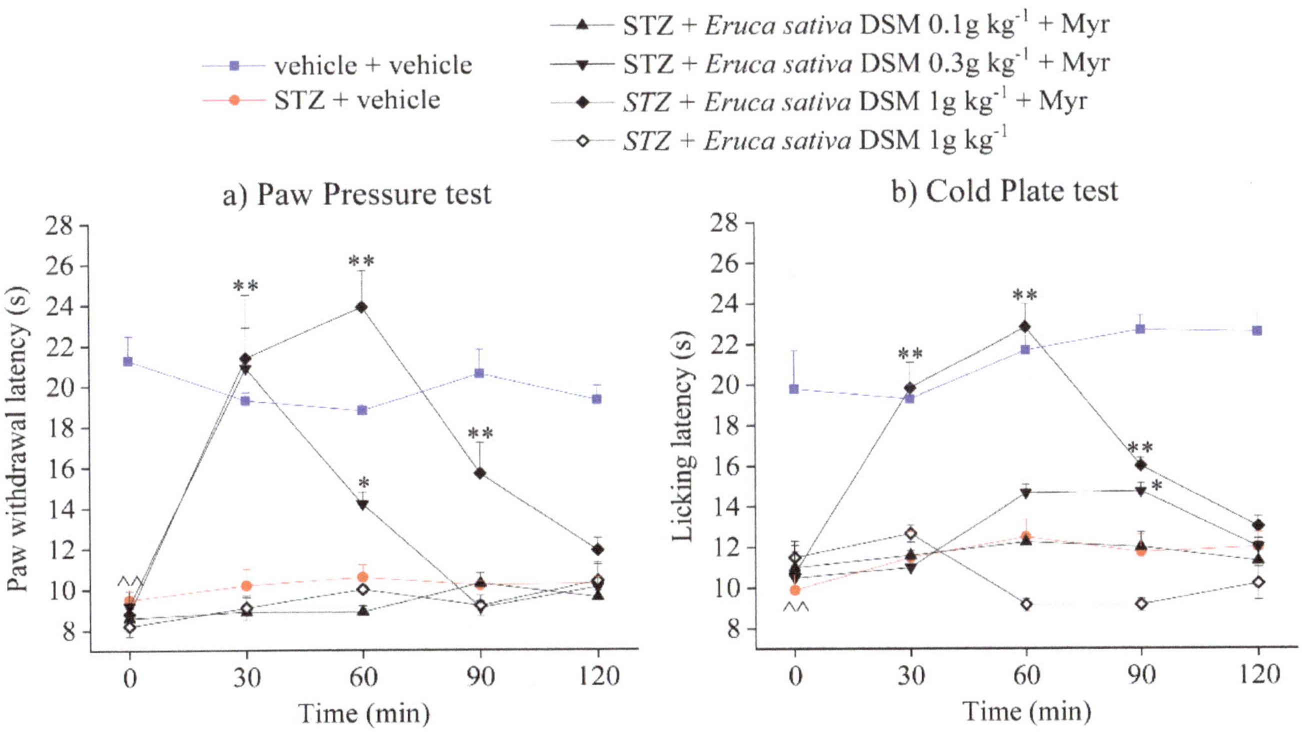

Figure 1. Effect of acute administration of bioactivated *Eruca sativa* defatted seed meal on streptozotocin (STZ)-induced neuropathic pain. The response to both a mechanical and a thermal stimulus was evaluated by measuring the latency (s) to pain-related behaviors; (**a**) withdrawal or (**b**) licking of the paw. *Eruca sativa* defatted seed meal (DSM) (0.1–1 g kg^{-1}) was bioactivated by adding 30 μL mL^{-1} of myrosinase (Myr) (32 U mL^{-1}) 15 min before the oral administration in STZ-treated animals. Tests were performed 30, 60, 90, and 120 min after the injection. ^^ $p < 0.01$ versus vehicle + vehicle-treated mice; * $p < 0.05$ and ** $p < 0.01$ versus STZ + vehicle-treated mice.

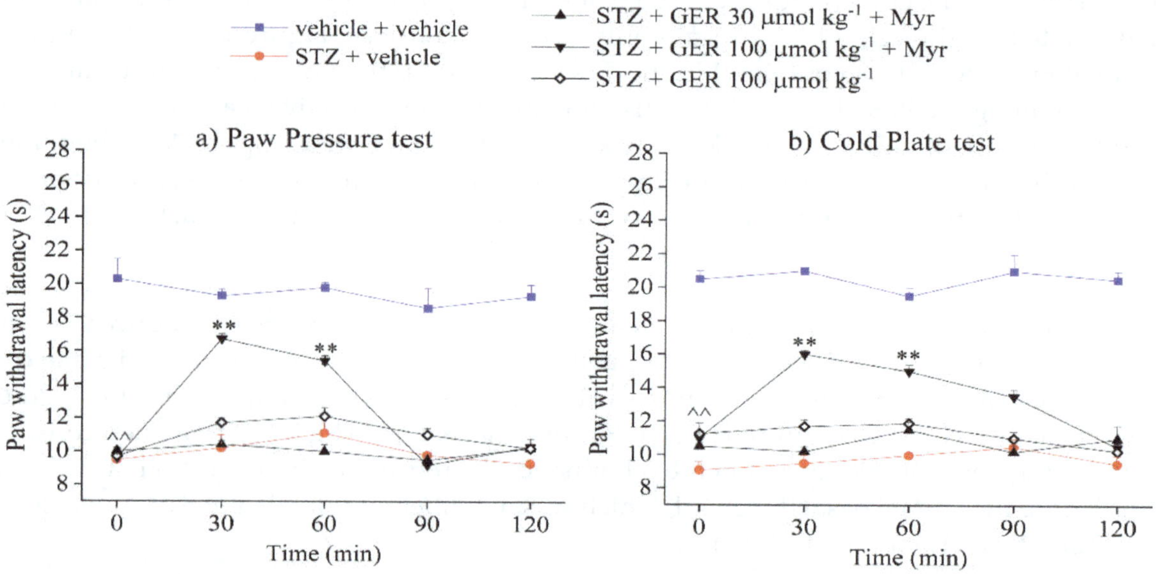

Figure 2. Effect of acute administration of bioactivated glucoerucin (GER) on streptozotocin (STZ)-induced neuropathic pain. The response to both a mechanical and a thermal stimulus was evaluated by measuring the latency (s) to pain-related behaviors; (**a**) withdrawal or (**b**) licking of the paw. GER (30–100 μkg^{-1}) was bioactivated by adding 30 $\mu L\ mL^{-1}$ of myrosinase (32 U mL^{-1}) 15 min before the oral administration in STZ-treated animals. Tests were performed 30, 60, 90, and 120 min after the injection. ^^ $p < 0.01$ versus vehicle + vehicle-treated mice; * $p < 0.05$ and ** $p < 0.01$ versus STZ + vehicle-treated mice.

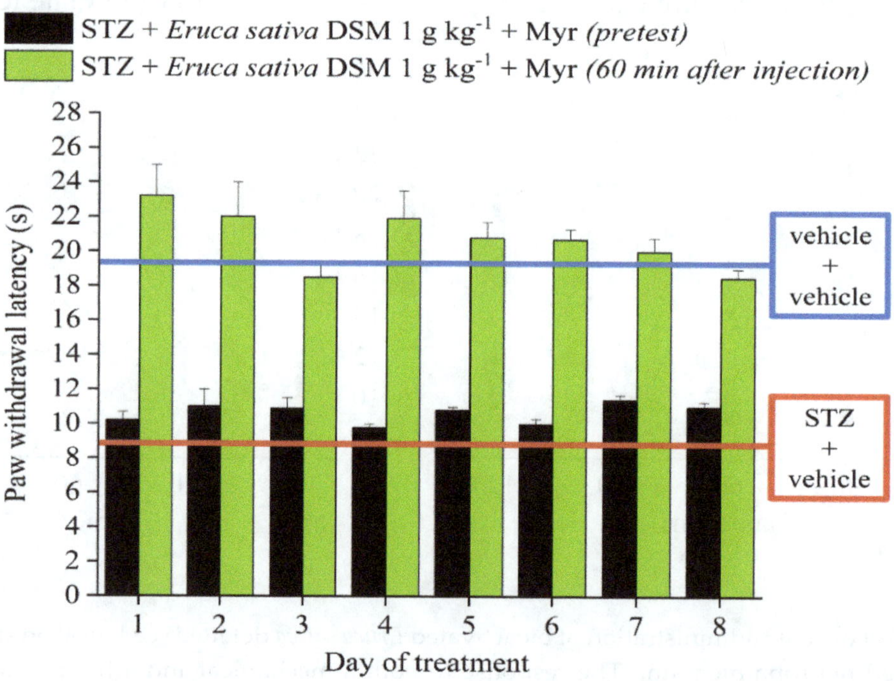

Figure 3. Effect of the repeated treatment with *Eruca sativa* defatted seed meal (DSM) on streptozotocin (STZ)-induced neuropathic pain. The response to a mechanical stimulus was evaluated by measuring the latency (s) to pain-related behaviors (paw withdrawal). The myrosinase (Myr)-bioactivated *Eruca sativa* DSM (1 g kg^{-1}) was administered once daily for 8 consecutive days in STZ-treated animals (once neuropathy was established) and pain threshold was assessed before and 60 min after the injection. ^^ $p < 0.01$ versus vehicle + vehicle-treated mice; * $p < 0.05$ and ** $p < 0.01$ versus STZ + vehicle-treated mice.

2.3. Role of Isothiocyanates and H_2S-Release in the Anti-Hyperalgesic Effect of Eruca sativa Defatted Seed Meal and Glucoerucin

To evaluate the role of H_2S in the anti-hyperalgesic effect showed from *E. sativa* DSM and GER, we administered the compounds in mixture with oxidized glutathione (GSSG), a compound able to bind the isothiocyanates, preventing the release of H_2S [35–37], and hemoglobin (Hb), a molecule able to bind H_2S [38]. The co-administration with GSSG (20 mg kg^{-1} po) was able to fully prevent the anti-hyperalgesic effect of *E. sativa* DSM (1 g kg^{-1}) as well as that of GER (100 μmol kg^{-1}): the pain threshold of animals treated with both these substances in mixture with GSSG was not significantly different from that of STZ + vehicle-treated animals (Figure 4a,b). The same result was observed by systemically administering GSSG (20 mg kg^{-1} sc) in concomitance with the oral administration of *E. sativa* DSM and GER (Figure 4a,b). Both the oral and the subcutaneous administration of GSSG (20 mg kg^{-1}) in STZ-treated animals did not elicit effects on animal pain threshold (Figure S1). The effect of the tested compounds was also abolished by co-administering Hb (300 mg kg^{-1} po) to both products (Figure 4c,d).

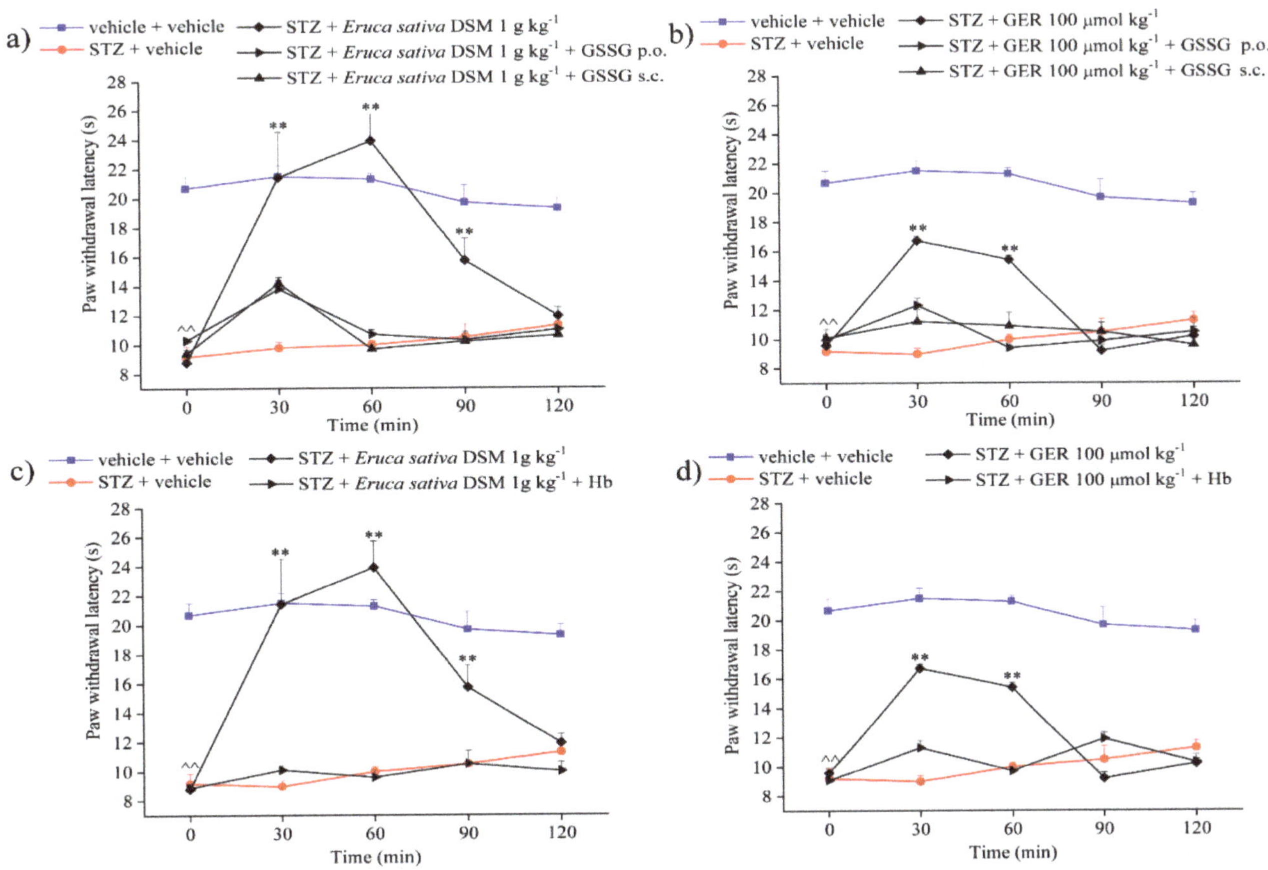

Figure 4. Role of H_2S in the pain-relieving effect of *Eruca sativa* defatted seed meal (DSM) and glucoerucin (GER). The response to a mechanical stimulus was evaluated by measuring the latency(s) to pain-related behavior (paw withdrawal). Oxidized glutathione (GSSG) (20 mg kg^{-1}) was orally and subcutaneously administered in concomitance with both (**a**) Myr-bioactivated *Eruca sativa* DSM (1 g kg^{-1}) and (**b**) GER (100 μmol kg^{-1}); tests were performed 30, 60, 90, and 120 min after injection. (**c**) Myrosinase (Myr)-bioactivated *Eruca sativa* DSM (1 g kg^{-1}) and (**d**) GER (100 μmol kg^{-1}) were orally administered alone or in mixture with human hemoglobin (Hb) (300 mg kg^{-1}); tests were performed 30, 60, 90, and 120 min after injection. ^^ $p < 0.01$ versus vehicle + vehicle-treated mice; * $p < 0.05$ and ** $p < 0.01$ versus streptozotocin (STZ) + vehicle-treated mice.

2.4. Involvement of Kv7 Potassium Channels in the Pain-Relieving Effect of Eruca sativa Defatted Seed Meal and Glucoerucin

To study the involvement of the Kv7 potassium channel in the anti-neuropathic effect of *E. sativa* DSM and GER, the selective Kv7 blocker, XE991, was intraperitoneally administered in concomitance with both the substances. Figure 5 shows the effect induced by *E. sativa* DSM (1g kg^{-1} po) and GER (100 μmol kg^{-1} po) on diabetes-induced neuropathic pain in comparison with that obtained by pre-treating the animals with XE991 (1 mg kg^{-1} ip). The anti-hyperalgesic effect of *E. sativa* DSM and GER was fully prevented by the intraperitoneal administration of XE991, as highlighted in Figure 5a,b, respectively.

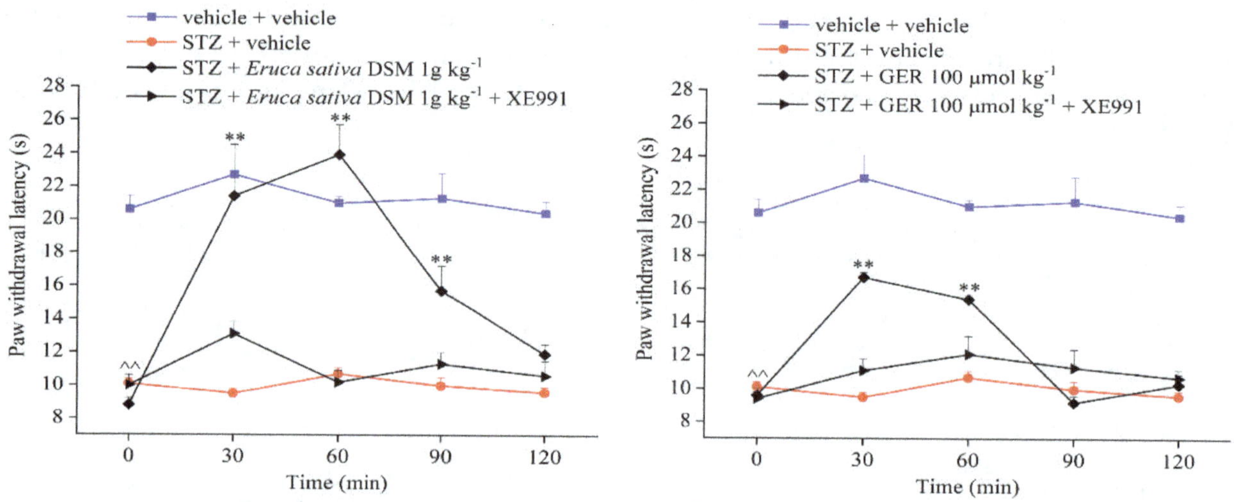

Figure 5. Involvement of Kv7 potassium channels in the pain-relieving effect of *Eruca sativa* defatted seed meal (DSM) and glucoerucin (GER). The response to a mechanical stimulus was evaluated by measuring the latency to pain-related behaviors (paw withdrawal). (**a**) Myrosinase (Myr)-bioactivated *Eruca sativa* DSM (1 g kg^{-1}) and (**b**) GER (100 μmol kg^{-1}) were orally administered in concomitance with XE991 (1 mg kg^{-1} ip); tests were performed 30, 60, 90, and 120 min after injection. ^^ $p < 0.01$ versus vehicle + vehicle-treated mice; * $p < 0.05$ and ** $p < 0.01$ versus streptozotocin (STZ) + vehicle-treated mice.

3. Discussion

This work, for the first time, highlighted the pain-relieving properties of *E. sativa*. In particular, we demonstrated that *E. sativa* DSM, along with its main GSL, GER, can counteract pain in animals affected by diabetic neuropathy induced by STZ. As in the case of other GSLs [18], the effect was mediated by H_2S release and the consequent activation of Kv7 potassium channels. However, the effect of the *E. sativa* DSM was not only attributable to the content of GER, suggesting a synergism between the GSLs and the other phytochemicals contained in this nutraceutical product.

Diabetic peripheral neuropathy is a distressing disease of the nerves in the hands and feet, it is a common complication of both type 1 and type 2 diabetes [1,39]. The symptoms most commonly experienced in these patients are burning, electric-shock type and sharp pains [39–41], while aching, itching, and cold pain are common but less prevalent manifestations [41,42]. These symptoms increase at night, predictably interfering with sleep [43]. In pre-clinical studies, the STZ model of diabetes has been shown to be associated with sensory changes including allodynia and hyperalgesia which develop starting in the few weeks following STZ administration [44,45].

The management of diabetic neuropathy involves maintaining good glycaemic control by drugs as well as by lifestyle modification, like diet and exercise [46–48]. Current therapies aiming to relieve neuropathy-related symptoms, such as pain, are helpful only in one-third of patients with 50% of efficacy [27], often achieved with troublesome side effects and low levels of satisfaction [47,49].

Evidence collected in the last few years supports a diet-based approach in the management of different types of diseases, including chronic pain syndromes [50–52]. Among the most largely studied nutraceutical products there are the GSLs, secondary metabolites that can be found in different concentrations among cruciferous vegetables [6,18]. It is thought that GSLs, together with myrosinase, are a part of a defense mechanism implemented by plants to protect themselves against biotic and abiotic stress [53]. Recently we discovered that GSLs along with their hydrolysis product, isothiocyanates, are strongly effective in relieving neuropathic pain induced by chemotherapy [18]. Interestingly, other natural and synthetic isothiocyanates-based compounds also showed broadly pain-relieving properties in animal models of persistent pain [4,5].

Eruca sativa is an edible plant indigenous of the Mediterranean area that has been traditionally used for its medicinal properties. Similar to other Brassicaceae, the characteristic pungent taste and odor of *E. sativa* leaves were attributed to GSLs. This plant has a high vitamin C content and is known for various health-promoting effects, including improvement of blood circulation, diuretic, and anti-inflammatory properties [27,54–56]. *Eruca sativa* DSM represents an enriched functional food formulated to modulate the release over time of GSLs degradation products, in order to obtain the most effective biological activity [28,57]. Accordingly, we found that the employment of *E. sativa* DSM led to a more strong and long-lasting effect in comparison with GER. The effect of both the compounds is dependent on the bioactivation mediated by myrosinase, indicating as being mainly responsible for pain relief the isothiocyanates derived from the hydrolysis of GER, erucin. The obtained result opened the way to two different hypotheses. The first is that the effect of *E. sativa* DSM is mediated not only by GSLs and the derived isothiocyanates but also by other constituents, as phenols and fatty acids. Indeed, the beneficial effects of antioxidant compounds, such as phenols, against neuropathic pain are well known [58–62]. On the other hand, the effect of *E. sativa* DSM is likely attributable to the GSL content [4,18], since its effect was completely abolished by co-administering the H_2S scavenger as well as by the oxidative cleavage of the isothiocyanate mediate by the disulfide GSSG. In particular, GSSG, systemically administered, was able to prevent the pain-relieving effect, indicating that the isothiocyanate erucin, once adsorbed in the gut, reaches the bloodstream where it probably releases H_2S. On the other hand, the administration of GSSG in a mixture with the bioactivated compounds could prevent its intestinal absorption.

The effect of *E. sativa* was also prevented blocking Kv7 potassium channels, confirming again the direct involvement of GSLs in the pain-relieving effect [4,18].

This evidence, which seems to diminish the importance of the other constituents of the meal own effect on pain modulation, actually move the attention to the second hypothesis, namely that this formulation could be able to modulate the release of the GSLs, improving their pharmacological profile. In fact, it is known that the efficacy of H_2S donors is closely linked to their pharmacokinetics—slower is the release of H_2S, higher is the efficacy [4,5]. This is mainly due to the bell-shape beneficial effect showed by H_2S in the organism [63]. In this context, the peculiar formulation of *E. sativa* DSM could determine a slow release of GSLs, allowing a sustained availability of isothiocyanates and consequently H_2S in vivo, and avoiding quick exhaustion of the pain-relieving effect.

A peculiar feature of GER is that it needs to be preventively bioactivated by myrosinase in solution before the administration in vivo. The same was observed with the *E. sativa* DSM, strengthening once again the importance of its glucosinolates content in the pain-relieving effect. This chemical property makes GER different from other GLSs, such as GRA. In fact, in our previous work, we tested the anti-hyperalgesic effect of this GLS and the derived isothiocyanate, SFN, in a model of neuropathic pain induced by chemotherapy [18]. In that case, we did not have to pre-treat the GLS with the enzyme myrosinase to get the effect. By mixing myrosinase with GER or *Eruca sativa* DSM, we are delivering the isothiocyanate erucin in vivo. It likely means that GER is ineffective. In the absence of myrosinase, GLS can be hydrolyzed to isothiocyanates by the bacteria that constitute the gut microflora. Nevertheless, it was found that the microbiome only supports poor hydrolysis, unless exposed to dietary GLSs for a period of days [64]. On the other hand, the microbiota could not have the time necessary to hydrolyze GER in the lumen if it is quickly absorbed or metabolized in different products in the gut. Anyway, the fact that these compounds need to be bioactivated does not preclude the possibility of using them but it is a point to take into account for the treatment protocol.

Another important point to consider is that the effect of *E. sativa* is eligible only after the acute administration and it does not show a therapeutic effect on the neuropathy, which also persists after the repeated treatment. By contrast, the analog, GRA, and the derived isothiocyanate, sSFN, were able to prevent the development of the neuropathy induced by chemotherapy [18]. This observation suggests that the administration of the GSLs can counteract the pathophysiological mechanisms that lead to the instauration of the neuropathies, such as the oxidative stress [5,65,66], but cannot revert it after its establishment. Anyway, in the case of diabetic neuropathy, it is difficult to apply a preventive treatment at clinical level since this type of disease is a long-term complication of uncontrolled hyperglycemia [2,39,40]. In fact, a proper treatment of hyperglycemia is the most effective and straight forward method to prevent neuropathy in diabetic patients. So, another interesting possibility could be to employ *E. sativa*-derived GLSs as a nutraceutical approach to manage pain in diabetes patients who have already developed the neuropathy, since it still represents a therapeutic problem [48,49]. Indeed, although *E. sativa* does not appear to be a resolving treatment for diabetic neuropathy, its acute anti-hyperalgesic efficacy joined to the characteristics of food supplements suggest its clinical use for treating neuropathic pain as monotherapy or in combination with drugs for sparing dosages and enhance efficacy.

In this perspective, *E. sativa* DSM proved to be a valid innovative formulation to guarantee proper delivery of GSLs in vivo and to enhance their therapeutic efficacy against pain, laying the bases for its rational use in patients affected by diabetic neuropathy.

4. Materials and Methods

4.1. *Eruca sativa* Defatted Seed Meal Production and Characterization

Eruca sativa Mill. Var. NEMAT was grown during the season 2014–2015, within a plot with a size of 1100 m^2, adopting a minimum agronomical input approach [23]. The cultivation was carried out at CREA experimental farm located at Budrio (Bologna) in the Po Valley area (Emilia Romagna region, 44°32′00″ N; 11°29′33″ E, altitude 28 m a.s.l.). The area was characterized by flat land with alluvial deep loamy soil with medium level content of total nitrogen and organic matter content. After harvesting, *E. sativa* seeds were accurately threshed with fixed small-scale threshing equipment and air-dried to reduce the high residual moisture content. *Eruca sativa* seeds were defatted using a small continuous seed crusher machine (Bracco Company model Elle.Gi type 0.90) at a temperature-controlled procedure, during which temperature was maintained at a maximum of 70 °C. *Eruca sativa* DSM was characterized by moisture, proteins, residual oil, GSL, total free phenolic content, and residual myrosinase activity according to the following methods:

(1) Moisture content was determined to evaluate the difference between its weight before and after oven-drying at 105 °C for 12 h.

(2) Proteins were determined from the total content of nitrogen determined using the elemental analyzer LECO CHN TruSpec according to the American Society for Testing Materials (ASTM D5373).

(3) Residual oil content was determined by the standard Soxhlet extraction method using hexane as a solvent and characterized for its fatty acid composition by the UNI EN ISO 5508 method (1998) [67]. Fatty acid composition of residual oil was analyzed after trans-methylation in 2N KOH methanol solution. Fatty acid methyl esters (FAMEs) were evaluated by gas chromatography and the internal normalization method [68] was used for determining the fatty acid profile.

(4) Glucosinolate content was determined following the ISO 9167-1 method with some minor modifications [69]. Briefly, 250 mg DSM were extracted in 70% ethanol at 80 °C. One milliliter of crude extract was loaded onto a DEAE Sephadex A-25 (GE Healthcare, Freiburg, Germany)

mini-column. After washing with 25 mM acetate buffer (pH 5.6), GSLs were desulfated by adding purified sulfatase (200 μL, 0.35 U/mL). The desulfo-GSLs were eluted in water (HPLC grade) and detected in HPLC-UV [69] monitoring their absorbance at 229 nm. They were identified with respect to their UV spectra and retention time, according to our library [70], and their amounts were estimated using sinigrin as an internal standard. Each extraction and analysis was performed in triplicate.

(5) Total free phenolic content was assayed with the Folin–Ciocalteu method according to [71]. Values are the mean ± SD of three independent extractions by four replicates for each measurement. *Eruca sativa* DSM extracts were obtained in acidified ethanol, ethanol/1 N HCl (85:15; *v*/*v*), after 30 min at 21 °C in 40 kHz ultrasonic bath (Sonica Sweep System, Soltec). The supernatants of a triple extraction procedure were collected and maintained at −20 °C in the dark for 48 h to facilitate macromolecule precipitation. Five serial dilutions of the filtered extracts were assayed at 765 nm, 20 °C, in an Infinite M200 NanoQuant Plate reader (Tecan, Switzerland). The slope of each calibration curve was compared to a standard gallic acid calibration curve (range 0.3–27 μg ml^{-1}, $r^2 = 0.9972$). The slope ratio of sample/standard curves was calculated, and results were expressed as mg of GAE per g of DSM.

(6) Myrosinase activity was determined by the pH-stat technique according to [28]. Briefly, 300 mg of *E. sativa* DSM were loaded in 15 mL of 1% NaCl into a reaction cell at 37 °C in a DL50 pH-Stat titrator (Mettler Toledo, Switzerland). The reaction started by adding 0.5 mL of 0.5 M sinigrin solution in distilled water, after 8–10 min of conditioning, and was monitored following NaOH additions used to maintain pH constant at 6.5, versus time in minutes. The assay was carried out in triplicate. One enzyme unit (U) corresponded to 1 μmol/g DSM of sinigrin transformed in 1 min.

4.2. Isolation of Glucoerucin

Glucoerucin was isolated starting from *E. sativa* seeds, as previously described [28]. Briefly, seeds of *E. sativa* from the Brassicaceae collection at CREA-CI, Bologna, Italy [36] were crushed in boiling 70% ethanol and the GSL was isolated as K^+ salt by two sequential steps, including ion exchange and size exclusion chromatography. Isolated GER preparation was analyzed by HPLC-UV after enzymatic desulfation according to [69] and it was identified by UV spectra and HPLC retention times according to our library [70]. The purity of GER was 97% as indicated by HPLC-UV chromatograms and 91 ± 2% on weight basis estimated using sinigrin as an internal standard. It was stored until use at −20 °C. Erucin was produced in-situ through myrosinase-catalyzed hydrolysis, as previously described [30]. Myrosinase (32 U/mL), was isolated from the seeds of *Sinapis alba* L. according to [72]. One unit of myrosinase activity is defined as the amount of enzyme capable of hydrolyzing 1 μmol sinigrin, per min, at pH 6.5 and 37 °C

4.3. Animals

Animals were male C57BL/6 mice (Envigo, Varese, Italy) weighing approximately 22–25 g at the beginning of the experimental procedure were used. Animals were housed in CeSAL (Centro Stabulazione Animali da Laboratorio, University of Florence) and used at least 1 week after their arrival. Ten mice were housed per cage (size = 26 × 41 cm); animals were fed with a standard laboratory diet and tap water ad libitum and kept at 23 ± 1 °C with a 12-hr light/dark cycle, with light at 7 a.m. All animal manipulations were carried out according to the Directive 2010/63/EU of the European Parliament and of the European Union council (September 22, 2010) on the protection of animals used for scientific purposes. The ethical policy of the University of Florence complies with the Guide for the Care and Use of Laboratory Animals of the U.S. National Institutes of Health (NIH Publication No. 85–23, revised 1996; University of Florence assurance number: A5278-01). Formal approval to conduct the described experiments was obtained from the Animal Subjects Review Board of the University of

Florence. Experiments involving animals have been reported according to ARRIVE guidelines [39]. All efforts were made to minimize animal suffering and to reduce the number of animals used.

4.4. Induction of Diabetic Neuropathy in Mice

Mice were intraperitoneally administered with STZ, (Sigma Aldrich, Milan, Italy) 100 mg kg^{-1}, followed three days after with a second dose of STZ 50 mg kg^{-1} [73]. Since streptozotocin has stability problems [74], the solution was prepared immediately before the injection. To maintain cleanliness and avoid the development of any infection due to excessive urination, animal bedding was changed frequently. Pain threshold was investigated each week after the injection of STZ and tests were performed once neuropathy was established in mice.

4.5. Assessment of Mechanical Hyperalgesia

Mechanical hyperalgesia was determined by measuring the latency in seconds to withdraw the paw away from a constant mechanical pressure exerted onto the dorsal surface [75]. A 15 g calibrated glass cylindrical rod (diameter = 10 mm) chamfered to a conical point (diameter = 3 mm) was used to exert the mechanical force. The weight was suspended vertically between two rings attached to a stand and was free to move vertically. A single measure was made per animal. A cut off time of 40 s was used.

4.6. Assessment of Thermal Allodynia

The animals were placed in a stainless-steel box (12 × 20 × 10 cm) with a cold plate as floor. The temperature of the cold plate was kept constant at 4 °C ± 1 °C. Pain-related behavior (licking of the hind paw) was observed, and the time (seconds) of the first sign was recorded. The cut-off time of the latency of paw lifting or licking was set at 30 s [76]. The results were expressed by the licking latency resulting from the compounds acute administration.

4.7. Compounds Administration

Eruca sativa DSM, GER, and myrosinase were produced according to the method described above. Compounds were acutely administered as follows. The doses of *E. sativa* DSM (0.1–1 g kg^{-1} po) were chosen based on previously published H_2S releasing and antinociceptive properties of synthetic and natural ITCs [4,5]. The doses of GER (30–100 μmol kg^{-1} po) used are equivalent to those contained in *E. sativa* DSM (0.3–1 g kg^{-1} po). Both *E. sativa* DSM and GER were bioactivated by adding 30 μL mL^{-1} of myrosinase (32 U mL^{-1}) 15 min before administering them in the animals. Behavioral tests were carried out 30, 60, 90, and 120 min after the injection. Afterward, repeated oral administrations of *E. sativa* DSM (0.3–1 g kg^{-1}) were carried out daily in the mice after the establishment of the diabetic neuropathy. Behavioral tests were performed once daily after the acute administration. In additional experiments, *E. sativa* DSM (1g kg^{-1}) and GER (100 μmol kg^{-1}) were administered in mixture with human hemoglobin 4.6 μmol kg^{-1} (300 mg kg^{-1}; Hb; Sigma-Aldrich, Italy) and with glutathione 65 μmol kg^{-1} (20 mg kg^{-1}; GSSG; Sigma-Aldrich, Milan, Italy). The effect of the subcutaneous administration of GSSG 15 min before *E. sativa* DSM (1g kg^{-1} po) and GER (100 μmol kg^{-1} po) was also evaluated. The Kv7 potassium channel blocker XE991 (Tocris Bioscience, Italy; 2.66 μmol kg^{-1}; 1 mg kg^{-1}; [77]) was dissolved in saline solution and intraperitoneally administered in concomitance with the tested compounds injection.

4.8. Statistical Analysis

Behavioral measurements were performed on 10 mice for each treatment carried out in two different experimental sets. Investigators were blind to all experimental procedures. Results were expressed as mean ± S.E.M. The analysis of variance of data was performed by one-way analysis of variance, and a Bonferroni's significant difference procedure was used as post hoc comparison. p values of less than 0.05 or 0.01 were considered significant. Data were analyzed using the "Origin 9" software (OriginLab, Northampton, MA, USA).

Author Contributions: L.L. and L.D.C.M. designed the experimental protocol. E.L. and C.P. performed the experiments. E.P. and R.M. provided the compounds used in the work and their characterization. L.T., A.M., and L.M. collaborated in the data analysis and in the conceptualization of the project. The main manuscript was written by E.L., L.D.C.M., and extended by E.P., C.G. and V.C. performed the statistical analysis and revised the manuscript.

References

1. Abbott, C.A.; Malik, R.A.; Van Ross, E.R.; Kulkarni, J.; Boulton, A.J. Prevalence and characteristics of painful diabetic neuropathy in a large community based diabetic population in the U.K. *Diabetes Care* **2011**, *34*, 2220–2224. [CrossRef] [PubMed]
2. Tesfaye, S.; Boulton, A.J.; Dickenson, A.H. Mechanisms and management of diabetic painful distal symmetrical polyneuropathy. *Diabetes Care* **2013**, *36*, 2456–2465. [CrossRef] [PubMed]
3. Boyle, J.; Eriksson, M.E.; Gribble, L.; Gouni, R.; Johnsen, S.; Coppini, D.V.; Kerr, D. Randomized, placebo-controlled comparison of amitriptyline, duloxetine, and pregabalin in patients with chronic diabetic peripheral neuropathic pain: Impact on pain, polysomnographic sleep, daytime functioning, and quality of life. *Diabetes Care* **2012**, *35*, 2451–2458. [CrossRef]
4. Di Cesare Mannelli, L.; Lucarini, E.; Micheli, L.; Mosca, I.; Ambrosino, P.; Soldovieri, M.V.; Martelli, A.; Testai, L.; Taglialatela, M.; Calderone, V.; et al. Effects of natural and synthetic isothiocyanate-based H_2S-releasers against chemotherapy-induced neuropathic pain: Role of Kv7 potassium channels. *Neuropharmacology* **2017**, *121*, 49–59. [CrossRef] [PubMed]
5. Lucarini, E.; Micheli, L.; Martelli, A.; Testai, L.; Calderone, V.; Ghelardini, C.; Di Cesare Mannelli, L. Efficacy of isothiocyanate-based compounds on different forms of persistent pain. *J. Pain Res.* **2018**, *11*, 2905–2913. [CrossRef] [PubMed]
6. Dinkova-Kostova, A.T.; Kostov, R.V. Glucosinolates and isothiocyanates in health and disease. *Trends Mol. Med.* **2012**, *18*, 337–347. [CrossRef] [PubMed]
7. Citi, V.; Martelli, A.; Testai, L.; Marino, A.; Breschi, M.C.; Calderone, V. Hydrogen sulfide releasing capacity of natural isothiocyanates: Is it a reliable explanation for the multiple biological effects of Brassicaceae? *Planta Medica* **2014**, *80*, 610–613. [CrossRef] [PubMed]
8. Mithen, R.; Ho, E. Isothiocyanates for Human Health. *Mol. Nutr. Food Res.* **2018**, *62*, 1870079. [CrossRef] [PubMed]
9. Ishida, M.; Hara, M.; Fukino, N.; Kakizaki, T.; Morimitsu, Y. Glucosinolate metabolism, functionality and breeding for the improvement of Brassicaceae vegetables. *Breed. Sci.* **2014**, *64*, 48–59. [CrossRef]
10. Fahey, J.W.; Wade, K.L.; Wehage, S.L.; Holtzclaw, W.D.; Liu, H.; Talalay, P.; Fuchs, E.; Stephenson, K.K. Stabilized sulforaphane for clinical use: Phytochemical delivery efficiency. *Mol. Nutr. Food Res* **2017**, *61*, 1600766. [CrossRef] [PubMed]
11. Guerrero-Beltran, C.E.; Calderon-Oliver, M.; Pedraza-Chaverri, J.; Chirino, Y.I. Protective effect of sulforaphane against oxidative stress: Recent advances. *Exp. Toxicol. Pathol.* **2012**, *64*, 503–508. [CrossRef] [PubMed]
12. Zhang, Y.; Kensler, T.W.; Cho, C.G.; Posner, G.H.; Talalay, P. Anticarcinogenicactivities of sulforaphane and structurally related synthetic norbornylisothiocyanates. *Proc. Natl. Acad. Sci. USA* **1994**, *91*, 3147–3150. [CrossRef]

13. Pu, D.; Zhao, Y.; Chen, J.; Sun, Y.; Lv, A.; Zhu, S.; Luo, C.; Zhao, K.; Xiao, Q. Protective effects of sulforaphane on cognitive impairments and ad-like lesions in diabetic mice are associated with the upregulation of Nrf2 transcription activity. *Neuroscience* **2018**, *381*, 35–45. [CrossRef] [PubMed]
14. Silva Rodrigues, J.F.; Silva, E.; Silva, C.; França Muniz, T.; De Aquino, A.F.; Neuza da Silva Nina, L.; Fialho Sousa, N.C.; Nascimento da Silva, L.C.; De Souza, B.G.G.F.; Da Penha, T.A.; et al. Sulforaphane Modulates Joint Inflammation in a Murine Model of Complete Freund's Adjuvant-Induced Mono-Arthritis. *Molecules* **2018**, *23*, 988. [CrossRef] [PubMed]
15. Tarozzi, A.; Angeloni, C.; Malaguti, M.; Morroni, F.; Hrelia, S.; Hrelia, P. Sulforaphane as a Potential Protective Phytochemical against Neurodegenerative Diseases. *Oxidative Med. Cell Longev.* **2013**, *2013*, 415078. [CrossRef] [PubMed]
16. Yanaka, A. Daily intake of broccoli sprouts normalizes bowel habits in human healthy subjects. *J. Clin. Biochem. Nutr.* **2018**, *62*, 75–82. [CrossRef] [PubMed]
17. Axelsson, A.S.; Tubbs, E.; Mecham, B.; Chacko, S.; Nenonen, H.A.; Tang, Y.; Fahey, J.W.; Derry, J.M.J.; Wollheim, C.B.; Wierup, N.; et al. Sulforaphane reduces hepatic glucose production and improves glucose control in patients with type 2 diabetes. *Sci. Transl. Med.* **2017**, *9*, 394. [CrossRef] [PubMed]
18. Lucarini, E.; Micheli, L.; Trallori, E.; Citi, V.; Martelli, A.; Testai, L.; De Nicola, G.R.; Iori, R.; Calderone, V.; Ghelardini, C.; et al. Effect of glucoraphanin and sulforaphane against chemotherapy-induced neuropathic pain: Kv7 potassium channels modulation by H_2S release in vivo. *Phytother. Res.* **2018**, *32*, 2226–2234. [CrossRef]
19. McDonnell, C.; Leánez, S.; Pol, O. The induction of the transcription factor Nrf2 enhances the antinociceptive effects of delta-opioid receptors in diabetic mice. *PLoS ONE* **2017**, *12*, e0180998. [CrossRef]
20. Redondo, A.; Chamorro, P.A.F.; Riego, G.; Leánez, S.; Pol, O. Treatment with sulforaphane produces antinociception and improves morphine effects during inflammatory pain in mice. *J. Pharmacol. Exp. Ther.* **2017**, *363*, 293–302. [CrossRef]
21. Martelli, A.; Testai, L.; Breschi, M.C.; Lawson, K.; McKay, N.G.; Miceli, F.; Taglialatela, M.; Calderone, V. Vasorelaxation by hydrogen sulphide involves activation of Kv7 potassium channels. *Pharmacol. Res.* **2013**, *70*, 27–34. [CrossRef] [PubMed]
22. Hedegaard, E.R.; Gouliaev, A.; Winther, A.K.; Arcanjo, D.D.; Aalling, M.; Renaltan, N.S.; Wood, M.E.; Whiteman, M.; Skovgaard, N.; Simonsen, U. Involvement of Potassium Channels and Calcium-Independent Mechanisms in Hydrogen Sulfide-Induced Relaxation of Rat Mesenteric Small Arteries. *J. Pharmacol. Exp. Ther.* **2016**, *356*, 53–63. [CrossRef] [PubMed]
23. Martelli, A.; Testai, L.; Citi, V.; Marino, A.; Bellagambi, F.G.; Ghimenti, S.; Breschi, M.C.; Calderone, V. Pharmacological characterization of the vascular effects of aryl isothiocyanates: Is hydrogen sulfide the real player? *Vasc. Pharmacol.* **2014**, *60*, 32–41. [CrossRef] [PubMed]
24. Platz, S.; Piberger, A.L.; Budnowski, J.; Herz, C.; Schreiner, M.; Blaut, M.; Hartwig, A.; Lamy, E.; Hanske, L.; Rohn, S. Bioavailability and biotransformation of sulforaphane and erucin metabolites in different biological matrices determined by LC-MS-MS. *Anal. Bioanal. Chem.* **2015**, *407*, 1819–1829. [CrossRef] [PubMed]
25. Valgimigli, L.; Iori, R. Antioxidant and pro-oxidant capacities of ITCs. *Environ. Mol. Mutagen.* **2009**, *50*, 222–237. [CrossRef] [PubMed]
26. Lazzeri, L.; Errani, O.; Leoni, M.; Venturi, G. *Eruca sativa* spp. oleifera: A new non-food crop. *Ind. Crops Prod.* **2004**, *20*, 67–73. [CrossRef]
27. Fuentes, E.; Alarcón, M.; Fuentes, M.; Carrasco, G.; Palomo, I. A novel role of *Eruca sativa* Mill. (Rocket) extract: Antiplatelet (NF-kB inhibition) and antithrombotic activities. *Nutrients* **2014**, *6*, 5839–5852. [CrossRef] [PubMed]
28. Sadiq, A.; Hayat, M.Q.; Mall, S.M. Qualitative and quantitative determination of secondary metabolites and antioxidant potential of *Eruca sativa*. *Nat. Prod. Chem. Res.* **2014**, *2*, 1000137. [CrossRef]
29. Sarwar Alam, M.; Kaur, G.; Jabbar, Z.; Javed, K.; Athar, M. *Eruca sativa* seeds possess antioxidant activity and exert a protective effect on mercuric chloride induced renal toxicity. *Food Chem. Toxicol.* **2007**, *45*, 910–920. [CrossRef]
30. Martelli, A.; Piragine, E.; Citi, V.; Testai, L.; Pagnotta, E.; Ugolini, L.; Lazzeri, L.; Di Cesare Mannelli, L.; Manzo, O.L.; Bucci, M.; et al. Erucin exhibits vasorelaxing effects and antihypertensive activity by H2 S-releasing properties. *Br. J. Pharmacol.* **2019**. [CrossRef]

31. Citi, V.; Piragine, E.; Pagnotta, E.; Ugolini, L.; Di Cesare Mannelli, L.; Testai, L.; Ghelardini, C.; Lazzeri, L.; Calderone, V.; Martelli, A. Anticancer properties of erucin, an H2 S-releasing isothiocyanate, on human pancreatic adenocarcinoma cells (AsPC-1). *Phytother. Res.* **2019**, *33*, 845–855. [CrossRef] [PubMed]
32. Clarke, J.D.; Hsu, A.; Riedl, K.; Bella, D.; Schwartz, S.J.; Stevens, J.F.; Ho, E. Bioavailability and inter-conversion of sulforaphane and erucin in human subjects consuming broccoli sprouts or broccoli supplement in a cross-over study design. *Pharmacol. Res.* **2011**, *64*, 456–463. [CrossRef] [PubMed]
33. Franco, P.; Spinozzi, S.; Pagnotta, E.; Lazzeri, L.; Ugolini, L.; Camborata, C.; Roda, A. Development of a liquid chromatography-electrospray ionization-tandem mass spectrometry method for the simultaneous analysis of intact glucosinolates and isothiocyanates in Brassicaceae seeds and functional foods. *J. Chromatogr. A* **2016**, *1428*, 154–161. [CrossRef] [PubMed]
34. Zaka, M.; Abbasi, B.H. Effects of bimetallic nanoparticles on seed germination frequency and biochemical characterisation of *Eruca sativa*. *IET Nanobiotechnol.* **2017**, *11*, 255–260. [CrossRef] [PubMed]
35. Oliviero, T.; Verkerk, R.; Dekker, M. Isothiocyanates from Brassica Vegetables—Effects of Processing, Cooking, Mastication, and Digestion. *Mol. Nutr. Food Res.* **2018**, *62*, 1701069. [CrossRef] [PubMed]
36. Dinkova-Kostova, A.T.; Fahey, J.W.; Kostov, R.V.; Kensler, T.W. KEAP1 and done? Targeting the NRF2 pathway with sulforaphane. *Trends Food Sci. Technol.* **2017**, *69*, 257–269. [CrossRef] [PubMed]
37. Rohwerder, T.; Sand, W. The sulfane sulfur of persulfides is the actual substrate of the sulfur-oxidizing enzymes from *Acidithiobacillus* and *Acidiphilium* spp. *Microbiology* **2003**, *149*, 1699–1710. [CrossRef]
38. Mishanina, T.V.; Libiad, M.; Banerjee, R. Biogenesis of reactive sulfur species for signaling by hydrogen sulfide oxidation pathways. *Nat. Chem. Biol.* **2015**, *11*, 457–464. [CrossRef]
39. Schreiber, A.K.; Nones, C.F.; Reis, R.C.; Chichorro, J.G.; Joice, M.; Cunha, J.M. Diabetic neuropathic pain: Physiopathology and treatment. *World J. Diabetes* **2015**, *6*, 432–444. [CrossRef]
40. Callaghan, B.C.; Cheng, H.T.; Stables, C.L.; Smith, A.L.; Feldman, E.L. Diabetic neuropathy: Clinical manifestations and current treatments. *Lancet Neurol.* **2012**, *11*, 521–534. [CrossRef]
41. Galer, B.S.; Gianas, A.; Jensen, M.P. Painful diabetic polyneuropathy: Epidemiology, pain description, and quality of life. *Diabetes Res. Clin. Pract.* **2000**, *47*, 123–128. [CrossRef]
42. Themistocleous, A.C.; Ramirez, J.D.; Shillo, P.R.; Lees, J.G.; Selvarajah, D.; Orengo, C.; Tesfaye, S.; Rice, A.S.; Bennett, D.L. The Pain in Neuropathy Study (PiNS): A cross-sectional observational study determining the somatosensory phenotype of painful and painless diabetic neuropathy. *Pain* **2016**, *157*, 1132–1145. [CrossRef] [PubMed]
43. Gore, M.; Brandenburg, N.A.; Dukes, E.; Hoffman, D.L.; Tai, K.S.; Stacey, B. Pain severity in diabetic peripheral neuropathy is associated with patient functioning, symptom levels of anxiety and depression, and sleep. *J. Pain Symptom Manag.* **2005**, *30*, 374–385. [CrossRef] [PubMed]
44. Malcangio, M.; Tomlinson, D.R. A pharmacologic analysis of mechanical hyperalgesia in streptozotocin/diabetic rats. *Pain* **1998**, *76*, 151–157. [CrossRef]
45. Murakami, T.; Iwanaga, T.; Ogawa, Y.; Fujita, Y.; Sato, E.; Yoshitomi, H.; Sunada, Y.; Nakamura, A. Development of sensory neuropathy in streptozotocin-induced diabetic mice. *Brain Behav.* **2013**, *3*, 35–41. [CrossRef] [PubMed]
46. Tesfaye, S. Recent advances in the management of diabetic distal symmetrical polyneuropathy. *J. Diabetes Investig.* **2011**, *2*, 33–42. [CrossRef]
47. Pop-Busui, R.; Boulton, A.J.; Feldman, E.L.; Bril, V.; Freeman, R.; Malik, R.A.; Sosenko, J.M.; Ziegler, D. Diabetic Neuropathy: A Position Statement by the American Diabetes Association. *Diabetes Care* **2017**, *40*, 136–154. [CrossRef]
48. Tesfaye, S.; Vileikyte, L.; Rayman, G.; Sindrup, S.H.; Perkins, B.A.; Baconja, M.; Vinik, A.I.; Boulton, A.J. The Toronto expert Panel on Diabetic Neuropathy. Painful diabetic peripheral neuropathy: Consensus recommendations on diagnosis, assessment and management. *Diabetes Metab. Res. Rev.* **2011**, *27*, 629–638. [CrossRef]
49. Tölle, T.; Xu, X.; Sadosky, A.B. Painful diabetic neuropathy: A cross-sectional survey of health state impairment and treatment patterns. *J. Diabetes Complicat.* **2006**, *20*, 26–33. [CrossRef]
50. Wang, A.; Leong, D.J.; Cardoso, L.; Sun, H.B. Nutraceuticals and osteoarthritis pain. *Pharmacol. Ther.* **2018**, *187*, 167–179. [CrossRef]

51. Crawford, C.; Boyd, C.; Berry, K.; Deuster, P. HERB Working Group. Dietary Ingredients Requiring Further Research Before Evidence-Based Recommendations Can Be Made for Their Use as an Approach to Mitigating Pain. *Pain Med.* **2019**. [CrossRef]
52. Brain, K.; Burrows, T.L.; Rollo, M.E.; Chai, L.K.; Clarke, E.D.; Hayes, C.; Hodson, F.J.; Collins, C.E. A systematic review and meta-analysis of nutrition interventions for chronic noncancer pain. *J. Hum. Nutr. Diet.* **2019**, *32*, 198–225. [CrossRef] [PubMed]
53. Martínez-Ballesta, M.C.; Moreno, D.A.; Carvajal, M. The Physiological Importance of Glucosinolates on Plant Response to Abiotic Stress in Brassica. *Int. J. Mol. Sci.* **2013**, *14*, 11607–11625. [CrossRef] [PubMed]
54. Hetta, M.H.; Owis, A.I.; Haddad, P.S.; Eid, H.M. The fatty acid-rich fraction of *Eruca sativa* (rocket salad) leaf extract exerts antidiabetic effects in cultured skeletal muscle, adipocytes and liver cells. *Pharm. Biol.* **2017**, *55*, 810–818. [CrossRef] [PubMed]
55. Khoobchandani, M.; Ojeswi, B.K.; Ganesh, N.; Srivastava, M.M.; Gabbanini, S.; Matera, R.; Iori, R.; Valgimigli, L. Antimicrobial properties and analytical profile of 850 traditional *Eruca sativa* seed oil: Comparison with various aerial and root plant extracts. *Food Chem.* **2010**, *120*, 217–224. [CrossRef]
56. Bennett, R.N.; Rosa, E.A.; Mellon, F.A.; Kroon, P.A. Ontogenic profiling of glucosinolates, flavonoids, and other secondary metabolites in *Eruca sativa* (salad rocket), *Diplotaxis erucoides* (wall rocket), *Diplotaxis tenuifolia* (wild rocket), and *Bunias orientalis* (Turkish rocket). *J. Agric. Food Chem.* **2006**, *54*, 4005–4015. [CrossRef] [PubMed]
57. Lazzeri, L.; Leoni, O.; Manici, L.M.; Palmieri, S.; Patalano, G. Use of Seed Flour as Soil Pesticide. U.S. Patent No. 7749549, 6 July 2010.
58. Rajanandh, M.G.; Kosey, S.; Prathiksha, G. Assessment of antioxidant supplementation on the neuropathic pain score and quality of life in diabetic neuropathy patients—A randomized controlled study. *Pharmacol. Rep.* **2014**, *66*, 44–48. [CrossRef] [PubMed]
59. Stepanović-Petrović, R.; Micov, A.; Tomić, M.; Pecikoza, U. Levetiracetam synergizes with gabapentin, pregabalin, duloxetine and selected antioxidants in a mouse diabetic painful neuropathy model. *Psychopharmacology (Berl.)* **2017**, *234*, 1781–1794. [CrossRef] [PubMed]
60. Aswar, M.; Patil, V. Ferulic acid ameliorates chronic constriction injury induced painful neuropathy in rats. *Inflammopharmacology* **2016**, *24*, 181–188. [CrossRef] [PubMed]
61. Hasanein, P.; Mohammad Zaheri, L. Effects of rosmarinic acid on an experimental model of painful diabetic neuropathy in rats. *Pharm. Biol.* **2014**, *52*, 1398–1402. [CrossRef] [PubMed]
62. Sun, J.; Chen, F.; Braun, C.; Zhou, Y.Q.; Rittner, H.; Tian, Y.K.; Cai, X.Y.; Ye, D.W. Role of curcumin in the management of pathological pain. *Phytomedicine* **2018**, *48*, 129–140. [CrossRef] [PubMed]
63. Wallace, J.L.; Wang, R. Hydrogen sulfide-based therapeutics: Exploiting a unique but ubiquitous gasotransmitter. *Nat. Rev. Drug Discov.* **2015**, *14*, 329–345. [PubMed]
64. Angelino, D.; Dosz, E.B.; Sun, J.; Hoeflinger, J.L.; van Tassell, M.L.; Chen, P.; Harnly, J.M.; Miller, M.J.; Jeffery, E.H. Myrosinase-dependent and–independent formation and control of isothiocyanate products of glucosinolate hydrolysis. *Front. Plant Sci.* **2015**, *6*, 1345. [CrossRef] [PubMed]
65. Vincent, A.M.; Russell, J.W.; Low, P.; Feldman, E.L. Oxidative stress in the pathogenesis of diabetic neuropathy. *Endocr. Rev.* **2004**, *25*, 612–628. [PubMed]
66. Di Cesare Mannelli, L.; Zanardelli, M.; Failli, P.; Ghelardini, C. Oxaliplatin-induced neuropathy: Oxidative stress as pathological mechanism. Protective effect of silibinin. *J. Pain.* **2012**, *13*, 276–284. [CrossRef] [PubMed]
67. UNI EN ISO. *Animal and Vegetable Fats 536 and Oils—Analysis by Gaschromatography of Methyl Esters of Fatty Acids, Oli E Grassi Animali E Vegetali—Analisi Gascromatografica Degli Esteri Metilici Degli Acidi Grassi*; Ente Nazionale Italiano di Unificazione: Milan, Italy, 1998.
68. ISO. *Animal and Vegetable Fats and Oils—Gas Chromatography of Fatty acid Methyl Esters—Part 4: Determination by Capillary Gas Chromatography*; International Organization for Standardization: Geneva, Switzerland, 2015.
69. Pagnotta, E.; Agerbirk, N.; Olsen, C.E.; Ugolini, L.; Cinti, S.; Lazzeri, L. Hydroxyl and Methoxyl Derivatives of Benzylglucosinolate in Lepidium densiflorum with Hydrolysis to Isothiocyanates and non-Isothiocyanate Products: Substitution Governs Product Type and Mass Spectral Fragmentation. *J. Agric. Food Chem.* **2017**, *65*, 3167–3178. [CrossRef] [PubMed]

70. Abdull Razis, A.F.; Bagatta, M.; De Nicola, G.R.; Iori, R.; Plant, N.; Ioannides, C. Characterization of the temporal induction of hepatic xenobiotic- metabolizing enzymes by glucosinolates and isothiocyanates: Requirement for at least a 6 h exposure to elicit complete induction profile. *J. Agric. Food Chem.* **2012**, *60*, 5556–5564. [CrossRef]
71. Singleton, V.L.; Orthofer, R.; Lamuela-Raventos, R.M. Analysis of total phenols and other oxidant substrates and antioxidants by mean of Folin-Ciocalteu reagent. *Methods Enzymol.* **1999**, *299*, 152–178.
72. Pessina, A.; Thomas, R.M.; Palmieri, S.; Luisi, P.L. An improved method for the purification of myrosinase and its physicochemical characterization. *Arch. Biochem Biophys.* **1990**, *280*, 383–389. [CrossRef]
73. Obrosov, A.; Shevalye, H.; Coppey, L.J.; Yorek, M.A. Effect of tempol on peripheral neuropathy in diet-induced obese and high-fat fed/low-dose streptozotocin-treated C57Bl6/J mice. *Free Radic Res.* **2017**, *51*, 360–367. [CrossRef]
74. Rakieten, N.; Rakieten, M.L.; Nadkarni, M.V. Studies on the diabetogenic action of streptozotocin. *Cancer Chemother. Rep.* **1963**, *29*, 91–98. [PubMed]
75. Russo, R.; D'Agostino, G.; Mattace Raso, G.; Avagliano, C.; Cristiano, C.; Meli, R.; Calignano, A. Central administration of oxytocin reduces hyperalgesia in mice: Implication for cannabinoid and opioid systems. *Peptides* **2012**, *38*, 81–88. [CrossRef] [PubMed]
76. Di Cesare Mannelli, L.; Maresca, M.; Farina, C.; Scherz, M.W.; Ghelardini, C. A model of neuropathic pain induced by sorafenib in the rat: Effect of dimiracetam. *Neurotoxicology* **2015**, *50*, 101–107. [CrossRef] [PubMed]
77. Blackburn-Munro, G.; Jensen, B.S. The anticonvulsant retigabine attenuates nociceptive behaviours in rat models of persistent and neuropathic pain. *Eur. J. Pharmacol.* **2003**, *460*, 109–116. [CrossRef]

3

Phenolic Content and Antioxidant Activity in *Trifolium* Germplasm from Different Environments

Aldo Tava [1,*], Łukasz Pecio [2], Roberto Lo Scalzo [3], Anna Stochmal [2] and Luciano Pecetti [1]

1 CREA Research Centre for Animal Production and Aquaculture, viale Piacenza 29, 26900 Lodi, Italy; luciano.pecetti@crea.gov.it
2 Department of Biochemistry and Crop Quality, Institute of Soil Science and Plant Cultivation, State Research Institute, ul. Czartoryskich 8, 24-100 Pulawy, Poland; lpecio@iung.pulawy.pl (Ł.P.); asf@iung.pulawy.pl (A.S.)
3 CREA Research Centre for Engineering and Agro-Food Processing, via G. Venezian 26, 20133 Milano, Italy; roberto.loscalzo@crea.gov.it
* Correspondence: aldo.tava@crea.gov.it;

Academic Editor: Pinarosa Avato

Abstract: Phenolics are important mediators in plant-environment interactions. The presence and concentration of phenolic compounds and their antioxidant activity were evaluated in leaves and flowers of a set of *Trifolium* species originating from contrasting environments encompassing lowland and mountain sites. The current germplasm proved a great reservoir of phenolic compounds, with different chemical structure and, possibly, diversified biological activity. Germplasm groups with specific phenolic composition were observed. In some cases, different patterns bore a taxonomic meaning. Lowland germplasm showed higher concentration of total phenolics in leaves than mountain accessions (50.30 vs. 34.19 mg/g dry matter (DM)), while the latter had higher concentration in flowers (114.16 vs. 57.44 mg/g DM). Outstanding concentration of isoflavones was observed in leaves of lowland germplasm (24.19 mg/g DM), and of both proanthocyanidins and flavonoids in flowers of mountain germplasm (53.81 and 56.62 mg/g DM, respectively). The pattern of phenolic composition in lowland and mountain germplasm was suggestive of different adaptive strategies. Three assays of antioxidant activity were tested, which were characterised by rather different reactivity towards phenolic composition. The scavenging activity was higher for leaf extracts of lowland germplasm, and for flower extracts of mountain germplasm. Besides identifying germplasm of interest, this study also suggested possible links between environmental factors and concentration and composition of phenolic compounds.

Keywords: antioxidant activity; flavonoids; isoflavones; phenolics; proanthocyanidins; *Trifolium*

---

1. Introduction

The genus *Trifolium* includes a large array of species. Some of them represent very important forage crops worldwide, such as white clover (*T. repens* L.), and red clover (*T. pratense* L.) [1,2]. Other species have an agronomic relevance in specific areas, such as berseem clover (*T. alexandrinum* L.) and subterranean clover (*T. subterraneum* L.) in Mediterranean environments [3]. Wild forms of these and other cultivated species, as well as populations of many other *Trifolium* species occur in natural grasslands of diversified environments, where they can represent valuable feed resources [4–6].

Besides being rich in proteins, *Trifolium* species have been reported to contain a wealth of biologically active secondary metabolites [7], of which phenolic compounds are one of the main classes. Phenolic compounds have a wide range of structures, but they generally share a remarkable antioxidant activity [8]. Flavonoids are an important class of phenolics that includes compound groups such as flavones, flavonols and isoflavones, all characterized by a phenylbenzopyran chemical structure [8].

In recent decades, there has been an increasing interest on flavonoids in medical research owing to their useful properties, such as anti-inflammatory, estrogenic, antimicrobial, antiallergenic and antitumor activities [9]. The antioxidant activity, determined by their ability of decreasing free radical formation and scavenging free radicals and reactive oxygen species (ROS), is an asset of major interest for flavonoids [10,11].

The role of flavonoids and other phenolic compounds as protective dietary constituents (nutraceuticals) with their antioxidant capacity has also become an increasingly important area of research [12]. The potential benefit that a dietary intake of phenolics may produce in the prevention or reduction of degenerative diseases such as cardiovascular diseases and cancer has been reported [13,14]. Isoflavones are a group of flavonoids typical of some legume species only. They exhibit estrogenic activity and represent the main phytoestrogens of current interest as nutraceuticals and dietary supplements [15,16]. An antioxidant activity of possible physiological relevance was also reported for isoflavones such as genistein and daidzein [17].

Phenolic compounds, including flavonoids, have often been used as chemotaxonomic markers in plants [18]. These compounds were also examined in the genus *Trifolium*. Oleszek et al. [19] characterized the phenolic composition of over 50 *Trifolium* species, emphasizing similarities and differences among taxa for the concentration pattern of the main groups of phenolics. More recently, the isoflavone prunetin was proposed as a possible chemotaxonomic marker in snow clover (*T. pratense* L. subsp. *nivale* (Koch) Arcang.) [20].

Phenolics play a fundamental role in the interaction of plants with the environment, including their defense mechanisms against biotic and abiotic stresses and other adaptation processes [21,22]. It is well known that the presence of phenolics in plants and the subsequent antioxidant capacity can also be subjected to significant variation due to environmental conditions and to biotic and abiotic stresses [23,24]. Hence, the current study evaluated the presence and concentration of phenolic compounds, as well as their antioxidant activity in a set of *Trifolium* species originating from different Italian environments. The main objectives of this investigation were to identify germplasm of interest as potential source of phenolic metabolites, also in view of their possible exploitation for medical/nutraceutical purposes, and to assess any possible role of the environment on the phenolic composition of the species.

2. Results

2.1. Germplasm Collection and Identification of Phenolics

The list of *Trifolium* species used in this investigation is reported in Table 1. Both cultivated and natural populations from different environments (lowlands and mountains) were analyzed for their phenolic content. Phenolics occurring in the extract of the 14 *Trifolium* samples under investigation were separated by UPLC method (see Materials and Methods) and UV spectra were obtained using a photo diode array detector. As an example, the UPLC chromatogram of leaf and flower extracts of *T. repens* var. *sylvestre* is shown in Figure 1. Six groups of phenolics were identified based on their characteristic absorption spectra (Figure 2), namely: phenolic acids (Figure 2A), clovamides (Figure 2B), flavanols (Figure 2C), flavones (Figure 2D), flavonols (Figure 2E) and isoflavones (Figure 2F).

A comparison was made of their retention times and mass spectral data obtained in positive and negative mode with those of standard compounds or with compounds previously reported in literature for *Trifolium* spp. [19,20,25–28]. A tentative identification of phenolics was performed based on key fragment ions and other MS observations. For flavonoids and their glycosyl derivatives the loss of 162 *m/z* was indicative of hexose (glucose or galactose), the loss of 146 *m/z* was indicative of rhamnose, the loss of 132 *m/z* was indicative of pentose (xylose or arabinose). Moreover, the loss of 44 *m/z* in the negative ion mode and the loss of 86 *m/z* were indicative of the presence of a malonate.

Table 1. List of *Trifolium* germplasm evaluated for the concentration of phenolic compounds and antioxidant activity.

#	Species	Common Name	Germplasm Type	Name/Origin	Adaptation to/Origin From
1	*T. alexandrinum*	Berseem clover	Experimental cultivar	Sintetica E/Italy	Lowlands
2	*T. pratense*	Red clover	Cultivar	Aiace/Italy	Lowlands
3	*T. pratense* subsp. *nivale*	Snow clover	Natural population	Rhaetian Alps	Mountains*
4	*T. repens*	White clover (non-Ladino large-leaved type)	Cultivar	Regal/USA	Lowlands
5	*T. subterraneum*	Subterranean clover	Natural population	Sardinia	Lowlands
6	*T. subterraneum*	Subterranean clover	Natural population	Sardinia	Lowlands
7	*T. pratense*	Red clover	Natural population	Po Valley	Lowlands
8	*T. repens* var. *giganteum*	White clover (Ladino type)	Natural population	Po Valley	Lowlands
9	*T. alpinum*	Alpine clover	Natural population	Graian Alps	Mountains
10	*T. badium*	Brown clover	Natural population	Graian Alps	Mountains
11	*T. ochroleucum*	Sulphur clover	Natural population	Cottian Alps	Mountains
12	*T. pratense* subsp. *nivale*	Snow clover	Natural population	Graian Alps	Mountains
13	*T. repens* var. *sylvestre*	White clover (small-leaved type)	Natural population	Graian Alps	Mountains
14	*T. thalii*	Thal clover	Natural population	Graian Alps	Mountains

* Collected as seed in a mountain area and grown *ex-situ* in a lowland site.

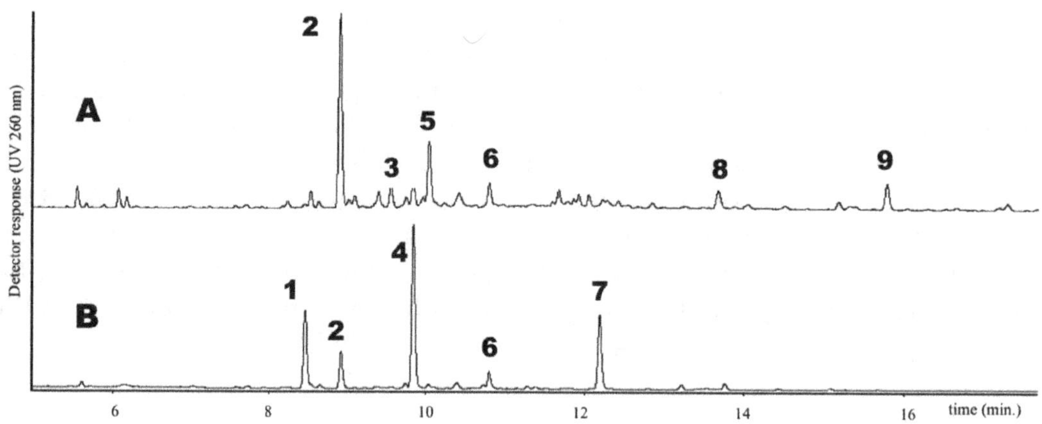

Figure 1. UPLC chromatogram of extracts from (**A**) leaves and (**B**) flowers of *T. repens* var. *sylvestre* (#13). **1**: myricetin-3-*O*-galactoside; **2**: quercetin-3-*O*-[xylosyl-(1→2)-galactoside]; **3**: kaempferol-3-*O*-[rhamnosyl-(1→6)-xylosyl-(1→2)-galactoside]; **4**: quercetin-3-*O*-galactoside; **5**: kaempferol-3-*O*-[xylosyl-(1→2)-galactoside]; **6**: kaempferol-3-*O*-galactoside; **7**: quercetin-3-*O*-galactoside-6′′-*O*-acetate; **8**: formononetin-7-*O*-glucoside; **9**: formononetin-7-*O*-glucoside-6′′-*O*-malonate.

Branched *C*-glycosides were also investigated by the presence of characteristic ions $[M-H-60]^-$, $[M-H-90]^-$, and $[M-H-120]^-$ [25–29].

Along with clovamide (*N*-caffeoyl-L-DOPA), phenolic acids were detected in almost all *Trifolium* extracts in low amount and were mostly constituted by glycosyl derivatives of caffeic acid, ferulic acid and coumaric acid.

Flavanols were identified in very low amount (< 0.3 mg g^{-1} dry matter) in some extracts, and identified as catechin/epicatechin and a catechin dimer. Flavones, flavonols and isoflavones represented the main bulk of flavonoid constituents of the extracts. The most abundant, tentatively identified, flavonoids in the 14 *Trifolium* samples are reported in Table 2 where their percentage amount in the whole extracts is indicated. All the identified compounds were quantitatively evaluated by appropriate standards (see Experimental).

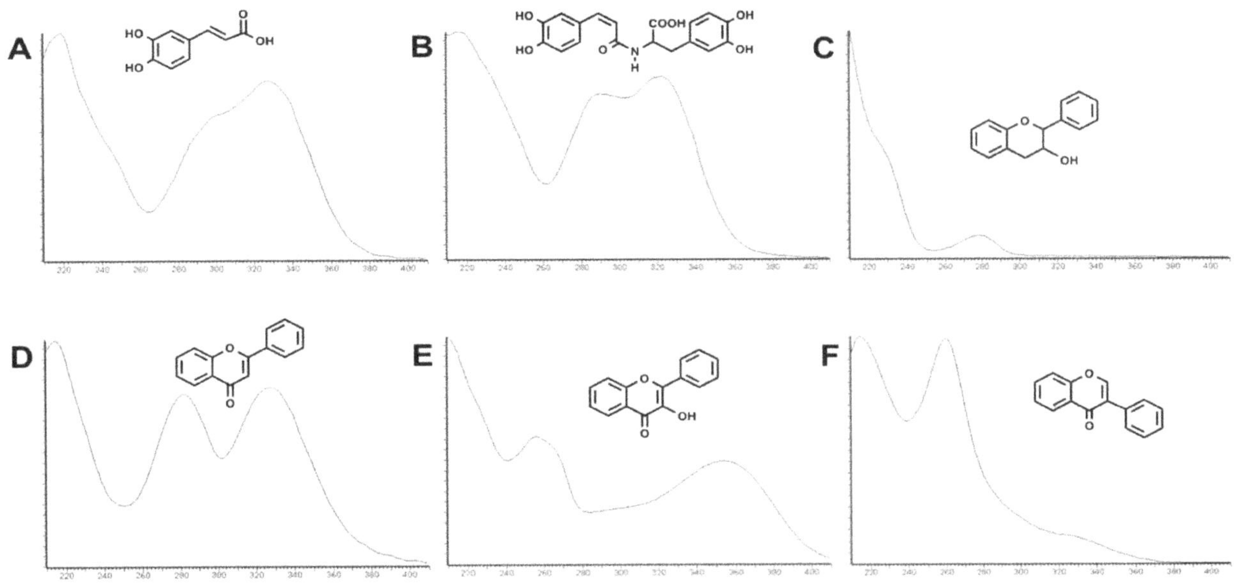

Figure 2. Characteristic UV spectra of the six groups of phenolics identified in *Trifolium* spp. **A**: phenolic acid; **B**: clovamide; **C**: flavanol; **D**: flavone, **E**: flavonol; **F**: isoflavone.

Glycosyl and glycosyl malonate derivative of luteolin, together with lower amount of derivatives of apigenin and of the isoflavone biochanin A, were the most abundant compounds identified in *T. alexandrinum* (#1) extracts. In flowers, large amounts of quercetin galactoside and quercetin glucoside were also detected. All these compounds were previously reported in the species [30–32]. High amounts of glycosyl and glycosyl malonate derivative of flavones (quercetin in leaves and quercetin and kaempferol in flowers) and isoflavones (biochanin A and formononetin in leaves and flowers) were detected in red clover (#2 and #7), as previously reported in this widely investigated *Trifolium* species [19,20,33–36]. In snow clover (#3 and #12) extracts, glycosyl and glycosyl malonate derivative of flavones (quercetin) and isoflavones (formononetin and prunetin) were detected in large amounts in both leaves and flowers. The abundant presence of prunetin was reported to be a characteristic feature of this clover species [20]. Leaf extracts of *T. repens* (#4, #8 and #13, see Figure 1) featured high content of di- and trisaccharide derivative of flavonols quercetin and kaempferol, together with other minor compounds, as already reported [37–40]. Flowers were characterized instead by high amount of quercetin galactoside and its acetyl derivative, together with lower content of myricetin galactoside. Subterranean clover (#5 and #6) leaves and flowers confirmed the large presence of isoflavones biochanin A, genistein and formononetin glycosides and glycosyl malonate derivatives [28]. *T. alpinum* (#9) extracts showed a complex mixture of flavonoids. In leaves, they were mainly constituted by mono and diglycosides of quercetin, while kaempferol glycosides were detected in flowers. The presence of glycosides of a quercetin isomer (MW=302) was also detected. The very low amount of isoflavones assessed in this *Trifolium* species was inconsistent with previous results [26]. Di- and tri-saccharide derivatives of quercetin were observed in *T. badium* (#10) extracts. An unidentified flavonoid (MW = 462) was abundant in leaves, while a monoglycoside of luteolin/luteolin isomer (MW = 286) was detected in large amount in flowers.

Leaves of *T. ochroleucum* (#11) mainly comprised mono- and di-saccharides of quercetin and, to a lesser extent, kaempferol. Quercetin and kaempferol glycosyl malonates were detected as the main constituents of flower extracts. Higher flavonoid content had been previously reported in *T. ochroleucum* leaves [19]. Quercetin and kaempferol diglycosides were abundant in *T. thalii* (#14) leaf extract, while the flower extract largely contained myricetin and quercetin glycosides. The isoflavone formononetin glycoside and its malonyl derivative were also detected in leaves.

Table 2. The most abundant, tentatively identified flavonoids in the 14 *Trifolium* samples and their quantitative evaluation (% dry matter, $n = 3$, mean value ± standard deviation) in leaves and flowers. See Table 1 for taxonomic classification, origin and adaptation of each sample.

#	UV λ_{max} (nm)	$[M + H]^+$ (*m/z*)	$[M - H]^-$ (*m/z*)	MW	Compound	Leaves	Flowers
1	253, 354	465, 303	463, 301	464	quercetin-3-*O*-galactoside	-	8.9 ± 0.5
	254, 354	465, 303	463, 301	464	quercetin-3-*O*-glucoside	-	10.2 ± 0.4
	255, 346	449, 287	447, 285	448	luteolin-7-*O*-glucoside	24.8 ± 1.6	8.7 ± 0.2
	266, 432	433, 271	431, 269	432	apigenin-7-*O*-glucoside	4.5 ± 0.3	0.5 ± 0.1
	254, 346	535, 449$[M - 86]^+$, 287	533, 489$[M - 44]^-$, 285	534	luteolin-7-*O*-glucoside-6″-*O*-malonate	17.8 ± 0.6	30.4 ± 0.9
	266, 337	519, 433$[M - 86]^+$, 271	517, 473$[M - 44]^-$, 269	518	apigein-7-*O*-glucoside-6″-*O*-malonate	3.8 ± 0.3	2.6 ± 0.4
	254, 344	287	285	286	luteolin	15.3 ± 0.2	3.7 ± 0.9
	260, 324	533, 285	531, 487$[M - 44]^-$, 283	532	biochanin A-7-*O*-glucoside-6″-*O*-malonate	7.4 ± 0.7	6.8 ± 0.9
2	253, 354	465, 303	463, 301	464	quercetin-3-*O*-galactoside	6.5 ± 0.2	5.5 ± 0.8
	256, 354	551, 303	549, 505$[M - 44]^-$, 301	550	quercetin-3-*O*-glucoside-6′′- *O*-malonate	6.2 ± 0.2	14.7 ± 0.5
	265, 344	535, 287	533, 489$[M - 44]^-$, 285	534	kaempferol-3-*O*-galactoside-6′′-*O*-malonate	-	11.7 ± 1.3
	251, 300	517, 269	515, 471$[M - 44]^-$, 267	516	formononetin-7-*O*-glucoside-6′′-*O*-malonate	14.5 ± 0.8	7.9 ± 0.7
	260, 324	533, 285	531, 487$[M - 44]^-$, 283	532	biochanin A-7-*O*-glucoside-6′′-*O*-malonate	20.9 ± 1.6	18.0 ± 1.7
3	253, 354	465, 303	463, 301	464	quercetin-3-*O*-galactoside	11.1 ± 0.4	15.1 ± 1.2
	256, 354	551, 303	549, 505$[M - 44]^-$, 301	550	quercetin-3-*O*-glucoside-6′′-*O*-malonate	9.0 ± 0.3	26.3 ± 1.4
	251, 300	431, 269	429, 267	430	formononetin-7-*O*-glucoside	3.1 ± 0.4	1.5 ± 0.2
	251, 300	517, 269	515, 471$[M - 44]^-$, 267	516	formononetin-7-*O*-glucoside-6′′-*O*-malonate	3.7 ± 0.1	1.7 ± 0.1
	260, 325	447, 285	445, 283	446	prunetin-4′-*O*-glucoside	7.6 ± 1.5	2.3 ± 0.9
	260, 325	355, 285	531, 487$[M - 44]^-$, 283	532	prunetin-4′-*O*-glucoside-6′′-*O*-malonate	20.0 ± 0.2	9.5 ± 1.2
4	266, 337	481, 319	479, 317	480	myricetin-3-*O*-galactoside	-	10.9 ± 0.2
	256, 347	743, 597, 303	741, 301	742	quercetin-3-*O*-{[rhamnosyl-(1→6)]-[xylosyl-(1→2)-galactoside]}	6.4 ± 0.6	2.0 ± 0.1
	256, 354	597, 465, 303	595, 301	596	quercetin-3-*O*-[xylosyl-(1→2)-galactoside]	22.6 ± 2.2	6.8 ± 0.1
	256, 344	727, 581, 449, 287	725, 285	742	kaempferol-3-*O*-{[rhamnosyl-(1→6)]-[xylosyl-(1→2)-galactoside]}	6.3 ± 0.4	1.1 ± 0.1
	253, 354	465, 303	463, 301	464	quercetin-3-*O*-galactoside	3.0 ± 0.2	24.5 ± 0.9
	265, 346	581, 449, 287	579, 285	580	kaempferol-3-*O*-[xylosyl-(1→2)-galactoside]	10.6 ± 0.7	1.5 ± 0.1
	256, 355	507, 303	505, 301	506	quercetin-3-*O*-galactoside-6′′-*O*-acetate	0.9 ± 0.1	23.0 ± 0.3
5	259, 325	433, 271	431, 269	432	genistein-7-*O*-glucoside	14.4 ± 0.7	
	265, 344	535, 287	533, 489$[M - 44]^-$, 285	534	orobol-7-*O*-glucoside-6′′-*O*-malonate	4.2 ± 0.1	
	259, 325	519, 271	517, 473$[M - 44]^-$, 269	518	genistein-7-*O*-glucoside-6′′-*O*-malonate	13.2 ± 0.2	
	260, 325	447, 285	445, 283	446	biochanin A-7-*O*-glucoside	13.5 ± 1.0	
	260, 325	533, 285	531, 487$[M - 44]^-$, 283	532	biochanin A-7-*O*-glucoside-6′′-*O*-malonate	35.8 ± 1.9	
6	259, 325	433, 271	431, 269	432	genistein-7-*O*-glucoside	11.4 ± 1.3	4.2 ± 0.8
	259, 325	519, 271	517, 473$[M - 44]^-$, 269	518	genistein-7-*O*-glucoside-6′′-*O*-malonate	13.6 ± 0.4	6.0 ± 0.4
	251, 300	431, 269	429, 267	430	formononetin-7-*O*-glucoside	4.9 ± 0.7	7.9 ± 1.8
	251, 300	517, 269	515, 471$[M - 44]^-$, 267	516	formononetin-7-*O*-glucoside-6′′-*O*-malonate	12.9 ± 0.4	25.5 ± 3.0
	260, 325	447, 285	445, 283	446	biochanin A-7-*O*-glucoside	8.3 ± 0.6	6.7 ± 1.2
	260, 325	533, 285	531, 487$[M - 44]^-$, 283	532	biochanin A-7-*O*-glucoside-6′′-*O*-malonate	23.9 ± 2.3	24.8 ± 2.7

Table 2. *Cont.*

7	253, 354	465, 303	463, 301	464	quercetin-3-*O*-galactoside	8.7 ± 0.5	8.5 ± 1.2
	256, 354	551, 303	549, 505[M − 44]$^-$, 301	550	quercetin-3-*O*-glucoside-6′′-*O*-malonate	8.9 ± 0.2	21.1 ± 0.3
	265, 344	535, 287	533, 489[M − 44]$^-$, 285	534	kaempferol-3-*O*-galactoside-6′′-*O*-malonate	-	14.1 ± 2.4
	251, 300	517, 269	515, 471[M − 44]$^-$, 267	516	formononetin-7-*O*-glucoside-6′′-*O*-malonate	8.3 ± 0.5	4.7 ± 0.6
	260, 324	533, 285	531, 487[M − 44]$^-$, 283	532	biochanin A-7-*O*-glucoside-6′′-*O*-malonate	18.9 ± 1.0	9.4 ± 0.9
8	266, 337	481, 319	479, 317	480	myricetin-3-*O*-galactoside	-	13.5 ± 0.6
	256, 347	743, 597, 303	741, 301	742	quercetin-3-*O*-{[rhamnosyl-(1→6)]-[xylosyl-(1→2)-galactoside]}	5.7 ± 0.5	2.1 ± 0.1
	256, 354	597, 465, 303	595, 301	596	quercetin-3-*O*-[xylosyl-(1→2)-galactoside]	22.3 ± 0.6	8.8 ± 0.3
	256, 344	727, 581, 449, 287	725, 285	742	kaempferol-3-*O*-{[rhamnosyl-(1→6)]-[xylosyl-(1→2)-galactoside]}	4.0 ± 0.3	1.3 ± 0.1
	253, 354	465, 303	463, 301	464	quercetin-3-*O*-galactoside	2.5 ± 0.3	29.9 ± 0.5
	256, 355	507, 303	505, 301	506	quercetin-3-*O*-galactoside-6′′-*O*-acetate	1.3 ± 0.1	21.7 ± 0.3
9	256, 354	627, 465, 303	625, 301	626	quercetin-hexose-hexose	11.4 ± 0.1	16.6 ± 0.4
	265, 344	611, 449, 287	609, 447, 285	610	kaempferol-hexose-hexose	-	3.6 ± 0.0
	255, 332	949, 625, 463, 303	947	948	302-hexose-hexose-hexose-hexose	10.1 ± 01	1.7 ± 0.1
	256, 355	465, 303	463, 301	464	quercetin-3-*O*-galactoside	0.7 ± 0.0	9.1 ± 0.1
	256, 355	465, 303	463, 301	464	quercetin-3-*O*-glucoside	1.3 ± 0.1	18.9 ± 0.1
	254, 332	833, 303	831, 301	832	302-hexose-hexose-hexose-acetate	6.0 ± 0.2	1.0 ± 0.0
	265, 341	449, 287	447, 285	448	kaempferol-3-*O*-glucoside	-	3.9 ± 0.1
10	256, 354	759	757, 595, 462, 301	758	quercetin-hexose-hexose-pentose	5.0 ± 0.1	-
	256, 354	773, 303	771, 609, 462, 301	772	quercetin-hexose-hexose-rhamnose	8.8 ± 0.2	1.0 ± 0.1
	282, 332	463	461, 285	462	unidentified	18.2 ± 0.7	-
	265, 348	449, 287	447, 285	448	luteolin-hexose	6.7 ± 0.4	60.1 ± 0.4
	256, 349	595	593, 447, 285	594	luteolin-rhamnose-hexose	8.7 ± 0.2	8.6 ± 0.1
11	256, 354	773, 611, 465, 303	771, 301	772	quercetin-hexose-hexose-rhamnose	3.9 ± 0.1	0.9 ± 0.1
	256, 354	627, 465, 303	625, 301	626	quercetin-hexose-hexose	5.8 ± 0.2	0.3 ± 0.0
	256, 354	611, 449, 303	609, 447, 301	610	quercetin-hexose-rhamnose	6.5 ± 0.2	0.9 ± 0.1
	256, 356	757, 611, 465, 303	755, 301	756	quercetin-hexose-rhamnose-rhamnose	26.7 ± 0.2	10.8 ± 0.5
	256, 355	465, 303	463, 301	464	quercetin-3-*O*-galactoside	8.9 ± 0.2	12.1 ± 0.8
	265, 344	741, 595, 449, 287	739, 593, 447, 285	740	kaempferol-hexose-rhamnose-rhamnose	9.6 ± 0.1	10.5 ± 0.2
	256, 354	551, 303	549, 505[M − 44]$^-$, 301	550	quercetin-3-*O*-glucoside-6′′-*O*-malonate	2.4 ± 0.1	26.1 ± 0.1
	265, 344	535, 287	533, 489[M − 44]$^-$, 285	534	kaempferol-3-*O*-galactoside-6′′-*O*-malonate	-	16.8 ± 1.9
12	253, 354	465, 303	463, 301	464	quercetin-3-*O*-galactoside	4.5 ± 0.3	21.6 ± 1.9
	256, 355	465, 303	463, 301	464	quercetin-3-*O*-glucoside	10.1 ± 2.0	1.1 ± 0.3
	256, 354	551, 303	549, 505[M − 44]$^-$, 301	550	quercetin-3-*O*-glucoside-6′′-O-malonate	27.2 ± 2.1	44.6 ± 2.6
	251, 300	431, 269	429, 267	430	formononetin-7-*O*-glucoside	1.8 ± 0.6	-
	260, 325	447, 285	445, 283	446	prunetin-4′-*O*-glucoside	8.7 ± 1.9	0.5 ± 0.0
	260, 325	355, 285	531, 487[M − 44]$^-$, 283	532	prunetin-4′-*O*-glucoside-6′′-O-malonate	17.4 ± 1.2	1.9 ± 0.1

Table 2. *Cont.*

13	266, 337	481, 319	479, 317	480	myricetin-3-*O*-galactoside	-	18.9 ± 0.2
	256, 354	597, 465, 303	595, 301	596	quercetin-3-*O*-[xylosyl-(1→2)-galactoside]	29.1 ± 0.3	8.1 ± 0.2
	256, 344	727, 581, 449, 287	725, 285	742	kaempferol-3-*O*-{[rhamnosyl-(1→6)]-[xylosyl-(1→2)-galactoside]}	3.3 ± 0.1	0.4 ± 0.1
	253, 354	465, 303	463, 301	464	quercetin-3-*O*-galactoside	3.9 ± 0.1	36.4 ± 0.4
	265, 346	581, 449, 287	579, 285	580	kaempferol-3-*O*-[xylosyl-(1→2)-galactoside]	11.0 ± 1.2	1.1 ± 0.2
	263, 351	449, 287	447, 285	448	kaempferol-3-*O*-galactoside	3.8 ± 0.5	6.3 ± 0.1
	256, 355	507, 303	505, 301	506	quercetin-3-*O*-galactoside-6′′-*O*-acetate	1.5 ± 0.3	17.8 ± 0.3
14	266, 337	481, 319	479, 317	480	myricetin-3-*O*-galactoside	-	23.4 ± 0.2
	256, 354	597, 465, 303	595, 301	596	quercetin-3-*O*-[xylosyl-(1→2)-galactoside]	46.2 ± 0.3	10.8 ± 0.3
	253, 354	465, 303	463, 301	464	quercetin-3-*O*-galactoside	4.2 ± 0.2	46.3 ± 0.6
	265, 346	581, 449, 287	579, 285	580	kaempferol-3-*O*-[xylosyl-(1→2)-galactoside]	9.6 ± 0.3	1.2 ± 0.1
	256, 355	523, 319	521, 317	522	myricetin-3-*O*-galactoside-6″-*O*-acetate	-	5.2 ± 0.1
	251, 300	431, 269	429, 267	430	formononetin-7-*O*-glucoside	4.8 ± 0.8	-
	251, 300	517, 269	515, 471[M − 44]$^-$, 267	516	formononetin-7-*O*-glucoside-6′′-*O*-malonate	6.0 ± 1.5	-

2.2. Evaluation of Phenolic Compounds in the Trifolium Species in Relation to Their Antioxidant Activities

To facilitate the assessment of the biological activity of the different *Trifolium* extracts and to evaluate their antioxidant properties in relation to the phytocomplex (whole extract), the detected compounds were grouped into four distinct classes based on their chemical structure and biological properties, namely, phenolic acids, clovamides, isoflavones, and other flavonoids, this latter including flavanols, flavonols, and flavones. The presence of a fifth group of phenolic compounds, namely proanthocyanidins (or condensed tannins) was assessed by the butanol/HCl method [41], and evaluated with pelargonidin as a standard. Although with some limitations, this method was reported to allow for the most effective detection of proanthocyanidins [42–44]. Pelargonidin was selected as a standard because of its presence in all samples among anthocyanidins obtained from the acid-catalysed cleavage of the condensed tannins. Preliminary investigation performed by a cellulose bidimensional thin layer chromatography (2D TLC) of the obtained anthocyanidin (data not reported), showed the presence of pelargonidin, cyanidin and delfinidin. In all the analyzed samples, variation was observed for these compounds, with pelargonidin being one of the most detected compounds.

Results of the quantitative evaluation of different phenolics in leaves and flowers of the 14 samples of clover under investigation are reported in Tables 3–5.

Flower tissues featured higher concentration of total phenolics compared to leaves across all accessions (Table 3). However, differences between plant organs for individual phenolic group concentrations were not consistent, with no difference for phenolic acids and clovamides, higher concentration in leaves for isoflavones, and higher concentration in flowers for other flavonoids and for proanthocyanidins. The antioxidant activity was higher in flower than in leaf extracts according to each of the three applied assays.

It is widely accepted that leaves have higher amount of phenolic compounds than flowers, owing to the abundance of pathway precursors in leaves due to photosynthesis [45,46]. However, the current result of higher concentration of total phenolics in flowers than in leaves had several precedents in different folk-medicine species, such as yarrow, *Achillea millefolium* L. [47], pomegranate, *Punica granatum* L. [48], or white-weed, *Ageratum conyzoides* L. [49]. The facts that pigments are composed of flavonoids in most flowers, and that proanthocyanidins are produced by closely related branches of the flavonoid pathway using the same metabolic intermediates, make of no surprise the finding that flowers in our germplasm collection were particularly rich in these groups of phenolics. Abeynayake et al. [50] reported that white clover plants accumulate higher level of proanthocyanidins in flowers than in vegetative tissues. In addition to a possible ultraviolet (UV)-screening effect exerted by phenolics [22], a role for flavonoids was reported in the development of functional pollen [51], which may also explain the abundance of these compounds in flower tissues. Total phenolic concentration in flowers, especially as proanthocyanidins, fully supported higher antioxidant activity of flower compared to leaf extracts, no matter the applied scavenging assay. Nonetheless, greater sensitivity of the peroxyl radical scavenging for proanthocyanidins was evident, confirming the results in Jayaprakasha et al. [52], thus accounting for the current outstanding difference between leaf and flower extracts for this assay.

The 14 *Trifolium* samples differed significantly ($P < 0.05$) for leaf phenolic concentrations and antioxidant activity according to ANOVA (Table 4). The red clover cultivar Aiace (#2) was rich in phenolic acids, followed by the snow clover population #3 and the berseem clover experimental cultivar #1. Clovamides were found in highest concentration in red clover samples (#2 and #7) and they were also present in the snow clover populations #3 and #12 and the berseem cultivar #1.

Table 3. Comparison between leaves and flowers (mean values across the 14 *Trifolium* samples reported in Table 1) for concentration of phenolic groups and antioxidant activity.

	Phenolic Group Concentration (mg/g Dry Matter)						Antioxidant Activity Assay		
Sample	Phenolic Acids	Clovamides	Isoflavones	Other Flavonoids	Proanthocyanidins	Total Phenolics	Fremy's Salt Scavenging *	Superoxide Anion Scavenging *	Peroxyl Radical Scavenging **
leaves	2.13 a	5.23 a	14.51 a	20.83 b	1.12 b	43.83 b	4.94 b	2.03 b	44.93 b
flowers	1.33 a	3.12 a	2.23 b	34.90 a	40.84 a	82.42 a	11.06 a	4.61 a	489.29 a

In each column, mean values followed by different letters (a or b) are different at $P < 0.05$ according to analysis of variance. * µmol gallic acid equivalents (GAE)/100 g freeze-dried matter;.** mmol Trolox equivalents (TE)/100 g freeze-dried matter.

Table 4. Concentration of phenolic groups and antioxidant activity determined on leaves of 14 *Trifolium* samples. See Table 1 for taxonomic classification.

	Phenolic Group Concentration (mg/g Dry Matter)						Antioxidant Activity Assay		
#	Phenolic acids	Clovamides	Isoflavones	Other Flavonoids	Proanthocyanidins	Total Phenolics	Fremy's Salt Scavenging *	Superoxide Anion Scavenging *	Peroxyl Radical Scavenging **
1	4.66	8.53	4.20	41.15	4.10	62.65	5.37	2.12	28.00
2	5.94	29.86	22.63	13.78	0.66	72.89	15.40	4.07	88.25
3	4.68	8.64	16.55	16.88	0.14	46.90	6.08	2.19	21.60
4	1.40	-	0.31	9.19	0.05	10.96	3.18	2.13	10.05
5	2.00	-	70.03	7.55	0.06	79.64	1.47	1.82	137.50
6	1.87	-	48.00	7.94	0.03	57.84	2.15	0.61	8.85
7	2.85	22.33	22.72	21.08	0.12	69.11	9.40	1.92	130.00
8	1.27	-	0.70	6.18	0.25	8.42	3.27	0.60	3.70
9	-	-	0.38	27.68	0.37	28.44	4.49	0.88	16.80
10	-	-	0.17	34.70	8.58	43.45	3.24	5.86	24.30
11	2.42	-	0.54	44.14	0.39	47.51	3.63	2.19	24.10
12	1.71	3.89	14.56	28.54	0.32	49.02	5.54	1.58	110.85
13	-	-	0.56	14.39	0.04	14.95	3.37	0.93	2.55
14	1.02	-	0.79	18.50	0.47	21.79	2.59	1.43	22.45
$LSD_{(P = 0.05)}$	1.17	0.48	2.72	2.79	0.18	4.18	2.43	1.60	30.04

* µmol gallic acid equivalents (GAE)/100 g freeze-dried matter; ** mmol Trolox equivalents (TE)/100 g freeze-dried matter.

Table 5. Concentration of phenolic groups and antioxidant activity determined on flowers of 13 *Trifolium* samples. See Table 1 for taxonomic classification.

#	Phenolic Group Concentration (mg/g Dry Matter)						Antioxidant Activity Assay		
	Phenolic Acids	Clovamides	Isoflavones	Other Flavonoids	Proanthocyanidins	Total Phenolics	Fremy's Salt Scavenging *	Superoxide Anion Scavenging *	Peroxyl Radical Scavenging **
1	2.23	6.88	1.15	19.12	29.14	58.53	5.04	4.41	46.30
2	2.63	11.99	10.91	23.70	42.94	92.18	6.20	1.13	423.40
3	2.83	7.29	5.17	22.58	39.03	76.90	5.06	1.00	394.40
4	0.85	-	0.14	15.47	24.10	40.82	9.96	2.69	436.80
6	0.46	-	4.57	0.74	4.96	10.73	2.35	0.76	4.10
7	2.89	10.50	5.44	25.58	37.39	81.81	6.37	1.92	190.00
8	0.44	-	0.08	21.21	30.53	52.27	11.35	1.72	34.60
9	-	-	0.22	27.81	33.31	61.51	8.56	5.48	150.20
10	-	-	-	80.29	81.28	161.57	16.75	9.93	696.00
11	2.56	-	-	44.12	30.30	76.99	7.42	5.31	1065.20
12	1.13	1.29	1.29	54.01	56.88	117.17	9.87	3.67	603.00
13	1.28	-	-	55.60	54.95	111.83	27.19	9.90	940.60
14	-	-	-	63.46	66.11	129.57	27.61	12.01	1376.50
$LSD_{(P = 0.05)}$	0.62	0.62	0.62	6.77	3.23	8.93	2.33	2.51	253.37

* µmol gallic acid equivalents (GAE)/100 g freeze-dried matter; ** mmol Trolox equivalents (TE)/100 g freeze-dried matter.

The subterranean clover populations #5 and #6 showed the highest concentration of isoflavones, followed by the two red clover samples (#2 and #7) and the two snow clover populations (#3 and #12). Three mountain species, namely, sulphur clover (#11), brown clover (#10) and alpine clover (#9) featured the highest concentration of other flavonoids, together with the berseem clover (#1). The two white clover accessions from lowlands (#4 and #8) and the two subterranean clover populations (#5 and #6) were characterized by the lowest concentration of other flavonoids. Proanthocyanidins were abundant in leaves of brown clover (#10) and berseem clover (#1) only. The leaf concentration of total phenolics exceeded the level of 60 mg g^{-1} dry matter in the two red clover accessions (#2 and #7), the subterranean clover population #5 and the berseem clover #1, while barely reaching the level of 10 mg g^{-1} dry matter in the two lowland white clover samples (#8 and #4).

Just as for the leaf samples, there was significant variation among accessions ($P < 0.05$) according to ANOVA for the flower phenolic concentrations and antioxidant activity (Table 5). However, accession patterns of phenolic concentrations were largely different in flowers compared to leaves. Only clovamides showed an outstanding consistency between flowers and leaves of exclusive presence in red clover (#2 and #7), snow clover (#3 and #12) and berseem clover (#1) germplasm (Tables 4 and 5). Concentration of phenolic acids was highest in flowers of the red clover samples (#2 and #7), the snow clover population #3, the sulphur clover population #11 and the berseem clover cultivar #1. Isoflavone concentration (much lower in flowers than in leaves, see Table 3) was highest in the red clover accessions (#2 and #7), the snow clover population #3 and the subterranean clover population #6. The subterranean clover population #5, featuring the highest isoflavone concentration in leaves, was missing in the flower analysis, owing to too few flowers to be used in the chemical determinations. The brown clover population #10 showed the highest concentration of other flavonoids, followed by the Thal clover population #14, while the subterranean clover population #6 had remarkably low concentration of these compounds. Somewhat similar was the pattern of proanthocyanidin concentration, with highest values in mountain accessions (brown clover #10, Thal clover #14, snow clover #12, and white clover #13) and lowest one in the subterranean clover #6. The very high concentration of proanthocyanidins in the mentioned mountain accessions clearly contributed to their highest concentrations of flower total phenolics, with values exceeding 100 mg/g dry matter, while the subterranean clover population #6 was bottom ranking for flower total phenolics with a concentration of about 10 mg/g dry matter (Table 5).

Oleszek et al. [19] partitioned their *Trifolium* collection into groups according to the patterns of leaf phenolic composition. The present germplasm also featured accession groups with specific phenolic composition. In some cases, these patterns bore a taxonomic meaning. *T. subterraneum* and *T. pratense* (the latter, both as red clover and as snow clover subspecies) were characterized by high leaf concentration of isoflavones. Clovamides were restricted to red clover and, to a lesser extent, snow clover and berseem clover. Most alpine species and berseem clover were rich in flavonoids other than isoflavones. White clover (across the three evaluated taxonomic forms) featured the lowest leaf phenolic concentration.

The richness of leaf isoflavones in subterranean clover confirms previous results on this species [28]. Red clover isoflavone extracts are commercially available as nutraceuticals and they have been proposed as an alternative to hormone-replacement therapy [53]. Subterranean clover may represent an interesting new source of isoflavones, with higher concentration of these compounds and more diverse pattern of isoflavone composition compared to red clover [28].

As emphasized [19], attention should be paid for exploitation to those species comprising good concentration of different phenolic groups, as the presence of these groups may provide synergistic health effects of plant extracts.

Accession rankings for the antioxidant activity of leaf extracts according to the three assays were quite inconsistent (Table 4). The highest activity was observed in the two red clover samples (#2 and #7) for the Fremy's salt scavenging, in the subterranean clover population #5, the red clover population #7 and the snow clover population #12 for the peroxyl radical scavenging, and in the brown clover population #10 and the red clover cultivar #2 for the superoxide anion scavenging. The inconsistency of accession ranking for the three assays was confirmed by the lack of significant pairwise correlation between assays based on leaf accession values (data not reported).

Unlike for the data on leaf extracts, there was some consistency of accession ranking between assays for the antioxidant activity of flower extracts (Table 5). In particular, the Thal clover population #14 and the subterranean clover population #6 were always top- and bottom-ranking, respectively, regardless of the scavenging assay. The mountain white clover population #13 also featured rather high antioxidant activity of flower extract with all three assays. Overall, there were moderately high positive pairwise correlations between scavenging assays, ranging from $r = 0.74$, $P < 0.01$ (Fremy's salt vs. peroxyl radical) to $r = 0.87$, $P < 0.01$ (Fremy's salt vs. superoxide anion).

The presence of diversified patterns of phytochemical composition, and the contemporary presence of structurally different groups of phenolics, such as isoflavones, other flavonoids and proanthocyanidins, that were likely to determine different responses to the antioxidant assays [54], justified the choice of three methods of antioxidant measurements. These assays were characterised, indeed, by rather different reactivity towards distinct free radical molecular probes, as successively confirmed by the results of the regression analysis described below.

Lowland accessions had higher concentration of phenolic acids, clovamides and isoflavones, and lower concentration of other flavonoids and proanthocyanidins, than mountain accessions consistently in leaves and flowers. However, lowland germplasm showed higher concentration of total phenolics in leaves, while mountain accessions had higher concentration of total phenolics in flowers (Table 6). This inconsistency was mostly due to outstanding concentration of isoflavones in leaves of lowland germplasm, and of both proanthocyanidins and flavonoids other than isoflavones in flowers of mountain germplasm. An inconsistency of rankings between germplasm provenances was also largely observed for the antioxidant activity. Lowland accessions had, on average, higher scavenging activity of leaf extracts in two assays out of three, whereas the scavenging activity of flower samples was higher in mountain than in lowland germplasm regardless of the assay (Table 6).

As already anticipated, the high concentration of flavonoids (other than isoflavones) and proanthocyanidins, associated with higher antioxidant capacities, in flower tissues of mountain germplasm can be a hint of the photoprotection effect recognized to flavonoids and other phenolics [55], possibly exerted on the sensitive reproductive system [23]. It is indeed well known that UV levels increase with altitude, and mountain species must be provided with adequate protection. Accumulation of flavonoids in response to UV-B exposition was reported in silver birch, *Betula pendula* Roth [56], while UV-stress-adapted germplasm displayed particularly high constitutive or elicited levels of flavonoids and other phenolics in *Arabidopsis thaliana* (L.) Heynh. [57] and in white clover [38]. UV absorption is one of the UV-protective properties ascribed to flavonoids, which also include energy dissipation and antioxidant activities [55]. A role of free-radical scavenging in response to UV exposure can be postulated [58].

The pattern of phenolic composition in lowland germplasm was suggestive of different adaptive strategies. The abundance of isoflavones in lowland leaves, in particular, may indicate natural selection to decreased palatability for herbivores, or increased defence systems against invertebrate pests [59].

Table 7 summarizes the best linear models predicted for leaf and flower samples from the multiple regression analysis of the antioxidant activity on mean concentrations of groups of phenolic compounds within the *Trifolium* germplasm. The concentration of 'other flavonoids' and that of 'proanthocyanidins' consistently proved affected by multicollinearity in flowers, and for that reason only the former was retained in the regressions on flower data. Regardless of the scavenging assay and the plant organ, the adjusted R^2 of the models was only moderate at most, with the exception of the good prediction of the Fremy's salt scavenging in leaves ($R^2 = 0.934$, $P < 0.001$). In both leaves and flowers, the peroxyl radical scavenging had a complex best fitting model, including most of the phenolic groups as regressors, whereas the Fremy's salt and the superoxide anion scavenging showed simpler models for both plant organ extracts.

Table 6. Mean values of concentration of phenolic groups and antioxidant activity in leaves and flowers of *Trifolium* samples originating from, and sampled in, either lowland. (#1, 2, 4, 5, 6, 7 and 8 in Table 1) or mountain areas (# 9, 10, 11, 12, 13 and 14 in Table 1).

Area of Germplasm Origin and Sampling	Phenolic Group Concentration (mg/g Dry Matter)						Antioxidant Activity Assay		
	Phenolic Acids	Clovamides	Isoflavones	Other Flavonoids	Proanthocyanidins	Total Phenolics	Fremy's Salt Scavenging *	Superoxide Anion Scavenging *	Peroxyl Radical Scavenging **
Leaves									
Lowlands	2.86 a	7.62 a	24.19 a	14.82 b	0.75 b	50.30 a	5.75 a	1.90 a	58.05 a
Mountains	0.86 b	0.65 b	3.00 b	27.99 a	1.70 a	34.19 b	3.81 b	2.15 a	33.51 b
Flowers									
Lowlands	1.65 a	5.34 a	4.04 a	11.84 b	28.18 b	57.44 b	6.88 b	2.11 b	189.18 b
Mountains	0.90 b	0.70 b	0.25 b	56.62 a	53.81 a	114.16 a	16.24 a	7.72 a	805.23 a

In each column within each plant organ, mean values followed by different letters (a or b) are different at $P < 0.05$ according to analysis of variance. * µmol gallic acid equivalents (GAE)/100 g freeze-dried matter; ** mmol Trolox equivalents (TE)/100 g freeze-dried matter.

Table 7. Prediction of antioxidant activity in leaves and flowers of *Trifolium* germplasm, based on multiple regression analysis of accession mean values of each antioxidant assay on accession mean concentrations of groups of phenolic compounds. Group concentrations in the models (in parentheses) are expressed as mg g^{-1} dry matter.

Antioxidant Activity Assay	Best Linear Model	Model F Probability	Adjusted R^2
Leaves			
Fremy's salt scavenging *	3.368 + 0.373 *(clovamides) – 0.026 *(isoflavones)	< 0.001	0.934
Superoxid anion scavenging *	1.194 + 0.059 *(clovamides) + 0.468 *(proanthocyanidins)	< 0.001	0.685
Peroxyl radical scavenging * *	−2.217 – 12.624 *(phenolic acids) + 4.012 *(clovamides) + 1.317 *(other flavonoids) + 1.765 *(isoflavones)	< 0.05	0.554
Flowers			
Fremy's salt scavenging *	5.444 – 1.886 *(phenolic acids) + 0.233 *(other flavonoids)	< 0.001	0.524
Superoxid anion scavenging *	0.887 – 0.230 *(clovamides) + 0.127 *(other flavonoids)	< 0.001	0.728
Peroxyl radical scavenging **	−242.1 + 217.8 *(phenolic acids) – 80.8 *(clovamides) + 16.5 *(other flavonoids) + 52.5 *(isoflavones)	< 0.05	0.601

* µmol gallic acid equivalents (GAE)/100 g freeze-dried matter; ** mmol Trolox equivalents (TE)/100 g freeze-dried matter

The concentration of clovamides had a consistent, positive regression coefficient in the three best models predicted for the antioxidant activity in leaves. Similarly, the concentration of the group of flavonoids other than isoflavones contributed positively to predicting the antioxidant activity with all assays in flowers (Table 7).

The multicollinearity between the concentrations of flavonoids and proanthocyanidins prevented their simultaneous assessment as regressors in the prediction of the antioxidant activity. However, when taken individually in a simple correlation analysis with the three scavenging assays, the mean flower concentration of proanthocyanidins also proved positively correlated with the antioxidant activity, with correlation ranging between $r = 0.63$ ($P < 0.05$) with the peroxyl radical and $r = 0.73$ ($P < 0.01$) with the superoxide anion scavenging.

Although claimed as interesting antioxidant compounds, clovamides proved to be important but not critical for the antioxidant activity in cocoa, *Theobroma cacao* L. [60]. Subsequent findings indicated them as potent bioactive compounds with anti-inflammatory activity in human cells [61]. In the current study, clovamides appeared to have a conditional, positive role in determining the antioxidant activity of leaf extracts in the genus *Trifolium*. Our results are in line with those by Kolodziejczyk et al. [62], who reported that clovamide-rich extract from *T. pallidum* reduced the damage induced by oxidative stress to blood platelets and plasma.

A key role in determining the antioxidant activity in flowers of *Trifolium* germplasm was exerted instead by the classes of flavonoids (isoflavones excluded) and proanthocyanidins, which was fully justified by the strong antioxidant properties reported for these compounds [11,52,63]. As already mentioned, flower pigmentation and UV screening contribute to the abundance of flavonoids and proanthocyanidins in flower tissues.

This investigation confirmed the genus *Trifolium* as a great reservoir of phenolic compounds, with different chemical structure and, possibly, largely diversified biological activity. Such a wealth of potentially important metabolites is available for clinical and nutraceutical utilization. It is worth reminding that, unlike other species claimed for extraction of biologically active compounds, most *Trifolium* species have a well-established agronomic technique for their cultivation. This study also suggested possible links between environmental factors (stresses, in particular) and concentration and composition of phenolic compounds.

3. Materials and Methods

3.1. Plant Material

Swards of red clover, white clover, subterranean clover, berseem clover and snow clover were sampled in the lowland site of Lodi [45°19′ N, 9°30′ E, 81 m above sea level (asl)], in the Po Valley plain, northern Italy (Table 1). Some of the materials belonging to these taxa were grown in plots at the experimental station of the Research Centre for Animal Production and Aquaculture (CREA-ZA). In particular, the red clover cultivar Aiace, the white clover cultivar Regal (a non-Ladino large-leaved type of *T. repens*) and one snow clover natural population from the Rhaetian Alps were sampled from one-year-old sown swards. Aiace and Regal are cultivars selected in Italy and the USA, respectively, and both are adapted to temperate, favorable climatic conditions, such as those experienced under the sub-continental climate of Lodi (847 mm long-term average annual rainfall, 12.2 °C average annual mean daily temperature, −1.3 °C average minimum daily temperature of the coldest month). Seed of the snow clover population from the Rhaetian Alps was collected at 1850 m asl and it was sown in the lowland site as part of a trial carried out in altitude-contrasting environments. Germplasm of the annual species berseem clover (the experimental cultivar Sintetica-E) and subterranean clover (two natural populations whose seed was originally collected in Sardinia) were sown at CREA-ZA for this study. As both species are specifically adapted to Mediterranean conditions, they were sown in Lodi at the end of the winter preceding the sampling season to avoid possible frost damages. Besides the plot-grown materials, two more populations were sampled from a century-old grassland in Lodi, belonging to locally-adapted ecotypes of red clover and Ladino white clover (*T. repens* L. var. *giganteum* Lagr.-Foss.), respectively. Other natural populations used in this investigation were identified and sampled in the Alpine region (Table 1). They included one small-leaved population of white clover (*T. repens* var. *sylvestre*), which encompassed, therefore, three different types in the study, and one population each of snow clover, alpine clover (*T. alpinum* L.), brown clover (*T. badium* Schreb.), sulphur clover (*T. ochroleucum* Huds.) and Thal clover (*T. thalii* Vill.). Identification of different taxa was made according to reference guides on the Alpine flora [64]. All the mountain populations except the sulphur clover were sampled in the Graian Alps above 1900 m asl. The sulphur clover population was sampled in the Cottian Alps at 1250 m asl.

All the materials were sampled at the same phenological stage of full bloom. This stage occurred in spring (May) in the lowland site of Lodi, and in summer (July) in the mountain locations. Two samples of leaves and flowers were collected, respectively, from each sward, refrigerated and immediately brought to the laboratory. Leaf and flower samples were separately freeze-dried, finely powdered, defatted with chloroform and then used for the subsequent extractions.

3.2. *Extraction and Purification of Total Phenolics*

Samples (100 mg) were extracted with 80% MeOH (10 mL) at 50 °C using an automated accelerated solvent extractor ASE 200 (Dionex, Sunnyvale, CA, USA) at a working pressure of 1500 psi. Extracts were evaporated to dryness under reduced pressure at 40 °C, re-dissolved in 5 mL of Milli-Q water (Millipore Corp., Billerica, MA, USA) and purified using a C18 Sep-Pak (360 mg, 55–105 μm) cartridge (Waters Associates, Milford, MA, USA) preconditioned with water. The cartridge was washed first with water (5 mL) to remove sugars and other water-soluble compounds, then with 80% MeOH (5 mL) to elute phenolics. Extracts were evaporated to dryness under reduced pressure at 40 °C, re-dissolved in 2 mL of 80% MeOH and then used for analysis. Three independent extraction and purification procedures were performed on each replicated sample, and the extracts were properly diluted before analysis. A portion of the extracts was also freeze-dried for subsequent antioxidant activity assays.

3.3. *Determination and Quantitation of Phenolic Composition*

A Waters ACQUITY UPLC system equipped with a binary pump system, sample manager, column manager, photo diode array (PDA) detector (Waters Corp.) and coupled to a Waters ACQUITY TQD (tandem quadrupole mass detector) with an electrospray ionization (ESI) source was used. All data were acquired and processed using Waters MassLynx 4.1 and QuanLynx software. Chromatographic runs were carried out with a Waters BEH C18 column (100 mm × 1.0 mm i.d., 1.7 μm particles, 13 nm pore size) under a linear gradient of solvent A (H_2O/0.1% HCOOH) and solvent B (CH_3CN/0.1% HCOOH) as follows: 0.0–0.5 min (7% B), 8.0 min (25% B), 11.5 min (60% B), 12.0 min (80% B), 20 min (80% B). The flow rate was 0.19 mL/min, and the column temperature was 50 °C. A sample of 0.5 μL was injected for analysis. For MS detection, positive and negative ESI were used as ionization modes. Nitrogen was used as the desolvation and cone gas with flow rates of 800 L/h and 80 L/h, respectively. Argon was used as the collision gas at a flow rate of 2 mL/min. The MS parameters were as follows: Capillary 2.8 kV; extractor and radiofrequency voltage fixed at 3.0 V and 0.1 V, respectively; source and desolvation temperatures of 140 °C and 350 °C, respectively [20,28].

Phenolic compounds were identified by comparison of their UV absorption spectra, retention times and mass spectral data (positive and negative mode) with those of standard compounds, as well as with previously identified phenolic constituents of *Trifolium* spp. reported in the literature [19,20,25–28]. Individual compounds were quantified against reference standards at 260 nm. Astragalin, hyperoside, cymaroside, isoquercitrin, genistin, ononin, sissotrin, kaempferol, quercetin, apigenin, luteolin, myricetin, genistein, biochanin A, formononetin catechin, epicatechin were from Sigma-Aldrich (Milano, Italy). Concentration of glycoside malonates and acetates were calculated using the standard curves of the corresponding glycosides. Concentration of isoflavonoids without standards were calculated using the standard curves of ononin, while the concentration of other flavonoids was calculated using the calibration curves of isoquercitrin. Chlorogenic acid from Sigma-Aldrich was used to quantify clovamides and phenolic acids. For calibration curves, all standards were injected in triplicate in the range from 4.5 to 300 ng injection.

Proanthocyanidins (condensed tannins) were assessed by the butanol/HCl method [41], and evaluated with pelargonidin hydrochloride from Sigma-Aldrich as a standard.

All samples were extracted in triplicate and results expressed in mg g^{-1} dry matter as mean of three independent analyses ± standard deviation. As an indication of the relative abundance of the main tentatively identified compounds, the percentage values of their content in the whole extracts were reported in Table 2.

3.4. *Antioxidant Activity*

The purified freeze-dried extracts were subsequently treated at room temperature with 2.5 mL MeOH, 2.5 mL water, and acidified with 0.05 mL of 1N HCl. The mixture was vortexed for 60 s and centrifuged (5000× *g*, 5 min) and the supernatant directly used for antioxidant assays. The antioxidant activity was assessed by three different methods, aimed at understanding the potential action of the different groups of antioxidant compounds isolated and thoroughly characterized in *Trifolium* extracts. The three methods, described as follows, were the Fremy's salt scavenging and the superoxide anion scavenging, both carried out by Electron Paramagnetic Resonance (EPR), and the scavenging of peroxyl radicals, performed with a spectrophotometric approach.

3.4.1. Fremy's Salt Scavenging

This EPR assay was performed using Fremy's salt, potassium nitrosodisulfonate $[(KSO_3)_2NO]$, a persistent water-soluble free radical that was successfully used in previous experiments investigating the antioxidant potential of fruit juices [65]. The reaction mixture contained 380 μL of 0.1 M acetate buffer, pH 4.5, and 100 μL of plant extract with 20 μL of 5.96 mM Fremy's salt solution dissolved in acetate buffer, final concentration 0.24 mM. Blank reaction was composed as before, by replacing the plant extract by the pure extracting solution. The mixture was stirred and transferred into a 100-μL glass capillary tube, and the EPR spectra were recorded after 3 min at 25 °C using a MS 200 EPR spectrometer (Miniscope, Berlin, Germany) operating on the X-band. The instrument settings were the following: field modulation 100 KHz, modulation amplitude 1500 mG, field constant 60 s, center field 3350 G, sweep width 99.70 G, X-band frequency 9.64 GHz, MW attenuation 7 dB, and gain 5. Under these conditions, the typical triplet Fremy's salt spectrum (1:1:1) was observed. The intensity of the EPR signal was measured at the height of the first line, with the resonance at 3336.6 G. The system was calibrated with solutions of gallic acid at known concentrations, hence the results were given as μmol of gallic acid equivalents (GAE)/100 g dried extract.

3.4.2. Superoxide Anion Scavenging

The antioxidant potential towards $O_2^{-\bullet}$ was based on the spin trapping of the radical generated by potassium superoxide (KO_2) in dimethyl sulfoxide (DMSO) with the addition of 18-crown-6 ether to complex K^+, using the previously performed and validated method by Picchi et al. [66], with some modifications. The spin trap reagent was 5,5-dimethylpyrroline-N-oxide (DMPO). Under these conditions, a typical DMPO-OOH adduct (1:1:1:1) was observed. The scavenging reaction mixture was 18-crown-6 ether/KO_2 (1:1, 20 mM) dissolved in DMSO. A blank solution contained 100 μL of a 100 mM DMPO phosphate buffer solution 0.1 M, pH 7.4, 130 μL of superoxide solution and 10 μL of extracting solution. The solution with the scavenging compound was composed exactly as the blank, by replacing 10 μL of extracting solution with the equivalent volume of the *Trifolium* extract. The reaction time was 60 sec at 25 °C. EPR recording conditions were as follows: field set, 3350 G; scan range, 70 G; scan time, 120 s; modulation amplitude, 1200 mG; microwave attenuation, 5 dB; receiver gain, 8 × 100. The intensity of the EPR signal was measured at the height of the first spectrum line, with the resonance at 3326.1 G. The system was calibrated with solutions of gallic acid at known concentrations, hence the results were given as mmol of gallic acid equivalents (GAE)/100 g dried extract.

3.4.3. Peroxyl Radical by Enzymatic Degradation of Linoleic Acid

In this method, the enzymatic peroxidation of linoleic acid, generating peroxyl radicals, was obtained by the addition of lipoxygenase (EC 1.13.11.12) with some modifications of the method described by Grossman and Zakut [67], successively checked and validated by Lo Scalzo et al. [68]. The peroxidation of linoleic acid was analyzed in the absence (blank) and presence (sample) of the assayed extracts by recording the increase in absorbance at 234 nm over 2 min at 25 °C after a 30 sec delay. The substrate was prepared by dissolving 40 μL of linoleic acid in 2 mL of absolute ethanol under nitrogen, followed by the addition of 10 μL of Tween 20. The solution was slowly mixed, then 40 mL of 0.05 M K_2HPO_4 were added, and the pH was adjusted to 9.0 with 0.05 M NaOH, the final substrate concentration resulting 3.21 mM. The lipoxygenase solution was freshly prepared by dissolving 11 mg of a lipoxygenase standard soybean extract (Sigma, St. Louis, MO, USA) in 16 mL of 0.1 M phosphate buffer (pH 7.0). In the sample test, the reaction solution was composed of 2.0 mL of 0.1 M phosphate buffer (pH 7.0), 0.2 mL of substrate (0.27 mM final concentration), 0.15 mL of scavenging solution, and 0.05 mL of lipoxygenase solution. In the blank test, the scavenging solution was substituted by 0.15 mL of pure extracting solution. The reaction was spectrophotometrically monitored at 234 nm to follow peroxyl radical conjugate diene formation. The antioxidant activity of enzymatically mediated linoleic acid peroxidation (LIPOX–LINOL) was expressed as the protection percentage monitored by the absorbance at 234 nm, by interpolating the data with those of a calibration curve obtained from standard solutions of Trolox (6-hydroxy-2,5,7,8-tetramethylchromane-2-carboxylic acid). The results were thus reported as mmol of Trolox equivalents (TE)/100 g dried extract.

3.5. Statistical Analyses

The general term 'accession' commonly used in germplasm collections was adopted throughout this work to equally indicate cultivated forms (cultivars), ecotypes, or natural populations of any evaluated species. Each replication of leaf and flower samples represented the basic experimental unit of each accession.

An analysis of variance (ANOVA) tested the differences between leaves and flowers (across all accessions and replications) for the mean concentration of each of the five groups of phenolics identified in this study and their total, and the mean antioxidant activity determined by three assays (Fremy's salt scavenging, superoxide anion scavenging and peroxyl radical scavenging). A second ANOVA assessed the differences among the 14 accessions (phenolic concentrations and antioxidant activity assays) for leaves and flowers, individually using the accession × replication variance as the error term. Differences between the areas of origin/sampling of the germplasm (lowlands vs. mountains) were assessed by another ANOVA for leaves and flowers, individually, testing the variance of the 'area' factor over the pooled variance of the nested factor 'accession within area'. In this analysis, the snow clover population #3, originating from the Alps but sampled in the lowland site, was excluded.

Given the diverse range of *Trifolium* taxa encompassed by the current germplasm, an attempt was made to predict by multiple regression the antioxidant activity in the genus based on the recorded concentrations of phenolic groups. Accession mean values of each of the three antioxidant assays and of the five groups of phenolics were used as dependent variable and independent variables, respectively, in the regressions separately run for leaf and flower data. Prior to the choice of the best predicting models, the presence of multicollinearity between regressors was verified by different indexes, namely, the variance inflation factor, the condition number and the eigenvalues [69]. The choice of the best predicting regression model for each antioxidant assay in leaves and flowers was made examining different methods, namely, the stepwise procedure, the adjusted R^2, the C(p) index and the Press number, and choosing the most consistent model accordingly [69]. All statistical analyses were carried out using the Proc GLM and Proc Reg of the SAS software.

Author Contributions: A.T. and L.P. (Luciano Pecetti) designed the experiment, analysed the data, wrote and revised the paper; A.T., Ł.P. (Łucas Pecio) and R.L.S. performed the analyses; A.S. commented the data and the draft manuscript. All authors have red and approved the manuscript.

Acknowledgments: Technical support from A. Ursino and B. Pintus of CREA-ZA Lodi, Italy, is gratefully acknowledged.

References

1. Abberton, M.T.; Marshall, A.H. White clover. In *Fodder Cops and Amenity Grasses*; Handbook of Plant Breeding Series; Volume 5, Boller, B., Posselt, U.K., Veronesi, F., Eds.; Springer: New York, NY, USA, 2010; pp. 457–476.
2. Boller, B.; Schubiger, F.X.; Kölliker, R. Red clover. In *Fodder Cops and Amenity Grasses*; Handbook of Plant Breeding Series; Volume 5, Boller, B., Posselt, U.K., Veronesi, F., Eds.; Springer: New York, NY, USA, 2010; pp. 439–456.
3. Piano, E.; Pecetti, L. Minor legume species. In *Fodder Cops and Amenity Grasses*; Handbook of Plant Breeding Series; Volume 5, Boller, B., Posselt, U.K., Veronesi, F., Eds.; Springer: New York, NY, USA, 2010; pp. 477–500.
4. Woodgate, K.; Maxted, N.; Bennet, S. A generic conspectus for the forage legumes of the Mediterranean basin. In *Genetic Resources of Mediterranean Pasture and Forage Legumes*; Bennett, S.J., Cocks, P.S., Eds.; Kluwer Academic Publishers: Dordrecht, The Netherlands, 1999; pp. 182–226.
5. Cavallero, A.; Aceto, P.; Gorlier, A.; Lombardi, G.; Lonati, M.; Martinasso, B.; Tagliatori, C. *I Tipi Pastorali delle Alpi Piemontesi*; Alberto Perdisa Editore: Bologna, Italy, 2007.
6. Rognli, O.A.; Fjellheim, S.; Pecetti, L.; Boller, B. Semi-natural grasslands as a source of genetic diversity. In *The Role of Grasslands in a Green Future. Grasslands Science in Europe*; Algadóttir, Á., Hopkins, A., Eds.; Prentsmiđjan Oddi: Reykjavík, Iceland, 2013; Volume 18, pp. 303–313.
7. Sabudak, T.; Guler, N. *Trifolium* L.—A review on its phytochemical and pharmacological profile. *Phytoter. Res.* **2009**, *23*, 439–446. [CrossRef]
8. Pereira, D.M.; Valentão, P.; Pereira, J.A.; Andrade, P.B. Phenolics: From chemistry to biology. *Molecules* **2009**, *14*, 2202–2211. [CrossRef]
9. Tapas, A.R.; Sakarkar, D.M.; Kakde, R.B. Flavonoids as nutraceuticals: A review. *Tropic. J. Pharm. Res.* **2008**, *7*, 1089–1099. [CrossRef]
10. Wang, H.; Cao, R.L.; Prior, J. Total Antioxidant Capacity of Fruits. *J. Agric. Food Chem.* **1996**, *44*, 701–705. [CrossRef]
11. Pietta, P.G. Flavonoids as antioxidants. *J. Nat. Prod.* **2000**, *63*, 1035–1042. [CrossRef] [PubMed]
12. Dillard, C.J.; German, J.B. Phytochemicals: Nutraceuticals and human health. *J. Sci. Food Agric.* **2000**, *80*, 1744–1756. [CrossRef]
13. Hertog, M.G.; Feskens, E.J.; Hallman, P.C.; Katan, M.B.; Kromhout, D. Dietary antioxidant flavonoids and risk of coronary heart disease: The Zutphen Elderly Study. *Lancet* **1993**, *342*, 1007–1011. [CrossRef]
14. Bobe, G.; Weinstein, S.J.; Albanes, D.; Hirvonen, T.; Ashby, J.; Taylor, P.R.; Virtamo, J.; Stolzenberg-Solomon, R.Z. Flavonoid intake and risk of pancreatic cancer in male smokers (Finland). *Cancer Epidemiol. Biomark. Prev.* **2008**, *17*, 553–562. [CrossRef] [PubMed]
15. Cornwell, T.; Cohick, W.; Raskin, I. Dietary phytoestrogen and health. *Phytochemistry* **2004**, *65*, 995–1016. [CrossRef] [PubMed]
16. Hidalgo, L.A.; Chedraui, P.A.; Morocho, N.; Ros, S.; San Miguel, G. The effect of red clover isoflavones on menopausal symptoms, lipid and vaginal cytology in menopausal women: A randomized, double-blind, placebo-controlled study. *Gynecol. Endocrinol.* **2005**, *21*, 257–264. [CrossRef]
17. Rüfer, C.E.; Kulling, S.E. Antioxidant activity of isoflavones and their major metabolites using different in vitro assays. *J. Agric. Food Chem.* **2006**, *54*, 2926–2931. [CrossRef] [PubMed]
18. McRae, J.M.; Yang, Q.; Crawford, R.J.; Palombo, E.A. Chemotaxonomic applications of flavonoids. In *Nutrition and Diet Research Progress Series: Flavonoids: Biosynthesis, Biological Effects and Dietary Sources*; Keller, R.B., Ed.; Nova Science Publisher: Hauppauge, NY, USA, 2009; Chapter 11; pp. 291–299.
19. Oleszek, W.; Stochmal, A.; Janda, B. Concentration of isoflavones and other phenolics in the aerial parts of *Trifolium* species. *J. Agric. Food Chem.* **2007**, *55*, 8095–8100. [CrossRef] [PubMed]

20. Tava, A.; Pecio, Ł.; Stochmal, A.; Pecetti, L. Clovamide and flavonoids from leaves of *Trifolium pratense* and *T. pratense* subsp. *nivale* grown in Italy. *Nat. Prod. Comm.* **2015**, *10*, 933–936.
21. Di Ferdinando, M.; Brunetti, C.; Fini, A.; Tattini, M. Flavonoids as antioxidants in plants under abiotic stresses. In *Abiotic Stress Responses in Plants: Metabolism, Productivity and Sustainability*; Ahmad, P., Prasad, M.N.V., Eds.; Springer Science+Business Media, LLC: New York, NY, USA, 2012; pp. 159–180.
22. Cheynier, V.; Comte, G.; Davies, K.M.; Lattanzio, V.; Martens, S. Plant phenolics: Recent advances on their biosynthesis, genetics, and ecophysiology. *Plant Physiol. Biochem.* **2013**, *72*, 1–20. [CrossRef] [PubMed]
23. Winkel-Shirley, B. Biosynthesis of flavonoids and effect of stress. *Curr. Opin. Plant Biol.* **2002**, *5*, 218–223. [CrossRef]
24. Blokhina, O.; Virolainen, E.; Fagerstedt, K.V. Antioxidants, oxidative damage and oxygen deprivation stress: A review. *Ann. Bot.* **2003**, *91*, 179–194. [CrossRef]
25. de Rijke, E.; Out, P.; Niessen, W.M.A.; Ariese, F.; Gooijer, C.; Brinkman, U.A.T. Analytical separation and detection methods for flavonoids. *J. Chromatogr. A* **2006**, *1112*, 31–63. [CrossRef]
26. Polasek, J.; Queiroz, E.F.; Hostettmann, K. On-line identification of phenolic compounds of *Trifolium* species using HPLC-UV-MS and post-column UV-derivatization. *Phytochem. Anal.* **2007**, *18*, 13–23. [CrossRef]
27. Kowalska, I.; Jedrejek, D.; Ciesla, L.; Pecio, L.; Masullo, M.; Piacente, S.; Oleszek, W.; Stochmal, A. Isolation, chemical and free radical scavenging characterization of phenolics from *Trifolium scabrum* L. aerial parts. *J. Agric. Food Chem.* **2013**, *61*, 4417–4423. [CrossRef]
28. Tava, A.; Stochmal, A.; Pecetti, L. Isoflavone content in subterranean clover germplasm from Sardinia. *Chem. Biodiv.* **2016**, *13*, 1038–1045. [CrossRef]
29. Stobiecki, M.; Kachlicki, P.; Wojakowska, A.; Marczak, L. Application of LC/MS systems to structural characterization of flavonoid glycoconjugates. *Phytochem. Lett.* **2015**, *11*, 358–367. [CrossRef]
30. Shehata, M.N.; Hassan, A.; El-Shazly, K. Identification of the oestrogenic isoflavones in fresh and fermented berseem clover (*Trifolium alexandrinum*). *Aust. J. Agric. Res.* **1982**, *33*, 951–956. [CrossRef]
31. Ahmed, Q.U.; Kaleem, M.; Parveen, N.; Khan, N.U. Phytochemical and pharmacological investigations of Egyptian colver, *Trifolium alexandrinum* L. Sustainable Management and Utilization of Medicinal Plant Resources. In Proceedings of the International Conference Medicinal Plants, Kuala Lumpur, Malaysia, 5–7 December 2005; pp. 219–226.
32. Sharaf, M. Chemical constituents from the seeds of *Trifolium alexandrinum*. *Nat. Prod. Res.* **2008**, *22*, 1620–1623. [CrossRef] [PubMed]
33. Lin, L.Z.; He, X.G.; Lindenmaier, M.; Yang, J.; Cleary, M.; Qui, S.X.; Cordell, G.A. LC-ESI-MS study of the flavonoid glycoside malonates of red clover (*Trifolium pratense*). *J. Agric. Food Chem.* **2000**, *48*, 354–365. [CrossRef] [PubMed]
34. Klejdus, B.; Vitamvasova-Sterbova, D.; Kuban, V. Identification of isoflavone conjugates in red clover (*Trifolium pratense*) by liquid chromatography-mass spectrometry after two-dimensional solid-phase extraction. *Anal. Chim. Acta* **2001**, *450*, 81–97. [CrossRef]
35. Tsao, R.; Papadopoulos, Y.; Yang, R.; Young, J.C.; McRae, K. Isoflavone profiles of red clovers and their distribution in different parts harvested at different growing stages. *J. Agric. Food Chem.* **2006**, *54*, 5797–5805. [CrossRef] [PubMed]
36. Saviranta, N.M.M.; Julkunen-Tiitto, R.; Oksanen, E.; Karjalainen, R.O. Leaf phenolic compounds in red clover (*Trifolium pratense* L.) induced by exposure to moderately elevated ozone. *Environ. Poll.* **2010**, *158*, 440–446. [CrossRef] [PubMed]
37. Foo, L.Y.; Lu, Y.; Molan, A.L.; Woodfield, D.R.; McNabb, W.C. The phenols and prodelphinidins of white clover flowers. *Phytochemistry* **2000**, *54*, 539–548. [CrossRef]
38. Hofmann, R.W.; Swinny, E.E.; Bloor, S.J.; Markham, K.R.; Ryan, K.G.; Campbell, B.D.; Jordan, B.R.; Fountain, D.W. Responses of nine *Trifolium repens* L. populations to ultraviolet-B radiation: Differential flavonol glycoside accumulation and biomass production. *Ann. Bot.* **2000**, *86*, 527–537. [CrossRef]
39. Carlsen, S.C.K.; Mortensen, A.G.; Oleszek, W.; Piacente, S.; Stochmal, A.; Fomsgaard, S. Variation in flavonoids in leaves, stem and flowers of white clover cultivars. *Nat. Prod. Comm.* **2008**, *3*, 1299–1306.
40. Kicel, A.; Wolbis, M. Study of the phenolic constituents of the lowes and leaves of *Trifolium repens* L. *Nat. Prod. Res.* **2012**, *26*, 2050–2054. [CrossRef] [PubMed]
41. Porter, L.J.; Hrstich, L.N.; Chan, B.G. The conversion of procyanidins and prodelphinidins to cyanidin and delphinidin. *Phytochemistry* **1986**, *25*, 223–230. [CrossRef]

42. Schofield, P.; Mbugua, D.M.; Pell, A.N. Analysis of condensed tannins: A review. *Anim. Feed Sci. Technol.* **2001**, *91*, 21–40. [CrossRef]
43. Wolfe, R.M.; Terrill, T.H.; Muir, J.P. Drying method and origin of standard affect condensed tannin (CT) concentrations in perennial herbaceous legumes using simplified butanol-HCl CT analysis. *J. Sci. Food Agric.* **2008**, *88*, 1060–1067. [CrossRef]
44. Kardel, M.; Taube, F.M.; Schulz, H.; Schütze, W.; Gierus, M. Different approaches to evaluate tannin content and structure of selected plant extracts—Review and new aspects. *J. Appl. Bot. Food Qual.* **2013**, *86*, 154–166.
45. Davies, K.M.; Schwinn, K.E. Molecular biology and biotechnology of flavonoids. In *Flavonoids Chemistry, Biochemistry and Applications*; Andersen, O.M., Markham, K.R., Eds.; CRC Press, Tylor & Francis Group: Boca Raton, FL, USA, 2006; Chapter 3; pp. 143–218.
46. Saboonchian, F.; Jamedi, R.; Sarghein, S.H. Phenolic and flavonoid content of *Elaeagnus angustifolia* L. (leaf and flower). *Avic. J. Phytomed.* **2014**, *4*, 231–238.
47. Dokhani, S.; Cottrell, T.; Khajeddin, J.; Mazza, G. Analysis of aroma and phenolic components of selected Achillea species. *Plant Food Hum. Nutr.* **2005**, *60*, 55–62. [CrossRef]
48. Mekni, M.; Azez, R.; Tekaya, M.; Mechri, B.; Hammami, M. Phenolic, non-phenolic compounds and antioxidant activity of pomegranate flower, leaf and bark extracts of Tunisian cultivars. *J. Med. Plants Res.* **2013**, *7*, 1100–1107.
49. Dores, R.G.R.; Guimaraes, S.F.; Braga, T.V.; Fonseca, M.C.M.; Martinus, P.M.; Ferreira, T.C. Phenolic compounds, flavonoids and antioxidant activity of leaves, flowers and roots of white-weed. *Hortic. Brasil.* **2014**, *32*, 486–490. [CrossRef]
50. Abeynayake, S.W.; Panter, S.; Chapman, R.; Webster, T.; Rochfort, S.; Mouradov, A.; Spangenberg, G. Biosynthesis of proanthocyanidins in white clover flowers: Cross talk within the flavonoid pathway. *Plant Physiol.* **2012**, *158*, 666–678. [CrossRef]
51. van der Meer, I.M.; Stam, M.E.; van Tunen, A.J.; Mol, J.N.M.; Stuitje, A.R. Antisense inhibition of flavonoid biosynthesis in petunia anthers results in male sterility. *Plant Cell* **1992**, *4*, 253–262. [CrossRef] [PubMed]
52. Jayaprakasha, G.K.; Singh, R.P.; Sakariah, K.K. Antioxidant activity of grape seed (*Vitis vinifera*) extracts on peroxidation models in vitro. *Food Chem.* **2001**, *73*, 285–290. [CrossRef]
53. Beck, V.; Rohr, U.; Jungbauer, A. Phytoestrogen derived from red clover: An alternative to estrogen replacement therapy? *J. Steroid Biochem. Mol. Biol.* **2005**, *94*, 499–518. [CrossRef] [PubMed]
54. Cao, G.; Sofic, E.; Prior, R.L. Antioxidant and prooxidant behavior of flavonoids: Structure-activity relationship. *Free Radic. Biol. Med.* **1997**, *22*, 749–760. [CrossRef]
55. Agati, G.; Brunetti, C.; Di Ferdinando, M.; Ferrini, F.; Pollastri, S.; Tattini, M. Funcional roles of flavonoids in photoprotection: New evidence, lessons from the past. *Plant Physiol. Biochem.* **2013**, *72*, 35–45. [CrossRef]
56. Morales, L.O.; Tegelberg, R.; Brosché, M.; Keinänen, M.; Lindfors, A.; Aphalo, P.J. Effects of solar UV-A and UV-B radiation on gene expression and phenolic accumulation in *Betula pendula* leaves. *Tree Physiol.* **2010**, *30*, 923–934. [CrossRef]
57. Bieza, K.; Lois, R. An *Arabidopsis* mutant tolerant to lethal ultraviolet-B levels shows constitutively elevated accumulation of flavonoids and other phenolics. *Plant Physiol.* **2001**, *126*, 1105–1115. [CrossRef]
58. Jansen, M.A.K.; Gaba, V.; Greenberg, B.M. Higher plants and UV-B radiation: Balancing damage, repair and acclimatation. *Trends Plant Sci.* **1998**, *3*, 131–135. [CrossRef]
59. Nichols, P.G.H.; Foster, K.J.; Piano, E.; Kaur, P.; Ghamkhar, K.; Pecetti, L.; Collins, W.J. Genetic improvement of subterranean clover (*Trifolium subterraneum* L.). 1. Germplasm, traits and future prospects. *Crop Pasture Sci.* **2013**, *64*, 312–346. [CrossRef]
60. Arlorio, M.; Locatelli, M.; Travaglia, F.; Coisson, J.D.; Del Grosso, E.; Minassi, A.; Appendino, G.; Martelli, A. Roasting impact on the contents of clovamide (*N*-caffeoyl-*L*-DOPA) and the antioxidant activity of cocoa beans (*Theobroma cacao* L.). *Food Chem.* **2008**, *106*, 967–975. [CrossRef]
61. Zeng, H.; Locatelli, M.; Bardelli, C.; Amoroso, A.; Coïsson, J.D.; Travaglia, F.; Arlorio, M.; Brunelleschi, S. Anti-inflammatory properties of clovamide and *Theobroma cacao* phenolic extracts in human monocytes: Evaluation of respiratory burst, cytokine release, NF-κB activation, and PPARγ modulation. *J. Agric. Food Chem.* **2011**, *59*, 5342–5350. [CrossRef] [PubMed]
62. Kolodziejczyk, J.; Olas, B.; Wachowicz, B.; Szajwaj, B.; Stochmal, A.; Oleszek, W. Clovamide-rich extract from *Trifolium pallidum* reduces oxidative stress-induced damage to blood platelets and plasma. *J. Physiol. Biochem.* **2011**, *67*, 391–399. [CrossRef] [PubMed]

63. Bagchi, D.; Bagchi, M.; Stohs, S.J.; Das, D.K.; Ray, S.D.; Kuszynski, C.A.; Joshi, S.S.; Pruess, H.G. Free radical and grape seed proanthocyanidin extract: Importance in human health and disease prevention. *Toxicology* **2000**, *148*, 187–197. [CrossRef]
64. Pignatti, S. *Flora d'Italia*; Edagricole: Bologna, Italy, 1982.
65. Gardner, P.T.; White, T.A.C.; McPhail, D.B. The relative contribution of vitamin C, carotenoid and phenolics to the antioxidant potential of fruit juices. *Food Chem.* **2000**, *68*, 471–474. [CrossRef]
66. Picchi, V.; Migliori, C.; Lo Scalzo, R.; Campanelli, G.; Ferrari, V.; Di Cesare, L.F. Phytochemical content in organic and conventionally grown Italian cauliflower. *Food Chem.* **2012**, *130*, 501–509. [CrossRef]
67. Grossman, S.; Zakut, R. Determination of the activity of lipoxygenase. In *Method of Biochemical Analysis*; Glick, D., Ed.; Wiley-Interscience: New York, NY, USA, 1979; pp. 313–316.
68. Lo Scalzo, R.; Todaro, A.; Rapisarda, P. Methods used to evaluate the peroxyl (ROO·) radical scavenging capacities of four common antioxidants. *Eur. Food Res. Technol.* **2012**, *235*, 1141–1148. [CrossRef]
69. Donatelli, M.; Annicchiarico, P. *Nota Sull'analisi di Dati Sperimentali in Agricoltura Tramite il SAS (Statistical Analysis System)*, Seconda edizione; ISCI e ISCF: Bologna, Italy, 1999.

4

Formulations of Curcumin Nanoparticles for Brain Diseases

María L. Del Prado-Audelo [1], Isaac H. Caballero-Florán [2,3], Jorge A. Meza-Toledo [3,4], Néstor Mendoza-Muñoz [5], Maykel González-Torres [6,7], Benjamín Florán [2], Hernán Cortés [8,*] and Gerardo Leyva-Gómez [3,*]

1 Laboratorio de Posgrado en Tecnología Farmacéutica, FES-Cuautitlán, Universidad Nacional Autónoma de México, Cuautitlán Izcalli 54740, Mexico; ml.delprado@iim.unam.mx
2 Departamento de Fisiología, Biofísica & Neurociencias, Centro de Investigación y de Estudios Avanzados del Instituto Politécnico Nacional, Ciudad de México 07360, Mexico; hiram.qfohead@gmail.com (I.H.C.-F.); bfloran@fisio.cinvestav.mx (B.F.)
3 Departamento de Farmacia, Facultad de Química, Universidad Nacional Autónoma de México, Ciudad Universitaria, Circuito Exterior S/N, Del. Coyoacán, C.P. Ciudad de México 04510, Mexico; jamtoledo90@outlook.com
4 Escuela de Ciencias de la Salud, Universidad del Valle de México, Campus Coyoacán, Ciudad de México, 04910, Mexico
5 Facultad de Ciencias Químicas, Universidad de Colima, C.P. Colima 28400, México; nmendoza0@ucol.cmx
6 CONACyT-Laboratorio de Biotecnología, Instituto Nacional de Rehabilitación Luis Guillermo Ibarra Ibarra, Ciudad de México 14389, Mexico; mikegcu@gmail.com
7 Instituto Tecnológico y de Estudios Superiores de Monterrey, Campus Ciudad de México 14380, Mexico
8 Laboratorio de Medicina Genómica, Departamento de Genética, Instituto Nacional de Rehabilitación Luis Guillermo Ibarra Ibarra, Ciudad de México 14389, Mexico
* Correspondence: hcortes@inr.gob.mx or hcortes_c@hotmail.com (H.C.); gerardoleyva@hotmail.com (G.L.-G.);

Abstract: Curcumin is a polyphenol that is obtained from *Curcuma longa* and used in various areas, such as food and textiles. Curcumin has important anti-inflammatory and antioxidant properties that allow it to be applied as treatment for several emerging pathologies. Remarkably, there are an elevated number of publications deriving from the terms "curcumin" and "curcumin brain diseases", which highlights the increasing impact of this polyphenol and the high number of study groups investigating their therapeutic actions. However, its lack of solubility in aqueous media, as well as its poor bioavailability in biological systems, represent limiting factors for its successful application. In this review article, the analysis of its chemical composition and the pivotal mechanisms for brain applications are addressed in a global manner. Furthermore, we emphasize the use of nanoparticles with curcumin and the benefits that have been reached as an example of the extensive advances in this area of health.

Keywords: curcumin; nanoparticles; inflammation; protein aggregation; brain diseases; Alzheimer's disease; Parkinson's disease

---

1. Introduction

Curcumin is an active natural polyphenol component of *Curcuma longa*. Due to its chemical structure, this molecule could be applied in several different fields, such as food, textile, and the pharmaceutical industry. It has been shown that curcumin possess anti-inflammatory and antioxidant properties [1,2]. It also presents a spread spectrum of molecular targets such as transcription factors and their receptors, growth factors, cytokines, genes, and adhesion molecules. For example, curcumin could inhibit the cell signaling pathway of nuclear factor kappa B (NF-κB), which is an important cellular target of cancer cells [3–5]. Additionally, the blockade of NF-κB triggers the reduction in the expression of different NF-κB-regulated products, such as tumor necrosis factor alpha (TNF-α), interleukin 8 (IL-8), and cyclooxygenase 2 (COX-2), which play key roles in the inflammation process [6]. Furthermore, it has been recently demonstrated that curcumin may inhibit protein aggregation, such as amyloid-β (Aβ) protein, which is related to several neurological pathologies, such as Alzheimer's disease (AD) [7].

For these reasons, in recent years, there has been an increasing interest in curcumin-based treatments as managements for many disorders, such as brain diseases. However, its poor bioavailability, low solubility in aqueous media, instability in body fluids, and elevated degradation rate have limited the therapeutic applications of this drug. Different strategies, such as the use of nanotechnology, have emerged to tackle these problems. In general, nanoparticles-based drug delivery systems present important advantages, such as a long lifetime circulation, ability to improve the drug's aqueous solubility as well the bioavailability, and the capacity to overcome physiological barriers [8–10].

Many authors have demonstrated that curcumin-loaded nanoparticles comprise a very effective and attractive treatment for several diseases. Therefore, the main objective of this work is to present an extensive review of the properties of curcumin, the nanotechnology-based curcumin delivery systems, and its potential application for the treatment of brain diseases, particularly AD, Parkinson's disease (PD), and cancer.

2. Curcumin Chemical Information

Chemically, curcumin is a naturally polyphenol denominated (1E,6E)-1,7-bis(4-hydroxy-3-methoxyphenyl)-1,6-heptadiene-3,5-dione) (Figure 1), which is isolated from the rhizomes of *C. longa*. From a structural point of view, there are three chemical entities in the molecule: two aromatic ring systems containing *o*-methoxy phenolic groups linked by a seven-carbon spacer consisting of an α,β-unsaturated β-diketone moiety [11]. Therefore, the diketo group exhibits keto–enol tautomerism, meaning that curcumin can exist in equilibrium between the keto and the enol tautomer. However, nuclear magnetic resonance (NMR) studies carried out on a variety of solvents concluded that the enol form of curcumin is essentially the only form of this molecule in solution [12]. The relevance of the tautomerism was explored by Yanagizawa et al. [13]; these authors suggested that curcumin and its analogues exist predominantly in the enol form during binding to Aβ fibrils/aggregates, in turn suggesting that the enolization of curcumin derivatives is crucial for binding to Aβ aggregates in the treatment of AD. In this respect, some physicochemical properties are described below.

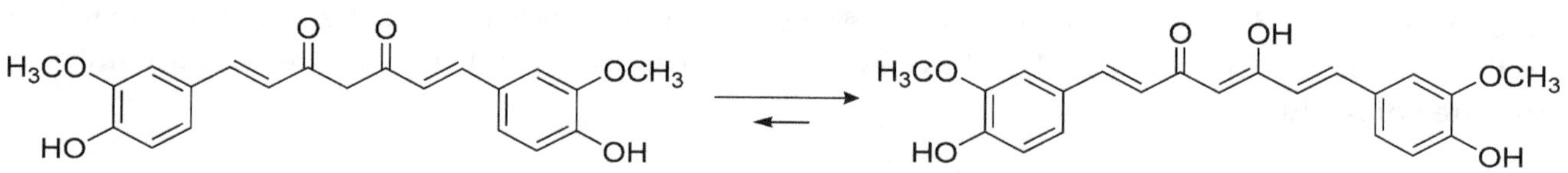

Figure 1. Chemical structure of curcumin and keto–enol tautomerism.

2.1. Thermal Analysis of Curcumin

Thermogravimetric analysis is a common complementary tool to describe this molecule. Therefore, we performed an evaluation of the thermal degradation of curcumin at a heating rate of 10 °C/min and under a nitrogen atmosphere. As can be observed in Figure 2a, the initial temperature of the mass loss is approximately 193 °C. This behavior results in the decomposition of the turmeric powder; below this temperature, weight loss in the curcumin follows a gradual decrease related to the loss of moisture. In a complementary way, a differential scanning calorimetry thermogram (Figure 2b) showed a melting temperature for curcumin of 174.05 °C, which is in agreement with data reported previously [14].

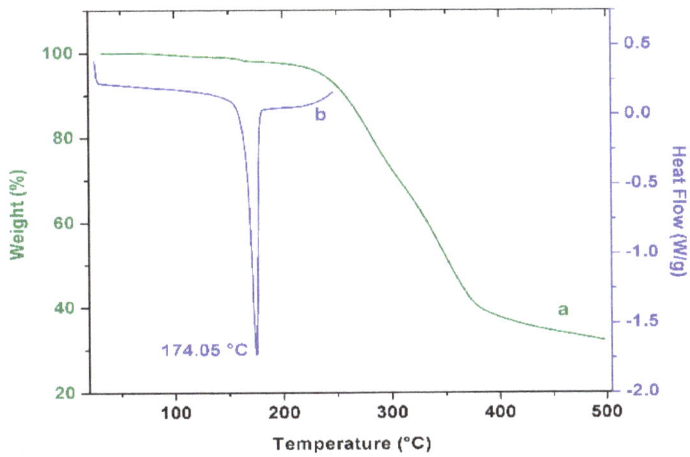

Figure 2. Thermal analysis of curcumin. Thermogravimetric analysis ((a), green line) and differential scanning calorimetry ((b), blue line). Melting point of curcumin is indicated at 174.05 °C.

2.2. Ultraviolet-Visible Spectrophotometric Analysis of Curcumin

The chemical reactivity and solubility of curcumin depends on the medium pH in which it is dissolved; that is, under acidic conditions, curcumin exhibits moderate solubility, and the solution maintains a yellow color (Figure 3A), whereas at a neutral pH, curcumin is not fully soluble, as can be observed in Figure 3B. On the other hand, within the basic pH range, curcumin is more water-soluble than in the neutral form, and the color of the solution changes to red (Figure 3C). The color change under alkaline conditions could be an effect deriving from the deprotonation. It is known that the photophysical and photochemical properties of curcumin are related to the solvents polarity because of the keto–enol structure of curcumin that involves intramolecular proton transfer [15]. Kharat M. et al. [16] mentioned the formation of condensation yellow products (such as feruloymethane) as a potential reason for this color increment under an alkaline environment.

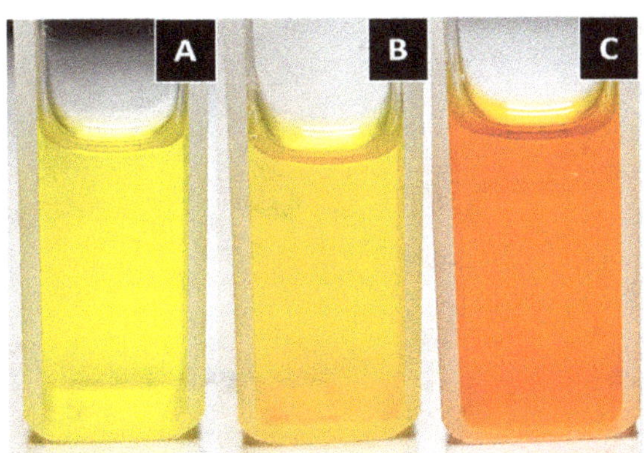

Figure 3. Curcumin dissolved in different mediums. (**A**) Curcumin in an acidic solution (pH 3.5); and (**B**) curcumin in a neutral solution (pH 7.4); both with the addition of 1% Tween 80 in order to increase solubility. (**C**) Curcumin in a basic solution (pH 12).

In order to corroborate the solubility of curcumin, we tested the drug incorporated in solvents with different pH levels (maintaining a concentration of eight mg/mL), through ultraviolet (UV)-vis spectrophotometry. Figure 4 depicts that at a neutral pH (lines a and b), the maximum absorption peak of curcumin was found at 420 nm, which is in agreement with the literature [17], while the maximum absorption in alkaline pH was found at 470 nm (Figure 4, line c). This result is in agreement with the reported by Priyadarsini [11], who reported that the maximum absorption peak of the fully deprotonated curcumin is found at 467 nm under alkaline conditions (>pH 10).

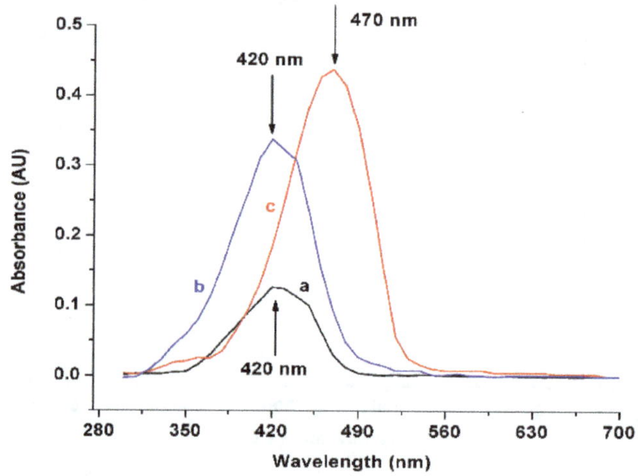

Figure 4. Ultraviolet-Visible spectrophotometric scanning of curcumin. (a) Absorption in methanol, maximum peak of absorption found at 420 nm; (b) Absorption in neutral medium, maximum peak of absorption found at 420 nm; and (c) Absorption in basic medium, maximum peak of absorption found at 470 nm.

2.3. Fourier Transform Infrared Spectroscopy of Curcumin

Infrared spectroscopy is commonly employed to study the molecules' chemical structure; a curcumin spectrum is shown in Figure 5. As depicted, the characteristic band of the O—H bond stretching appears at 3506 cm^{-1}. The infrared (IR) band at 2915 cm^{-1} and its doublet at 2847 cm^{-1} are due to the asymmetric and symmetric stretching vibrations of the C–H_2 group. For C–C stretching, a peak at 1624 cm^{-1} is found. The C=O stretching vibration of the carboxylic groups (methyl esters and triglycerides) can be attributed to the strong band at 1510 cm^{-1} [18]. In plane C–OH bending vibration can be assigned to the IR bands at 1375 cm^{-1}. Curcumin shows a peak at around 1270 cm^{-1}, which corresponds to the C—O stretching frequency of the ether group in curcumin. The peaks at 729 cm^{-1}, 806 cm^{-1}, and 955 cm^{-1} indicate the bending vibrations of the —CH bond of the alkene group [19].

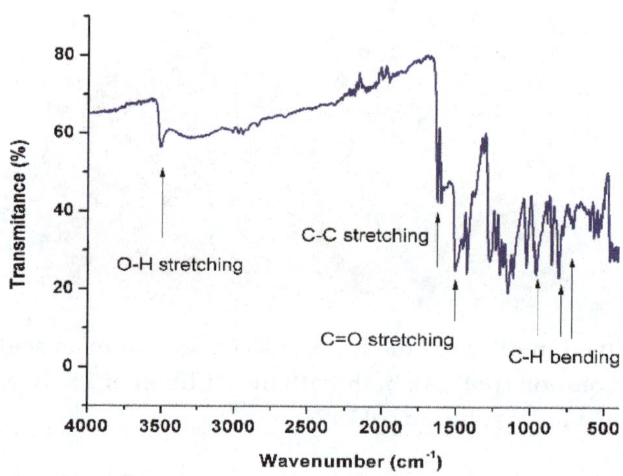

Figure 5. Fourier transform infrared spectroscopy of curcumin. Characteristic bands of the molecule are indicated with arrows.

2.4. Solubility

Curcumin has poor solubility in water (an estimated of 3.21 mg/L at 25 °C); however, it is soluble in ethanol, dimethyl sulfoxide (DMSO), methanol, acetonitrile, chloroform, and ethyl acetate [11,20]. The theoretical Hansen solubility parameters (HSP), which were calculated on the basis of the group contribution method, are δ_d = 17.46, δ_p = 3.66, δ_h = 13.84, and δ_{total} = 22.46 for the enol form of curcumin [21]. The first pKa_1 = 7.5–8.5 corresponds to the deprotonation of the enolic proton group, while pKa_2 = 8.5–10.4 and pKa_3 = 9.5–10.7 are for the phenolic protons, indistinctly [11]. The log octanol–water partition coefficient (log Kow) is 3.29 (estimated), conferring hydrophobic characteristics on the molecule [20].

Curcumin is unstable in aqueous and alcoholic solution, and it is more stable in acidic pH (1.2–6) than in alkaline pH (Figure 3); the degradation products found under hydrolytic conditions are: trans-6-(4′-hydroxy-3′-methoxyphenyl)-2,4-dioxo-5-hexenal, ferulic acid, ferulic aldehyde, feruloylmethane, and vanillin [22,23]. However, new evidence suggests that the major degradation product is bicyclopentadione, which is the result of the autoxidation of curcumin [24], and is formed by the oxygenation and double cyclization of the heptadienedione chain connecting the two methoxyphenol rings of curcumin [25]. Curcumin is also sensitive to light. It has been shown to decompose when it is exposed to UV/visible light, both in solution and in the solid state [26].

3. Biological Activity

Curcumin has a broad spectrum of biological activities. For example, it has been reported as possessing antioxidant, anti-AD, anticarcinogenic, antimutagenic, and anti-inflammatory properties (Figure 6).

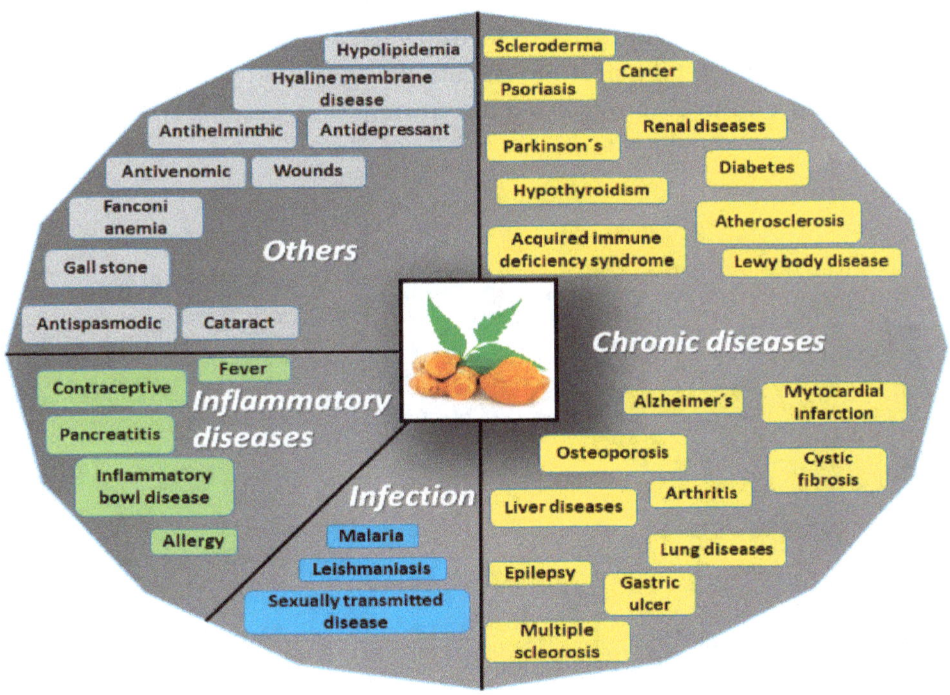

Figure 6. Potential applications of curcumin. Due to the structure of curcumin, this molecule could be applied as treatment for a wide range of disorders, such as chronic diseases, inflammatory disorders, infections of diverse etiology, and other conditions. Adapted with permission from [26].

With respect to antioxidant activity, evidence has shown that curcumin can directly scavenge several free radicals as the result of its two phenolic sites. Likewise, curcumin has been effective against the generation of reactive oxygen species (ROS) and reactive nitrogen species (RNS) in the cellular environment. Curcumin also reduces low-density lipoprotein (LDL), and inhibits the oxidation of proteins and DNA. At the enzymatic level, curcumin inhibits lipoxygenase/cyclooxygenase and xanthine dehydrogenase/oxidase, which are two enzymes related to the generation of ROS, and upregulates superoxide dismutase and glutathione peroxidase, which are two first-line enzymes of defense against oxygen-free radicals [22].

In AD, curcumin protects against Aβ-induced oxidative stress, prevents the formation and extension of Aβ fibrils, destabilizes Aβ fibrils, inhibits acetylcholinesterase, decreases neuroinflammation, and sequesters transition metals [22]. A variety of structure–activity studies have proven that the three moieties in the chemical structure of curcumin play different roles in its interaction with the Aβ peptide: one of the hydroxyl substitutions in the aromatic end group is necessary for inhibition, while the other one of the hydroxyl substitutions is required for activity. Finally, the diketo chain contributes to the flexibility and correct length between aromatic rings [27]. Curcumin has been extensively evaluated and possesses potential antioxidant and anti-inflammatory activity in AD. The most important mechanism of the anti-inflammatory action of curcumin is based on the inhibition of NF-kB, which leads to the decreased formation of cytochemokines and Aβ fibrils. Other molecular targets inhibited by curcumin are inducible nitric oxide synthase (iNOs), c-Jun N-terminal kinase (JNK) activation, and activating protein-1 (AP-1) [28].

In anticancer therapy, curcumin inhibits oxidative stress, reduces lipid peroxidation and DNA single-strand breakage, inhibits the COX-1 and COX-2 enzymes, suppresses NF-kB activation, and possesses antiproliferative effects. Moreover, it induces apoptosis by targeting mitochondria, and affects tumor protein p53 (p53)-related signaling [22]. The specific molecular targets for curcumin that are therapeutically important in cancer-signaling pathways include cyclin-dependent kinases (CDKs), p53, Ras, phosphoinositide 3-kinase (PI3K), Protein kinase B (Akt), Wnt/β-catenin, and mammalian target of rapamycin (mTOR) [29]. During angiogenesis, curcumin can inhibit and/or downregulate the expression of various pro-angiogenic growth factors such as the vascular endothelial growth factor (VEGF), fibroblast growth factor (FGF), and the endothelial growth factor (EGF) [30]. An overview of the molecular targets of curcumin is represented in Figure 7.

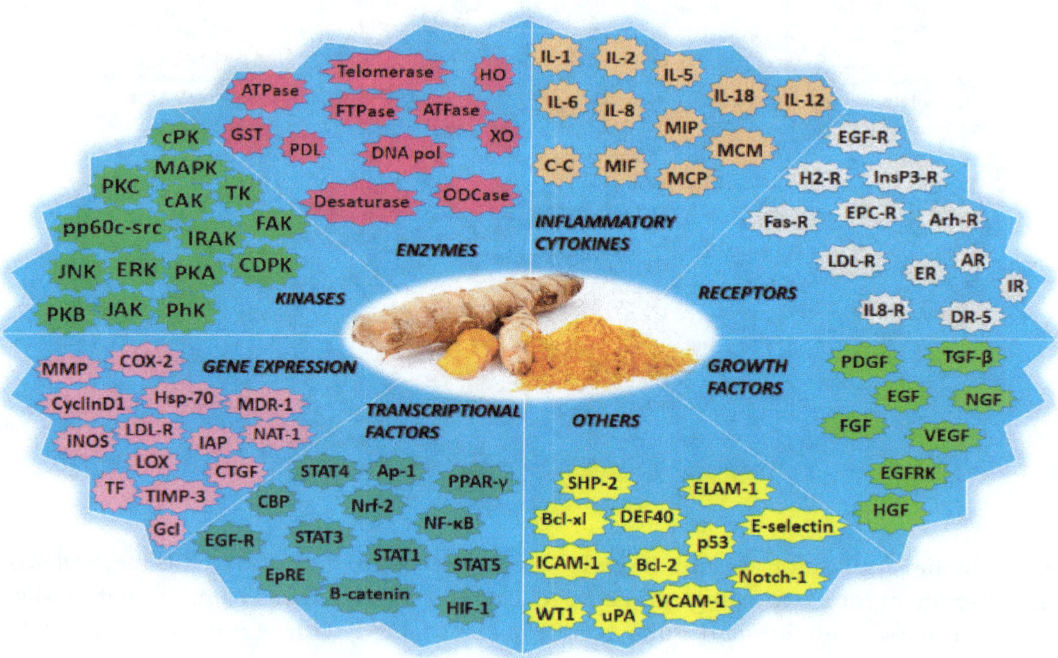

Figure 7. Curcumin is a pleiotropic agent with multiple molecular targets. This molecule could modify the expression of genes, inflammatory cytokines, transcriptional and growth factors, enzymes, and receptors, among others. Adapted with permission from [26].

3.1. *Effect of Curcumin on Aggregation Protein*

Protein aggregation is the process by which misfolded proteins assume a conformation that cause their polymerization into aggregates and organized fibrils. The adequate aggregation of protein is a precise progression that requires extensive guidance from an excellent control network, which comprises approximately 800 proteins in humans. Many neurodegenerative diseases are associated with inappropriate protein aggregation [31]. These neuronal diseases include disorders in which the aggregates may accumulate in the nucleus, such as for example in polyglutamine expansion diseases (such as spinocerebellar ataxias and Huntington's disease (HD)), which are pathologies that are characterized by inclusions in cytoplasm (for example, α-synuclein in PD), disorders in which the aggregates are found outside of the cell (prion diseases), or both intracellularly and extracellularly (such as Aβ in AD) [31].

The effect of curcumin on prion disease has been studied by several authors. Hafner-Bratkovič et al. [32] reported that the binding of curcumin to the α-intermediate could block conformational change into the β-structure, and that the binding of curcumin to prion fibrils could prevent further growth, thus, the formation of new seeds. Similarly, Caughey et al. [33] concluded in their work that curcumin inhibits prion protein resistance (PrP-Res) accumulation in neuroblastoma cells infected with the scrapie agent. In addition, these authors reported the partial inhibition of the conversion of PrP into PrP-res.

Additionally, Pandey et al. [34] analyzed the curcumin effect both in vitro and in cell culture models of α-synuclein aggregation. The authors concluded that curcumin induces the inhibition of α-synuclein aggregation in a dose-dependent manner. Also, their results suggested that curcumin increased α-synuclein solubility in cells containing aggregates.

The oligomerization of α-synuclein aggregates is structurally similar to the Aβ-protein aggregates of AD. Therefore, curcumin has been investigated as a potential AD treatment. Brahmkhatri et al. [35] reported that curcumin-loaded gold nanoparticles inhibited Aβ aggregation, and that these were capable of dissolving aggregates. Likewise, Mithu et al. [36] reported that curcumin disorganizes Aβ fibrils; the disruption of Aβ-fibrils was achieved by means of structural changes in the salt bridge region and near the C terminus. A more detailed report on the inhibition of Aβ aggregation revealed that, besides curcumin inhibiting fibril formation in vitro, it also inhibited the formation of Aβ oligomers and their toxicity in vivo [37].

It has been reported that amyloid formation could be limited by mechanisms such as metal chelation [38], and reducing the induction of the β-secretase enzyme (BACE1) by proinflammatory cytokines [39]. It has been suggested that BACE1 has a main role in the initiation of the formation of Aβ [40]; therefore, it is an attractive drug target for AD. The sequential proteolytic cleavage of the Aβ precursor protein (APP), which is a type I transmembrane protein, produced the formation of Aβ.

Zhang et al. [7] studied the interaction between curcumin and Aβ. These authors proposed the modulation of APP levels in the secretory pathway as the cellular mechanism by which curcumin reduces Aβ levels. In addition, they reported that the use of curcumin considerably increased the retention of immature APP in the endoplasmic reticulum. Furthermore, the authors suggested that APP endocytosis could be attenuated by treatment with curcumin.

In order to identify the chemical features that are most important for preventing Aβ accumulation, Reinke et al. [27] examined the effect of three features on the inhibition of amyloid aggregation: the presence of aromatic groups at both extremes of the molecule, the substitution pattern of these aromatics, and the distance and flexibility of the linker section. They demonstrated that the presence of just one single aromatic group did not decrease the protein aggregation; thus, the curcumin efficiency as an aggregation inhibitor could be related to its two phenyl groups. Also, their results suggested that the substitution of these aromatics groups is important for activity, since these are capable of taking part in hydrogen bonding. In addition, the authors reported the approximate distance between the docking sites, which are found between eight and 16 Å from each other; this is similar to the distance between the terminal aromatic regions of curcumin.

3.2. Effect of Curcumin in Neuroinflammation

In recent years, interest in the identification and application of natural compounds that limit neuroinflammation has been growing. The term neuroinflammation has been used to describe several different pathological events, from modifications in the morphology of glial cells to fully fledged tissue invasion and destruction by leukocytes. Neuroinflammation plays a key role in the progression of neurodegenerative diseases and in the invasion of central nervous system (CNS) parenchyma by leukocytes, it is one of its main characteristics, as well as a severe loss of the blood–brain barrier (BBB) integrity [6].

Due to the latter, lymphocytes and myeloid cells express cytokines in the tissue, increasing the inflammatory cascade. Interleukins such as IL-1β, IL-6, and IL-23, and cytokines such as TNF, interferon gamma (IFNγ), and granulocyte/macrophage colony-stimulating factor (GM-CSF), chemokines (such as CCL2, CCL5, and CXCL1), secondary messengers (nitric oxide and prostaglandins), and ROS are also mediators for the neuroinflammatory response [41]. The excessive production of these inflammatory mediators could cause neuronal damage and death. It has been demonstrated that curcumin reduces the expression of several inflammatory cytokines, including IL-1α, IL-1β, IL-6, TNF, IFNγ, and many others (Figure 8) [42,43].

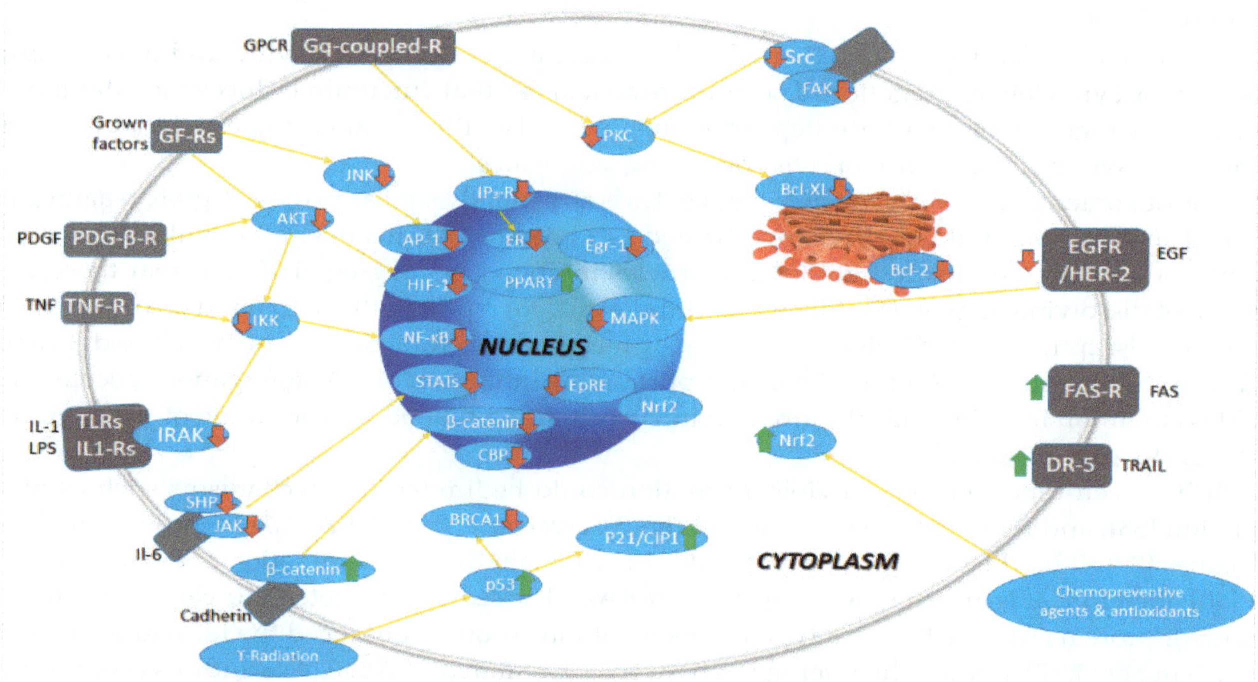

Figure 8. Signaling pathways modulated by curcumin. Up and green arrows indicate the intermediaries upregulated by curcumin; meanwhile, down and red arrows indicate the intermediaries downregulated by curcumin. Adapted with permission from [26].

Some authors have reported that curcumin suppresses the expression of IL-1β [44,45]. This mechanism suggests that curcumin inhibits the activation of the Nod-like receptor protein 3 (NLRP3) inflammasome, which is the most characterized inflammasome, and an important innate immune sensor. The NLRP3 inflammasome is activated by an extensive variety of signals of pathogenic, endogenous, and environmental origin. Some authors found that curcumin suppressed inflammation via a strong inhibition of NLRP3-dependent caspase-1 activation and IL-1 β secretion [44].

In the same manner, Devi et al. [46] reported that curcumin could exert a direct effect on constitutive signal transducer and activator of transcription 3 (STAT3) phosphorylation. These authors also mentioned that curcumin is a potent inhibitor of IL-6 expression in stromal cells. They suggested that this inhibition was related to the IκB kinase (IKK)/NF-κB pathway. Likewise, NF-κB is a ubiquitous transcription factor; its activation is linked with the promotion or inhibition of apoptosis, depending on the cell type and condition. Likewise, the inflammatory response induced by TNF-α is strongly linked to the activation of NF-kB.

On the other hand, TNF-α is a very important inflammatory mediator; thus, its reduction is a therapeutic target in several inflammatory diseases [47]. For the interaction of the TNF-α and curcumin, Wang et al. [4] found inhibition in the expression of this factor through downregulating the expression of NF-κB. These authors reported that curcumin reduced the transcription and secretion of TNF-α, and also IL-6, which is induced by palmitate, and induces the nuclear translocation of NF-κB in a concentration-dependent manner [48,49].

Similarly, the suppression of CCL2 function may decrease the attraction of cells of the immune system to the sites of inflammation, which could result in a slowdown of the advancement of inflammation [50]. Zhang et al. [51] investigated the inhibitory effect of curcumin on lipopolysaccharide (LPS)-induced chemokine CCL production. First, these authors induced the upregulation of CCL2 mRNA and protein in C6 cells, utilizing one μg/mL of LPS. After this, they probed three doses of curcumin as treatments (2.5 μM, 10 μM, and 25 μM), and found that the expression of CCL2 mRNA decreased with these concentrations in a dose-dependent manner. Moreover, their results suggested that in astrocytoma cells, curcumin induces the downregulation of CCL2 expression through the JNK pathway. However, it appears that CCL2 could be inhibited by curcumin through other pathways besides the JNK pathway. Herman et al. [52] suggested that curcumin downregulates CCL2 activity via the inhibition of protein kinase C (PKC) and matrix metalloproteinases.

On the other hand, IFN-γ exerts important effects on epithelial integrity, promotes barrier dysfunction, and increases epithelial permeability through numerous mechanisms. The loss of integrity in BBB is involved in neuronal diseases. For example, Midura-Kiela et al. [53] studied the interaction of IFN-γ and curcumin in epithelial cells. They concluded that curcumin induces the inhibition of the signaling of IFN-γ. Furthermore, curcumin also inhibits the COX-2 pathway. COX-2 is overexpressed in malignant tissues. Accordingly, its inhibition could be a key to cancer and tumor treatments.

3.3. Effect of Curcumin on Oxidative Stress

Although oxygen plays an important role in energy production processes in cells (ATP), this molecule could be transformed into very toxic forms in the cells, which are denominated ROS [54]. Antioxidant systems are complex and act in concert to decrease the ROS load. A process known as oxidative stress occurs if an imbalance between ROS and antioxidant systems takes place in favor of oxidants. Oxidative stress has been related to mechanisms leading to neuronal cell injury in various neuronal diseases.

Antioxidants are compounds that can prevent biomolecules from undergoing oxidative damage through free radical-mediated reactions [55]. The majority of the antioxidants present a phenolic group or a β-diketone group in their structure [56].

To explain the protective properties of phenolic groups in antioxidants, two different mechanisms have been proposed. In the first mechanism (Equation (1)), the free radical becomes a radical by hydrogen atom transfer from the antioxidant (ArOH). This antioxidant activity is related to phenolic O–H bond dissociation enthalpy (BDE); thus, if the O–H bond attraction is weak, free radical inactivation will be easier.

In the second mechanism, the free radical receives an electron from the antioxidant. The free radical becomes a radical cation, which could be reacting with another antioxidant molecule (Equations (2) and (3)). In terms of this mechanism, the important parameter to analyze for antioxidant activity is the ionization potential (IP). With a low IP, electron abstraction will be easier. In addition to BDE and IP, proton dissociation enthalpy, proton affinity (PA), and electron transfer enthalpy are important factors for evaluating antioxidant activity [55,57].

$$ArOH + R^* \rightarrow ArO^* + RH, \tag{1}$$

$$ArOH + R^* \rightarrow ArOH^* + R^-, \quad (2)$$

$$ArOH + R^- \rightarrow ArO^* + RH. \quad (3)$$

As previously mentioned, curcumin possesses a wide range of biological functions, including antioxidant activity. Curcumin contains a variety of functional groups, including phenolic rings that act as electron traps to prevent H_2O_2 production and scavenge superoxide radicals, the β-diketo group that is involved in metal–ligand complexation, and carbon–carbon double bonds (Figure 9) [56,58]; together, these provide the molecule with unique antioxidant properties.

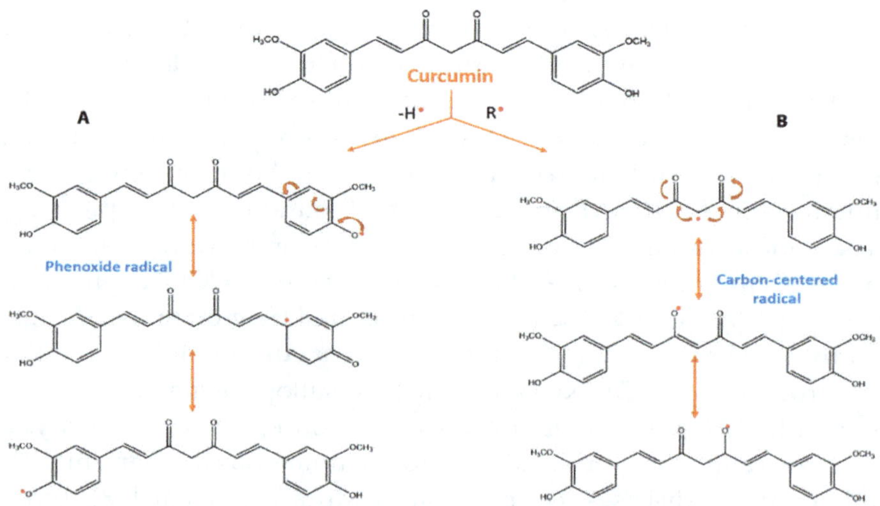

Figure 9. Antioxidant mechanism of curcumin. There are two mechanisms to form phenoxyl radicals. The first mechanism (**A**) begins by initial electron transfer to the free radical; thus, a radical cation is formed, which produces a phenoxyl radical by a proton loss. The second mechanism (**B**) is related to direct hydrogen abstraction. Based on the bond dissociation energies, many authors suggest that the most susceptible target for free radicals in curcumin is phenolic OH.

Under acidic to neutral conditions (pH = 3−7), the keto conformation is the major form. On the other hand, under basic conditions (pH > 8), the enol conformation is predominant, which presents powerful free radical-scavenger properties [59].

Using erythrocyte sedimentation rate (ESR), the reduction of ferric iron in aqueous medium, and intracellular ROS/toxicity assays, Barzegar et al. [60] analyzed the antioxidant properties of curcumin. Their results demonstrated that curcumin confers protection on the cells against the mortal effects of cumene hydroperoxide.

In addition, Zbarsky et al. [58] applied, in the unilateral 6-hydroxydopamine (6-OHDA) rat model of PD, natural compounds, with phenolic groups in their structure to evaluate the neuroprotection level. These authors reported that, with the sub-chronic administration of curcumin, the loss of dopaminergic neurons in the *substantia nigra pars compacta* was reduced significantly.

The antioxidant protective effect of curcumin was also evaluated against hemin-induced neuronal death. In 2013, González-Reyes et al. [61] evaluated the neuroprotection of curcumin in the primary cultures of the cerebellar granule neurons of rats. They concluded that the use of curcumin as a pretreatment induces antioxidant protection against hemin-induced neuronal death.

The antioxidant effect of curcumin has been evaluated in other applications in addition to neuronal pathologies. For example, Haryuna et al. [62] investigated the antioxidant action of curcumin against oxidative stress caused by diabetes mellitus. These authors worked with cochlear fibroblasts in rat models of diabetes mellitus, and reported that curcumin confers antioxidant protection via the increased expression of superoxide dismutase. These results showed that curcumin presents a wide range of applications.

4. Limitation of Chemical Properties and New Proposals

There are two main limitations when curcumin is formulated for therapeutic purposes: limited solubility in water and low permeability [63]. In addition, the low permeability is related to chemical degradation, a high rate of biotransformation, especially glucuronidation and sulfation [22], and rapid systemic elimination, resulting in low curcumin absorption and poor bioavailability. Therefore, curcumin can be classified as a BCS Class IV molecule. In fact, the majority of oral curcumin is excreted in the feces—about 90%—and the rest in urine (6%) after 72 hours in rats [64]. Consequently, high doses of curcumin are necessary to produce detectable plasma concentrations. For example, in a human clinical trial, 3.6 g of curcumin via the oral route was found to produce a plasma curcumin level of 11.1 nmol/L after one hour of dosing on days one, two, eight, and 29 of the administration [65]. Due to these limitations, novel drug delivery systems have been proposed to increase the bioavailability of curcumin.

5. New Formulations of Curcumin

As previously mentioned, one of the reasons that curcumin has poor bioavailability is due to its limited solubility in water; therefore, one of the directions in the development of new formulations for this molecule (as for other lipophilic compounds) is to increase solubility, following strategies such as modification of the solid state, reduction of particle size, the creation of supersaturated solutions, or the encapsulation into nanoparticles. Some new formulations are briefly described later.

Amorphous solid dispersions (ASD) are an interesting strategy of modification of the solid state to improve the rate of dissolution of drugs, and thus their bioavailability. Solid dispersion involves the incorporation of water-insoluble compounds into a hydrophilic carrier matrix. In a study performed by Gangurde et al. [66], the authors demonstrated that curcumin formulated in an Eudragit E (Evonik Nutrition & Care GmbH, Essen, Germany) polymeric matrix dissolved more rapidly (20–45% release after 60 min) than curcumin alone (2–5% release after 120 min) at pH 1.2. Solubility also was increased: with curcumin alone, solubility was 0.02%, whereas curcumin containing Eudragit E (Evonik Nutrition & Care GmbH) exhibited solubility of 40.29% and 18.78% by the spray-drying and rotoevaporation techniques, respectively. In other studies, curcumin revealed an increase of >1000 times when it was formulated as ASD in hydroxypropyl methylcellulose matrixes [67].

Nanosuspension is a carrier-free nanoparticle system containing only pure drug crystals, and is sometimes accompanied by a stabilizer. Nanosuspension can greatly increase the saturation solubility as well as the dissolution velocity (by increasing the superficial area). Curcumin has been formulated as a nanosuspension with good results. For example, Wang et al. [68] found an increase in the oral bioavailability of curcumin of about three to four times after the administration of curcumin in nanosuspensions in rats. Similarly, Li et al. [69] found an increase in bioavailability after the intravenous administration of a nanosuspension of about 4.2-fold compared to a curcumin solution.

Self-microemulsifying drug delivery systems (SMEDDS) are isotropic mixtures of oil, hydrophilic surfactant, and co-solvents that rapidly form oil-in-water (o/w) microemulsion upon gentle agitation followed by dilution in an aqueous medium [70]. This class of supersaturated systems has been effective in increasing the solubility of drugs at the absorption site. Formulated curcumin in SMEDDS has been proposed by Wu et al. [71]. The formulation, which is composed of 20% ethanol, 60% Cremophor RH40 (BASF Personal Care and Nutrition GmbH, Monhein, Germany) and 20% isopropyl myristate, improved the relative oral bioavailability of SMEDDS compared with the curcumin suspension by about 1213%. Similar studies conducted by other researches can be found in the references [72–74].

In addition, the encapsulation of curcumin into nanoparticles not only enhances its bioavailability and solubility (Figure 10), it also increases its stability by protecting it from the influence of the outside environment.

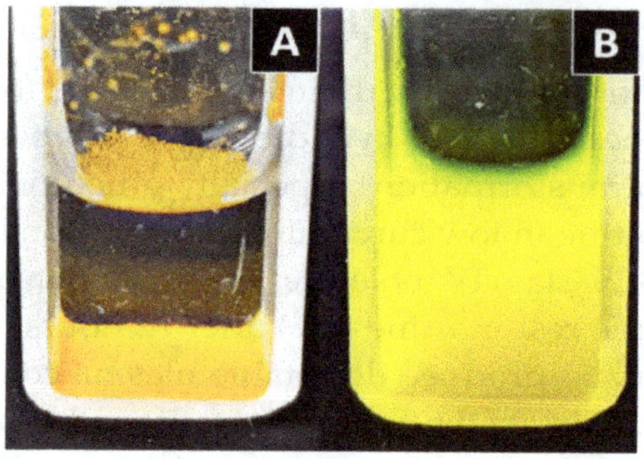

Figure 10. Curcumin solubility: (**A**) Curcumin showed poor solubility in aqueous medium; (**B**) the use of the nanoplatforms increased the drug solubility. Curcumin was entrapped in poly-ε-caprolactone nanoparticles stabilized by Pluronic F68 (Thermofisher, Whaltam, USA), with size of 170 nm and zeta potential of −7 mV.

Novel curcumin-nanoparticulated delivery approaches, including liposomes, polymeric nanoparticles, solid lipid nanoparticles, polymeric micelles, and others, are emerging as suitable and promising systems. This is because they can be designed and adapted to the desired size, chemical composition, surface charge, and surface functionalization, rendering them potent tools for the treatment of specific diseases such as neurodegenerative disorders and cancer [75,76]. In this review, a more detailed description on the development of formulations based on nanoparticles, specifically for neurodegenerative disorders are discussed in the following sections.

6. Formulations of Curcumin in Nanoparticles

Nanoparticles for medical purposes comprise a variety of drug transport systems; they traditionally have dimensions of fewer than 200 nm for brain applications, and are expandable up to 1000 nm, in concept. The small aggregation size confers a high degree of tissue penetration. Nanoparticles for medical and brain purposes are considered non-invasive systems. Although they are designed to flank and cross various tissues, their small size and composition guarantee, in the majority of cases, minimal invasion without risk. The main security provided comprises the chemical composition and the mechanisms of elimination and/or biodegradation. However, several research groups that have delved into this topic have always highlighted the need for a broad assessment in the area of nanotoxicology, because some materials, only by the change of size of aggregation from bulk to nanoparticles can increase their toxicity; contrariwise, other materials exhibit new and better properties.

Conventionally, nanoparticles for medical purposes arise from the combination of two master ideas: from Paul Ehrlich with the concept of magical bullets [77], and Richard Feynman with the notion of miniaturization [78]. However, the materialization of the investigation of new carriers for the transport of drugs to the brain with the use of nanoparticles dates from the first conceptions of Peter Speiser in 1969 [79]. Subsequently, J. Kreuter et al. [80] began the initial assessments on the coating of nanoparticles with polysorbate 80 to facilitate their passage into the CNS. These pioneering works set the standard for the development of polymeric nanoparticles. In parallel, R.H. Müller et al. [81] worked on the development of lipid nanoparticles that would later allow for wide applications in the same area.

The subsequent epochs were accompanied by pharmacokinetic and mechanistic studies at the cellular level with the intention of achieving greater degrees of vectorization. Therefore, some of the examples cited in the application of nanoparticles for the transport of curcumin to the CNS have employed as a strategy the coupling of ligands that permit targeting to the brain. Drug vectorization has advanced substantially, even to the achievement of reaching intranuclear levels in neurons. Some of the most commonly used systems for administering curcumin for the purpose of brain impairment are described below.

6.1. Polymeric Nanoparticles

Polymeric materials were the first to have been used to transport drugs to the brain, and a significant number of curcumin-carrying applications can be found in the literature. Some examples of traditional polymers include poly (butyl cyanoacrylate) (PBCA), poly (lactic-co-glycolic acid) (PLGA), and chitosan. In particular, the synthetic polymers PBCA and PLGA allow adequate control of the particle size, which results in highly reproducible production batches (Figure 11).

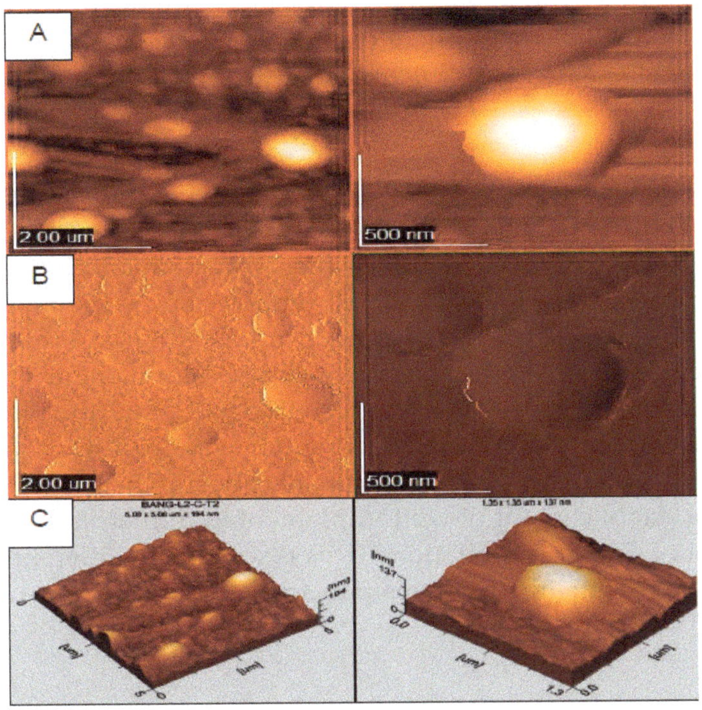

Figure 11. Atomic force microscopy (AFM) microscopy of curcumin poly-ε-caprolactone nanoparticles in two magnifications, left and right. Images in AFM (**A**), 2D (**B**) and 3D (**C**) mode.

Subsequent steps have been directed toward the synthesis of new polymers to couple different ligands that can permit adequate vectorization. Usually, these systems allow suitable stability with a zeta potential of at least –15 mV with polyvinyl alcohol (PVA), while with systems prepared with chitosan, although they appear very promising by the simple and rapid methods of ionic gelation, one of the disadvantages is usually the control of molecular weight. In general, PLGA polymer nanoparticles have shown adequate biocompatibility at the cellular level, and in studies in more complex biological models, even at high amounts up to one mg/mL at a cell density of 1×10^4. However, other studies have indicated that the degradation of PLGA could induce cellular damage by the generated acidic medium, although this is restricted to the amount of polymer that was administered [82].

6.2. Lipid Nanoparticles

Even when a broad demonstration of the biocompatibility of polymeric systems is available, doubt remains concerning their possible effects in prolonged administrations, due to the possible interactions within the nanometric range with biological systems or accumulation in some tissues. One of the main alternatives to the possible effects deriving from polymers are lipid nanoparticles. This term includes solid lipid nanoparticles and nanostructured lipid carriers. One of the great advantages of these systems is the use of lipids with high biocompatibility and biodegradation. The majority of lipid matrices are constituted of glyceride derivatives that are easily assimilated by our metabolism. We can imagine that several of these are also present in foods, and that they follow the same route of biotransformation. Therefore, this aspect is crucial in the choice of the type of nanoparticle matrix for the transport of curcumin, and it is reflected in a considerable percentage of the published information for brain diseases. The majority of production methods employ temperatures above the melting point of the lipids used. One aspect to be considered is the possible stability of lipid nanoparticles in aqueous dispersion and the exchange between polymorphic structures that can promote the expulsion of the drug. Interestingly, some lipids exhibit biological properties in addition to the nutritional aspect, and their applications are enhanced when handled in the nanometer state. Some of these demonstrate novel biological properties due to an increase in interaction with the biological environment, and to the high degree of distribution and penetration in tissues. If this were the case, the new properties that were exhibited can be complemented with the drugs encapsulated in the same system.

6.3. Liposomes

Liposomes are spherical vesicles with one or several layers of phospholipids with an internal aqueous compartment. They usually have a size of less than 100 nm. Due to the high percentage of phospholipids, they are also recognized as highly biocompatible and biodegradable systems. The difference with the previous systems, besides the composition, is the type of architecture. Lipid nanoparticles derive from a solid and compact matrix, and the liposomes do not; even there are some variants that confer flexibility to the structure. The development and evaluation of liposomes is evidenced by a long history in pharmaceutical technology. In fact, the first drug approved by the Food and Drug Administration (FDA) in the nano order was with liposomes, i.e., Doxil (Janssen, Titusville, FL, USA) for the treatment of certain types of cancer [83]. The long trajectory in liposome research also confers the establishment of well-implemented industrial processes that facilitate the subsequent development of similar formulations. This is somewhat different from the polymeric and lipid systems, in which there remain critical systems to be reinforced, especially when they involve high agitation speeds.

6.4. Cyclodextrins

Cyclodextrins are glucopyranose structures in the form of a glass with a hydrophobic interior and a hydrophilic exterior by the exposure of hydroxyl units [84]. Cyclodextrins can be used to transport drugs to different organs, and can also be derivatized to increase their vectorization. They have shown high biocompatibility for deriving from the starch. Unlike previous systems, cyclodextrins are prefabricated carriers for the direct incorporation of the cargo. In theory, competition is mentioned between the liquid medium inside the vessel and the new molecule that one wishes to enter. Therefore, it is necessary to know the constants of affinity and dissociation. As with a traditional glass, when transported to the table, the interior can spill. In the case of drugs, the cargo may also get in the way. The hydrophobic characteristic allows some lipid extraction at the BBB level, which could also facilitate passage into the brain region. Even in other pathologies, effects can be found with empty cyclodextrins due to the effect generated in lipophilic components.

6.5. Tools for Drug Targeting of Curcumin

The BBB is a highly sophisticated barrier that is designed to maintain the integrity and homeostasis of the brain. From a technological point of view, it is a great challenge to direct different carriers toward the brain region under the concept of "non-invasive". Some strategies that have been employed include the surface coupling of the nanoparticles of ligands to specific receptors, the coupling of transporter substrates overexpressed in the BBB, and transport by adsorption through the interaction of opposite electrical charges (negative of the endothelial cell membrane and positive of the carrier). In other situations, various pathologies related with neuroinflammation produce a relative opening of the narrow junctions, therefore increasing the probability of the passage of carriers into the nanoparticle architecture. Intentional opening has not comprised a viable option because of the risk involved. Other strategies include furtive aggressive participation. The use of peptides, some of these from virus fragments or modified versions to ensure efficacy without toxicity, is a highly effective option. The transactivating-transduction peptide (TAT) has been a classic example of this type of mechanism.

It is noteworthy that the presence of surface agents substantially modifies the targeting capacity of the curcumin nanoparticles toward the CNS. However, a study in the literature mentions the formulation of PLGA nanoparticles with curcumin obtained by flash nanoprecipitation without a stabilizing agent. These authors demonstrated a 20-fold reduction in the administered dose compared with bulk curcumin (see Table 1). It is even more important to point out that the majority of the studies mentioned in Table 1, some of these that have been widely extended in biological elucidation mechanisms do not involve the application of highly sophisticated systems. In other brain pathologies, it has become a challenge to possess the most sophisticated. On the other hand, some formulations of curcumin in nanoparticles even include the combination of two active molecules, such as puerarin and dexanabinol. In addition, in the search for multifunctional systems, or theranostics, curcumin has been conjugated in magnetic nanoparticles for the detection of Aβ plaques in AD and in combination with gold–iron oxide nanocomposite systems for brain-cancer theranostics (see Table 1 for details).

Table 1. Examples of nanoparticle formulation for transport of curcumin to the brain.

Carrier	Composition	Ligand/Stabilizer	Size, PI and Ψ (mV)	% of EE and DL	Model of Evaluation	Reference
Solid lipid nanoparticles	Polyoxyethylene stearate, stearic acid	Lecithin	60, Ψ = −21.7	DL = 21.61	Major depression (in vitro and in vivo models)	[85]
	Compritol 888 ATO (Gattefossé, Saint-Priest, France)	Tween 80, soya lecithin	136	81.9, 92.3	Cerebral ischemic injury (in vivo model)	[86]
	Stearic acid	Lecithin, taurocholate	148	EE = 93.2	Huntington's disease (in vivo model)	[87]
	Glyceryl monooleate	Pluronic F-68, vitamin E TPGS	93, Ψ = −30.9	EE = 65	Rotenone-induced mouse model of Parkinson's disease (in vitro and in vivo models)	[88]
	Palmitic acid, cholesterol	N-trimethyl Chitosan vitamin E TPGS	412, 0.26, Ψ = 35.7	93, 4	Biodistribution (in vitro and in vivo models)	[89]
	Compritol 888 ATO	Tween 80, soya lecithin	136	81.9, 92.3	Aluminum-induced behavioral (in vivo model)	[90]
Solid lipid nanoparticles (SLNs) and nanostructured lipid carriers (NLCs)	Cetyl palmitate (SLN), cetyl palmitate + oleic acid (NLC)	Tween 80	204.7, 0.194 and 117.36, 0.188	SLN = 83.98, 4.54 NLC = 82.60, 4.67	Pharmacokinetic (in vivo model)	[91]
Nanostructured lipid carriers	Precirol, capmul MCM	Tween 80, soya lecithin	146, 0.18, Ψ = −21.4	EE = 90.86	Astrocytoma-glioblastoma (in vitro and in vivo models)	[92]
	Glyceryl monostearate, soy lecithin, medium chain triglycerides	Poloxamer 188	129, 0.25 Ψ = −27.8	95.9, 4.21	Pharmacokinetic and biodistribution (in vivo model)	[93]
	Phosphatidyl choline, cholesterol oleate, glycerol trioleate	Lactoferrin	103.8, PI = 0.15, Ψ = −5.80	96.51, 2.60	Alzheimer´s disease (in vitro and in vivo models)	[94]
	PC, cholesterol oleate, glycerol trioleate	Polysorbate 80	90.5, 0.14, Ψ = −20.3	EE = 94.39, DL = 3.29	Biodistribution (in vitro and in vivo models)	[95]
Polymeric nanoparticles	PLGA	Lipid monolayer	193.4, PI=0.115, Ψ = −43.8	13.23, 2.31	Inflammation model (*in vitro* model)	[96]
	Poly(butyl) cyanoacrylate	Apolipoprotein E3	197, 0.18, Ψ = −22.44	-	Beta amyloid induced cytotoxicity in neuroblastoma cells (*in vitro* model)	[97]
	Poly(butyl) cyanoacrylate	Apolipoprotein E3	197, 0.18, Ψ = −22.44	EE = 77.85	Anticancer activity in neuroblastoma cells (*in vitro* model)	[98]
	PLGA	-	100	94.7, 47.3	Bioavailability in the CNS (*in vivo* model)	[99]
	PLGA	PVA	163, 0.053, Ψ = −12.5	EE = 46.9	Pharmacokinetic (*in vivo* model)	[100]
	PLGA	-	-	-	Opioid tolerance and dependence (*in vivo* model)	[101]
	Chitosan	Tween 80	10, Ψ = −16.8	-	Arsenic toxicity (*in vivo* model)	[102]
	Chitosan-alginate	-	50	-	Epilepsy (*in vivo* model)	[103]
	Chitosan	Bovine serum albumin	143.5, 0.021, Ψ = −10.8	EE = 95.4	Phagocytosis of the Aβ peptide (*in vitro* model)	[104]
	PLGA	PVA	200, Ψ = −19	EE = 77	Neurogenesis (*in vitro* and *in vivo* models)	[105]

Table 1. *Cont.*

Carrier	Composition	Ligand/Stabilizer	Size, PI and Ψ (mV)	% of EE and DL	Model of Evaluation	Reference
	PLGA	PVA	153, 0.15	90, 9.5	Pain (*in vivo* model)	[106]
	PLGA	Tet-1	150-200, Ψ = −30 to −20	-	Amyloid aggregates (*in vitro* model)	[107]
	PLGA	PEG-B6 peptide	150, Ψ = 3.8	DL = 15.6	Alzheimer transgenic mice (*in vitro* and *in vivo* models)	[108]
	PLGA	PEG, cyclic hexapeptide	97.3, 0.16	EE = 80.5	Glioma tumor cells (*in vitro* and *in vivo* models)	[109]
	PLGA	PEG, transferrin receptor-binding peptide T7	130, Ψ = −15.9	EE = 18	Brain tumor (*in vitro* and *in vivo* models)	[110]
	PLGA	1,2-distearoyl-glycerol-3-phospho-ethanolamine-N-[methoxy (polyethylene glycol)-2000	169, 0.22	EE = 35	Glioblastoma (*in vitro* and *in vivo* models)	[111]
	PLGA	PVA	220, Ψ = −20.6	81.7, 16.3	Subarachnoid hemorrhage-induced BBB disruption (*in vivo* model)	[112]
	PLA–PEG	PVP	55, 0.09, Ψ = −0.29	EE = 99	Alzheimer's Disease Tg2576 Mice (*in vitro* and *in vivo* models)	[113]
	Hyaluronic acid/chitosan	-	207, Ψ = 25.3	89.9, 6.5	Glioma cells (*in vitro* model)	[114]
Polymeric micelle	Oleoyl chloride, polyethylene glycol 400	-	142, 0.4, Ψ = −7	EE = 87	Glioblastoma cells (*in vitro* model)	[115]
Nanoemulsion	Labrafac Lipophile WL 1349, Solutol HS 15, Transcutol HP	Tween 80, Tween 20	67, 0.137, Ψ = −37	-	Malignant glioma cells (*in vitro* model)	[116]
	Labrafac Lipophile	Cremophor RH40	114, 0.25, Ψ = −21.8	-	Biodistribution (*ex vivo* and *in vivo* models)	[117]
	Castor oil	Soybean lecithin, PEG 660-stereate	20.7, 0.19, Ψ = −9.7	EE ≥ 99	Permeation in Franz cells (*ex vivo* model)	[118]
Metallic nanoparticles	Au	PEG	-	-	Lipopolysaccharide-induced inflammation (*in vitro* and *in vivo* models)	[119]
Magnetic nanoparticles	Iron (II) sulfate heptahydrate	PEG-PLA	94, 0.14, Ψ = −0.01	EE = 99	Detection of amyloid plaques in Alzheimer's (*in vitro* and *in vivo* models)	[120]
	Gold-iron oxide	Glutathione	40, 0.185, Ψ = −16	EE = 70, 0.7	Brain cancer (*in vitro* model)	[121]
	Fe3O4	-	185, Ψ = −37.5,	EE = 75	Schizophrenic rats (*in vivo* model)	[122]
	Iron oxide. SPIO nanoparticles, 10,12-pentacosadiynoic acid	PVA, Lactoferrin	100	EE = 90.3	Orthotopic Brain Tumor-Bearing Rat (*in vitro* and *in vivo* models)	[123]
Liposomes	1,2-dipalmitoyl-sn-glycerol-3-phosphatidylcholine, cholesterol	-	207, 0.25, Ψ = −10.5	-	Amyloid peptide plaques (*in vivo* model)	[124]
β-cyclodextrin (BCD), nanoliposome (NL)	β-cyclodextrin, phosphatidylcholine: cholesterol (5:1)	Tween 80 for liposome	133.49, −31.76 and 121.81, −7.91	BCD = 76.6, 19.73 NL = 88.2, 4.13	Dimethylhydrazine induced poison (*in vivo* model)	[125]

PVA: polyvinyl alcohol, PLGA: poly (lactic-co-glycolic acid), PVP: polyvinylpyrrolidone, PI: polidispersity index, PEG: polyethylene glycol, EE: entrapment efficiency, DL: drug load, D-α-tocopheryl polyethylene glycol 1000 Succinate: vitamin E TPGS, CNS: central nervous system, BBB: blood–brain barrier.

7. Applications of Curcumin in Nanoparticles

7.1. Alzheimer's Disease

Alzheimer's disease is the most frequent neurodegenerative disorder worldwide; it is characterized by extracellular Aβ aggregation, intracellular neurofibrillary tangles, tau hyperphosphorylation, and progressive neuron loss. Its main clinical features are memory loss, behavioral changes, and cognitive impairment [126,127]. At present, the limited efficacy of the available therapies has encouraged the search for new treatments. In this regard, recent investigations undertaken in diverse experimental models have suggested that curcumin could be helpful for AD treatment. However, limitations in the bioavailability of curcumin have hindered its use and promoted the search for suitable vehicles to improve its pharmacological activity, such as nanoparticle formulations.

In recent years, the development of nanocarriers to transport curcumin to the brain in AD models has increased considerably; however, the efficacy, safety, and suitability of these formulations is still a main concern. Thus, in addition to the cellular uptake, the evaluation of cell viability has become pivotal to demonstrate the biocompatibility of these formulations.

It has been suggested that aluminum is involved in the etiology of AD; thus, in an early study, the neuroprotective effect of solid lipid nanoparticles loaded with curcumin (SLN-Cur) was proved in an AD mouse model induced by 100 mg/kg of aluminum chloride [91]. The results showed that treatment with SLN-Cur (50 mg/kg) produced a 73% recovery in acetylcholinesterase and a 97.46% recovery in membrane lipids with respect to the group treated with aluminum chloride alone. In addition, mice treated with SLN-Cur underwent less learning impairment and cognition loss, as measured by the Morris water maze test, which suggests the potential of SLN-Cur as an alternative therapeutic for AD.

Similarly, evidence for a reduction of neurogenesis in AD has been shown, which suggests that the induction of this neuronal process mediated by endogenous neuronal stem cells (NSC) would be a probable therapeutic target. In this regard, Tiwari et al. [105] explored the effect of PLGA nanoparticles loaded with curcumin (PLGA–NP–Cur) on neuronal differentiation and NSC proliferation. Through transmission electron microscopy (TEM) analysis, these authors showed that PLGA-NP-Cur had the ability to internalize into NSC derived from the hippocampus. Moreover, Alamar blue reduction and MTT assays suggested that PLGA-NP-Cur (0.001–50 μM) increased NSC proliferation and cell viability, with the highest effect at 0.5 μM. It is noteworthy that bulk curcumin enhanced NSC proliferation only at 0.5 μM, whereas PLGA-NP-Cur significantly increased NSC proliferation at much lower doses (0.001 μM, 0.01 μM, 0.1 μM, and 0.2 μM). Likewise, the results demonstrated that PLGA-NP-Cur reversed deficits in hippocampal neurogenesis and in learning and memory dysfunction in an AD rat model induced by the brain injection of Aß. Interestingly, a more pronounced effect was exhibited by PLGA-NP-Cur when compared with bulk curcumin. Collectively, the results suggested that PLGA-NP-Cur could offer an alternative for the treatment of AD and regenerative medicine.

On the other hand, diverse evidences suggest that oxidative stress participates in the pathophysiology of AD; thus, Djiokeng Paka et al. [128] evaluated the antioxidant and anti-inflammatory activities of curcumin-loaded PLGA nanoparticles (Cur–PLGA–NP) in SK-N-SH cells, which are human neuroblastoma-derived cells. Through assays of radical scavenging activity, the authors found that Cur-PLGA-NP exhibited 1.5-fold and 2.2-fold greater antioxidant activity against peroxyl radical than curcumin alone and empty NP, respectively. They also showed that Cur-PLGA-NP prevented Tau phosphorylation and Akt activity, which have been shown as altered in AD brains. Therefore, the authors suggested that Cur-PLGA-NP could be potentially useful for treating AD.

In another study, Meng et al. [94] developed a low-density lipoprotein-mimic nanocarrier attached to lactoferrin encapsulated in curcumin (Lf–mNLC–Cur) and evaluated its effect on the progression of disease in a rat model of AD. The rat model was generated by means of an intraperitoneal injection of D-gal (0.3 mL/100 g/d for six weeks) and a bilateral injection of $A\beta_{1-42}$ in the dorsal hippocampus (one mg/mL; 5 μL). Through fluorescence images, it was shown that Lf-mNLC-Cur had the ability to cross the BBB, to penetrate into the brain, and to release curcumin. In order to evaluate the therapeutic effect of the formulation, histological preparations to examine the state of the nerve cells in the hippocampal region after the administration of Lf-mNLC-Cur and measurements of malondialdehyde (MDA) in blood were performed. Hematoxylin–eosin staining revealed a lower damage in the treatment with Lf-mNLC-Cur, and the content of MDA was reduced with respect to the control, which suggested that the formulation was effective for decreasing the oxidative stress associated with the progression of AD [94].

Similarly, Barbara et al. [129] designed and engineered a curcumin-encapsulated PLGA nanoparticle bound to peptide g7 (Cur-NP-g7) to promote BBB crossing. The authors demonstrated that Cur-NP-g7 can internalize hippocampal neurons, and that concentrations to around 200 μM were not toxic. Furthermore, the authors determined the effect of Cur-NP-g7 on Aβ aggregation, employing an in vitro AD model generated in the primary hippocampal culture derived from the rat brain. The results revealed an important decrease of Aβ; thus, they concluded that their formulation represent a promising tool for the treatment of AD.

On the other hand, a recent study demonstrated the anti-inflammatory effects of curcumin-loaded spherical polymeric nanoparticles (Cur-SPN). In that study, it was demonstrated that Cur-SPN (10 μM) reduced cytokines IL-1ß, IL-6, and TNF-α expression in macrophages stimulated by Aβ fibrils (2 μM). Likewise, cell viability assays revealed that Cur-SPN did not induce apoptosis, and no evidence of toxicity was detected. Based on their findings, the authors claimed that this approach could be helpful for the amelioration of inflammation observed in AD [94].

In a study undertaken by Huang et al. [130], PLGA nanoparticles were designed conjugated with the S1 peptide (an inhibitor of Aβ generation), brain-targeting calreticulin (CRT) (a peptide that binds to the transferrin receptor), and curcumin (as a therapeutic substance to tackle the disorder). The results revealed that the nanocarrier (S1-CRT-NP+Cur) was taken up into a cellular model of the BBB (brain microvascular bEnd.3 cells), suggesting that it can permeate across the BBB. In support of this hypothesis, S1-CRT-NP+Cur was distributed in mouse brain after intravenous administration, as demonstrated by in vivo bioluminescence imaging system and post-mortem studies. The therapeutic effect of S1-CRT-NP+Cur was explored by means of a Y-maze and a new object recognition test, the determination of astrogliosis and microgliosis, and the measurement of cytokines, superoxide dismutase (SOD), and ROS levels in a transgenic AD mouse model (APP/PS1dE9). Interestingly, S1-CRT-NP+Cur attenuated cognitive deficits, reduced astrogliosis and microgliosis, increased the number of synapses, decreased inflammatory cytokines, enhanced SOD levels, and reduced ROS levels. These findings highlight S1-CRT-NP+Cur as a promising approach for future use in AD treatment.

Finally, in a recent report, PLGA–PEG nanoparticles attached to the B6 peptide with curcumin encapsulated (PLGA/PEG-B6-Cur) were designed [108]. PLGA–PEG was employed to enhance the bioavailability, and the B6 peptide was employed to permit BBB crossing. In order to explore their potential usefulness in AD treatment, PLGA/PEG-B6-Cur were proven in HT22 cells and an AD rodent model (APP/PS1 transgenic mice). Cytotoxicity studies in HT22 cells demonstrated that PLGA/PEG-B6-Cur did not affect cell viability up to 500 μg/mL. To evaluate the effect of PLGA/PEG-B6-Cur on memory capability and spatial learning, the Morris water maze test was performed in animals intraperitoneally injected with the nanocarrier. The experimental results revealed that PLGA/PEG-B6-Cur significantly improved cognitive performance, which correlated with a decrease in tau phosphorylation and Aβ production in the hippocampus. Altogether, these findings suggest that PLGA/PEG-B6-Cur may represent a promising alternative for treating AD.

7.2. Parkinson's Disease

Parkinson's disease is the second most frequent neurodegenerative disorder and is characterized by abnormalities in the control of voluntary movements. The pathological hallmarks of PD include neuronal cell death, oxidative stress, mitochondrial dysfunction, and the accumulation of α-synuclein. The gold standard for the treatment of PD is L-Dopa; however, its chronic employment leads to a severe collateral problem known as dyskinesia. Therefore, the lack of a permanent cure has triggered the search for novel treatments. In this respect, curcumin has shown good effects in different experimental models; thus, it could be a key molecule for developing new strategies to reach a definitive treatment.

In this regard, in a first approach, alginate–curcumin nanoparticles (Alg-NP-Cur) were developed, and their probable therapeutic actions were evaluated in a PD Drosophila model. Alg-NP-Cur exhibited antioxidant power by the reduction of the lipid peroxidation in the PD Drosophila brain after a diet supplemented with the nanocarrier for 24 days. The effective prevention of the progression of the Parkinsonian symptoms in the PD flies was evidenced by the inhibition of the loss of climbing ability in flies with respect to PD flies without exposure to Alg-NP-Cur. Therefore, this report provided a rationale for employing curcumin-encapsulated nanoparticles in preclinical and clinical studies [131].

In this respect, in another study, Kundu et al. [88] designed glyceryl monooleate nanoparticles loaded with piperine and curcumin (GMO-NP-Pip/Cur). The anti-aggregate and anti-fibrillar effects of GMO-NP-Pip/Cur on α-synuclein oligomers were evaluated employing atomic force microscopy (AFM). The results showed that GMO-NP-Pip/Cur produced a pronounced inhibition of α-synuclein aggregation. Similarly, GMO-NP-Pip/Cur were able to ameliorate motor dysfunction when co-administered with rotenone in a PD mouse model. Interestingly, GMO-NP-Pip/Cur exhibited anti-apoptotic and antioxidant activities with no evidence of cytotoxicity. Therefore, GMO-NP-Pip/Cur could be an interesting approach for the treatment of PD.

In another study, Bollimpelli et al. [132] elaborated lactoferrin nanoparticles by sol-oil chemistry, which were loaded with curcumin (Lf-NP-Cur). The potential neuroprotective usefulness of this formulation was evaluated against toxicity induced by rotenone in SK-N-SH cells, employing microscopy, a lactate dehydrogenase (LDH) release assay, and an MTT assay. The findings suggested that Lf-NP-Cur protect the cells from the toxicity of rotenone, more than curcumin alone; thus, these may be a suitable drug-delivery strategy against PD.

Finally, nanoparticles with Polysorbate 80 are widely used to improve the BBB permeability of the nanoparticles; thus, Zhang et al. [133] developed curcumin-loaded polysorbate 80-modified cerasomes (PS80-NP-Cur). The formulation was able to modify the release time of curcumin monitored in C57BL/6 mice, producing a prolonged circulation time in the blood. Furthermore, PS80-NP-Cur produced a remarkable reduction of PD symptoms in a PD mouse model induced by 1-methyl-4-phenyl-1,2,3,6-tetrahydropyridine (MPTP), when these were administered concomitantly with ultrasound-targeted microbubble destruction (UTMD). Despite these promising results, the utilization of techniques such as UTMD should be evaluated to a greater extent, because its employment for prolonged times could lead to severe undesirable effects.

7.3. Huntington's Disease

Huntington's disease is a genetic neurodegenerative disorder whose clinical manifestations include involuntary movements and anxiety. To date, there is no specific medication to treat the disease; however, since mitochondrial impairment appears to contribute to neuronal death in HD, approaches to decrease mitochondrial dysfunction could represent a therapeutic alternative. In this regard, it has been reported that dietary curcumin possesses beneficial effects in HD. Therefore, Sandhir et al. [87] fabricated solid lipid nanoparticles loaded with curcumin (SLNP-Cur) and explored their neuroprotective effectiveness in a HD rat model induced by 3-nitropropionic acid (3-NP). The administration of SLNP-Cur was able to restore SOD activity and glutathione levels. Furthermore, SLNP-Cur decreased ROS, protein carbonyls, and lipid peroxidation. In addition, the formulation reduced the motor impairment induced by the treatment with 3-NP. Therefore, these results indicate that SLNP-Cur could be helpful for the treatment of HD.

8. Conclusions

Curcumin is an example of an ancestral phytochemical whose health benefits have been confirmed and new applications have been discovered with a high impact for incurable diseases. The study of curcumin is one of the few cases of broad applications demonstrated under methodological principles and in a reproducible manner. Recently, the greatest impacts of this molecule are due to the novel technological proposals for its biological administration. In particular, the use of nanoparticles has made it possible to demonstrate benefits at the brain level, which can even revolutionize medicine. However, as with any chemical substance, it is convenient to emphasize toxicity issues in order to ensure the safety of all clinical trials. In addition to the clear results in brain models, the increase in benefits can be addressed with an improvement in the functioning of nanotechnological carriers.

Author Contributions: Conceptualization, G.L.-G. and H.C.; Methodology, M.L.D.P.-A.; Software, J.A.M.-T.; Validation, B.F., M.G.-T. and I.H.C.-F.; Formal Analysis, M.L.D.P.-A.; Investigation, I.H.C.-F., N.M.-M.; Writing—Original Draft Preparation, N.M.-M., M.L.D.P.-A., G.L.-G., H.C.; Writing–Review and Editing, M.L.D.P.-A., G.L.-G., H.C.; Visualization, G.L.-G.; Supervision, G.L.-G. and H.C.

Acknowledgments: The authors would like to thank Carlos Flores-Morales for his assistance with AFM assessment, Miguel Ángel Canseco-Martínez for the help providing FTIR analysis, Karla Eriseth Reyes-Morales for her technical assistance with thermal tests.

Abbreviations

AD	Alzheimer disease
AP-1	activating protein-1
APP	amyloid-β precursor protein
AR	androgen receptor
Arh-R	aryl hydrocarbon receptor
AS	α-synuclein
ASD	Amorphous solid dispersions
Aβ	amyloid-β
BACE1	β-secretase enzyme
BBB	blood–brain barrier
BCS	Biopharmaceutics Classification System
cAK	autophosphorylation-activated protein kinase
CBP	CREB-binding protein
CDPK	Ca^{2+}-dependent protein kinase cellular src kinase
CNS	central nervous system
COX-2	cyclooxygenase-2
cPK	protamine kinase
CTGF	connective tissue growth factor
DFF40	DNA fragmentation factor; 40-kd subunit
DL	drug loading
DR-5	death receptor-5
EE	entrapment efficiency
EGF	epidermal growth Factor
EGF-R	EGF receptor
EGFRK	EGF receptor-kinase
Egr-1	early growth response gene-1
ELAM-1	endothelial leukocyte adhesion molecule-1; Bcl-2, B-cell lymphoma protein 2
EPC-R	endothelial protein C-receptor
EpRE	electrophile
ERK	extracellular receptor kinase
ER-α	estrogen receptor-α
FAK	focal adhesion kinase
Fas-R	Fas receptor
FDA	Food and Drug Administration
FGF	fibroblast growth factor
FPTase	farnesyl protein transferase
Gcl	Glutamate–cysteine ligase
GM-CSF	granulocyte-macrophage colony-stimulating factor
GST	glutathione-S-transferase
H2-R	histamine (2)-receptor

HGF	hepatocyte growth factor
HO	heme oxygenase
HSP-70	heat shock protein 70
IAP	inhibitory apoptosis protein
IARK	IL-1 receptor-associated kinase
ICAM-1	intracellular adhesion molecule-1
IFNγ	interferon gamma
IKK	IκB kinase
IL	interleukin
IL-8-R	interleukin-8-receptor
iNOS	inducible nitric oxide synthase
Inos	matrix inducible nitric oxide synthase
InsP3-R	inositol 1,4,5-triphosphate receptor
IR	Fourier transform infrared spectroscopy
IR	integrin receptor
JAK	janus kinase
JNK	c-jun N-terminal kinase
LDL-R	low-density lipoprotein-receptor
LOX	lipoxygenase
LPS	lipopolysaccharide
MAPK	mitogen-activated protein kinase
MCP	monocyte chemoattractant protein
MDR	multidrug resistance
MIF	migration inhibition protein
MIP	macrophage inflammatory protein
MMP	matrix metalloproteinase
Mv	Millivolts
NAT	arylamine N-acetyltransferases
NF-κB	nuclear factor-κB
NGF	nerve growth factor
NMR	nuclear magnetic resonance
Nrf-2	nuclear factor erythroid 2-related factor
PBCA	poly (butyl cyanoacrylate)
PDGF	platelet-derived growth factor
PhK	phosphorylase kinase
PKA	protein kinase A
PKB	protein kinase B
PKC	protein kinase C
PLGA	poly lactic-co-glycolic acid
pp60c-src	non-receptor protein tyrosine kinase c-Src
PPARγ	peroxisome proliferator-activated receptor-γ
PrP	prion protein
PrP-Res	prion protein resistance
PVA	polyvinyl alcohol
SHP-2	Src homology 2 domain containing tyrosine phosphatase 2
SMEDDS	Self-microemulsifying drug delivery systems
STAT	signal transducers and activators of transcription
TAT	transactivating–transduction peptide
TGF-β1	transforming growth factor-β1
TIMP	tissue inhibitor of metalloproteinase-3
TK	protein tyrosine kinase
TNF	tumoral necrosis factor
TNF-α	tumor necrosis factor-α
uPA	urokinase-type plasminogen activator

VCAM-1	vascular cell adhesion molecule-1
VEGF	vascular endothelial growth factor
Ψ	zeta potential

References

1. Aggarwal, B.B.; Harikumar, K.B. Potential therapeutic effects of curcumin, the anti-inflammatory agent, against neurodegenerative, cardiovascular, pulmonary, metabolic, autoimmune and neoplastic diseases. *Int. J. Biochem. Cell Biol.* **2009**, *41*, 40–59. [CrossRef] [PubMed]
2. Alsamydai, A.; Jaber, N. Pharmacological aspects of curcumin: Review article. *Int. J. Pharmacogn.* **2018**, *5*, 313–326.
3. Bengmark, S. Curcumin, an atoxic antioxidant and natural NFκB, cyclooxygenase-2, lipooxygenase, and inducible nitric oxide synthase inhibitor: A shield against acute and chronic diseases. *J. Parenter. Enter. Nutr.* **2006**, *30*, 45–51. [CrossRef]
4. Wang, S.L.; Ying, L.; Ying, W.; Chen, Y.F.; Na, L.X.; Li, S.T.; Sun, C.H. Curcumin, a potential inhibitor of Up-regulation of TNF-alpha and IL-6 induced by palmitate in 3T3-L1 adipocytes through NF-κB and JNK pathway. *Biomed. Environ. Sci.* **2009**, *22*, 32–39. [CrossRef]
5. Guo, Y.Z.; He, P.; Feng, A.M. Effect of curcumin on expressions of NF-κBp65, TNF-α and IL-8 in placental tissue of premature birth of infected mice. *Asian Pac. J. Trop. Med.* **2017**, *10*, 175–178. [CrossRef] [PubMed]
6. Becher, B.; Spath, S.; Goverman, J. Cytokine networks in neuroinflammation. *Nat. Rev. Immunol.* **2017**, *17*, 49–59. [CrossRef] [PubMed]
7. Zhang, C.; Browne, A.; Child, D.; Tanzi, R.E. Curcumin decreases amyloid-β peptide levels by attenuating the maturation of amyloid-β precursor protein. *J. Biol. Chem.* **2010**, *285*, 28472–28480. [CrossRef]
8. Fonseca-Santos, B.; Gremião, M.P.; Chorilli, M. Nanotechnology-based drug delivery systems for the treatment of Alzheimer's disease. *Int. J. Nanomed.* **2015**, *10*, 4981–5003. [CrossRef]
9. Li, J.; Sabliov, C. PLA/PLGA nanoparticles for delivery of drugs across the blood-brain barrier. *Nanotechnol. Rev.* **2013**, *2*, 241–257. [CrossRef]
10. Bhatia, S. Nanoparticles types, classification, characterization, fabrication methods and drug delivery applications. In *Natural Polymer Drug Delivery Systems*; Nanoparticles, Plants, and Algae; Springer International Publishing: Cham, Switzerland, 2016; pp. 33–85.
11. Priyadarsini, K. The Chemistry of Curcumin: From Extraction to Therapeutic Agent. *Molecules* **2014**, *19*, 20091–20112. [CrossRef]
12. Payton, F.; Sandusky, P.; Alworth, W.L. NMR study of the solution structure of curcumin. *J. Nat. Prod.* **2007**, *70*, 143–146. [CrossRef] [PubMed]
13. Yanagisawa, D.; Shirai, N.; Amatsubo, T.; Taguchi, H.; Hirao, K.; Urushitani, M.; Morikawa, S.; Inubushi, T.; Kato, M.; Kato, F.; et al. Relationship between the tautomeric structures of curcumin derivatives and their Aβ-binding activities in the context of therapies for Alzheimer's disease. *Biomaterials* **2010**, *31*, 4179–4185. [CrossRef] [PubMed]
14. Chen, Y.; Wu, Q.; Zhang, Z.; Yuan, L.; Liu, X.; Zhou, L. Preparation of curcumin-loaded liposomes and evaluation of their skin permeation and pharmacodynamics. *Molecules* **2012**, *17*, 5972–5987. [CrossRef] [PubMed]
15. Subramani, P.A.; Panati, K.; Lebaka, V.R.; Redd, D.D.; Narala, V.R. Nanostructures for curcumin delivery: Posibilities and challenges. In *Nano and -Micro Drug Delivery Systems*; Andrew, W., Ed.; Elsevier Science Ltd Desing and Fabrication: Amsterdam, The Netherlands, 2017; pp. 393–418.
16. Kharat, M.; Du, Z.; Zhang, G.; Mcclements, D.J. Physical and Chemical Stability of Curcumin in Aqueous Solutions and Emulsions: Impact of pH, Temperature, and Molecular Environment. *J. Agric. Food Chem.* **2017**, *65*, 1525–1532. [CrossRef] [PubMed]
17. Sharma, K.; Agrawal, S.S.; Gupta, M. Development and validation of UV spectrophotometric method for the estimation of curcumin in bulk drug and pharmaceutical dosage forms. *Int. J. Drug Dev. Res.* **2012**, *4*, 375–380.
18. Benassi, R.; Ferrari, E.; Lazzari, S.; Spagnolo, F.; Saladini, M. Theoretical study on Curcumin: A comparison of calculated spectroscopic properties with NMR, UV-vis and IR experimental data. *J. Mol. Struct.* **2008**, *892*, 168–176. [CrossRef]

19. Athira, G.K.; Jyothi, A.N. Preparation and characterization of curcumin loaded cassava starch nanoparticles with improved cellular absorption. *Int. J. Pharm. Pharm. Sci.* **2014**, *6*, 171–176.
20. O'Neil, M.J. (Ed.) *The Merck Index, An Encyclopedia of Chemicals, Drugs, and Biologicals*, 15th ed.; Royal Society of Chemistry: Cambridge, UK, 2013.
21. Doktorovova, S.; Souto, E.B.; Silva, A.M. Hansen solubility parameters (HSP) for prescreening formulation of solid lipid nanoparticles (SLN): In Vitro testing of curcumin-loaded SLN in MCF-7 and BT-474 cell lines. *Pharm. Dev. Technol.* **2018**, *23*, 96–105. [CrossRef]
22. Shen, L.; Ji, H.F. The pharmacology of curcumin: Is it the degradation products? *Trends Mol. Med.* **2012**, *18*, 138–144. [CrossRef]
23. Wang, Y.-J.; Pan, M.-H.; Cheng, A.-L.; Lin, L.-I.; Ho, Y.-S.; Hsieh, C.-Y.; Lin, J.-K. Stability of curcumin in buffer solutions and characterization of its degradation products. *J. Pharm. Biomed. Anal.* **1997**, *15*, 1867–1876. [CrossRef]
24. Schneider, C.; Gordon, O.N.; Edwards, R.L.; Luis, P.B. Degradation of Curcumin: From Mechanism to Biological Implications. *J. Agric. Food Chem.* **2015**, *63*, 7606–7614. [CrossRef] [PubMed]
25. Griesser, M.; Pistis, V.; Suzuki, T.; Tejera, N.; Pratt, D.A.; Schneider, C. Autoxidative and cyclooxygenase-2 catalyzed transformation of the dietary chemopreventive agent curcumin. *J. Biol. Chem.* **2011**, *286*, 1114–1124. [CrossRef] [PubMed]
26. Aggarwal, B.B.; Sundaram, C.; Malani, N.; Haruyo, I. Curcumin: The Indian solid gold. In *The Molecular Targets and Therapeutics Uses of Curcumin in Health and Disease*; Aggarwal, B.B., Surh, Y.-J., Shishodia, S., Eds.; Springer Science: Boston MA, USA, 2007; Volume 595, pp. 1–75.
27. Reinke, A.A.; Gestwicki, J.E. Structure-activity relationships of amyloid beta-aggregation inhibitors based on curcumin: Influence of linker length and flexibility. *Chem. Biol. Drug Des.* **2007**, *70*, 206–215. [CrossRef] [PubMed]
28. Ray, B.; Lahiri, D.K. Neuroinflammation in Alzheimer's disease: Different molecular targets and potential therapeutic agents including curcumin. *Curr. Opin. Pharmacol.* **2009**, *9*, 434–444. [CrossRef] [PubMed]
29. Kasi, P.D.; Tamilselvam, R.; Skalicka-Woźniak, K.; Nabavi, S.F.; Daglia, M.; Bishayee, A.; Pazoki-Toroudi, H.; Nabavi, S.M. Molecular targets of curcumin for cancer therapy: An updated review. *Tumor Biol.* **2016**, *37*, 13017–13028. [CrossRef] [PubMed]
30. Zhou, H.; Beevers, C.S.; Huang, S. The targets of curcumin. *Curr. Drug Targets* **2011**, *12*, 332–347. [CrossRef]
31. Aguzzi, A.; O'Connor, T. Protein aggregation diseases: Pathogenicity and therapeutic perspectives. *Nat. Rev. Drug Discov.* **2010**, *9*, 237–248. [CrossRef]
32. Hafner-Bratkovič, I.; Gašperšič, J.; Šmid, L.M.; Bresjanac, M.; Jerala, R. Curcumin binds to the α-helical intermediate and to the amyloid form of prion protein -A new mechanism for the inhibition of PrPSc accumulation. *J. Neurochem.* **2008**, *104*, 1553–1564. [CrossRef]
33. Caughey, B.; Raymond, L.D.; Raymond, G.J.; Maxson, L.; Silveira, J.; Baron, G.S. Inhibition of protease-resistant prion protein accumulation in vitro by curcumin. *J. Virol.* **2003**, *77*, 5499–5502. [CrossRef]
34. Pandey, N.; Strider, J.; Nolan, W.C.; Yan, S.X.; Galvin, J.E. Curcumin inhibits aggregation of α-synuclein. *Acta Neuropathol.* **2008**, *115*, 479–489. [CrossRef]
35. Brahmkhatri, V.; Sharma, N.; Punnepalli, S.; D'Souza, A.; Raghothama, S.; Atreya, H.S. Curcumin nanoconjugate Inhibits aggregation of N-terminal region (Aβ-16) of an amyloid beta peptide. *New J. Chem.* **2018**, *42*, 19881–19892. [CrossRef]
36. Mithu, V.S.; Sarkar, B.; Bhowmik, D.; Das, A.K.; Chandrakesan, M. Curcumin Alters the Salt Bridge-containing Turn Region in amyloid β(1-42) aggregates. *J. Biol. Chem.* **2014**, *289*, 11122–11131. [CrossRef] [PubMed]
37. Yang, F.; Lim, G.P.; Begum, A.N.; Ubeda, O.J.; Simmons, M.R.; Ambegaokar, S.S.; Chen, P.; Kayed, R.; Glabe, C.G.; Frautschy, S.A.; et al. Curcumin Inhibits Formation of Amyloid β Oligomers and Fibrils, Binds Plaques, and Reduces Amyloid in vivo. *J. Biol. Chem.* **2005**, *280*, 5892–5901. [CrossRef] [PubMed]
38. Huang, X.; Atwood, Æ.C.S.; Moir, Æ.R.D.; Hartshorn, M.A.; Tanzi, Æ.R.E.; Bush, A.I. Trace metal contamination initiates the apparent auto-aggregation, amyloidosis, and oligomerization of Alzheimer's Aβ peptides. *J. Biol. Inorg. Chem.* **2004**, *9*, 954–960. [CrossRef] [PubMed]
39. Cole, G.M.; Teter, B.; Frautschy, S.A. Neuropretective effects of curcumin. In *The Molecular Targets and Therapeutic Uses of Curcumin in Health and Disease*; Aggarwal, B.B., Surh, Y.J., Shishodia, S., Eds.; Springer: Boston, MA, USA, 2007; Volume 595, pp. 197–212.

40. Vassar, R. Bace 1 The β-secretase enzyme in alzheimer's disease. *J. Mol. Neurosci.* **2004**, *23*, 105–113. [CrossRef]
41. DiSabato, D.J.; Quan, N.; Godbout, J.P. Neuroinflammation: The Devil is in the Details. *J. Neurochem.* **2016**, *139*, 136–153. [CrossRef] [PubMed]
42. Karlstetter, M.; Lippe, E.; Walczak, Y.; Moehle, C.; Aslanidis, A.; Mirza, M.; Langmann, T. Curcumin is a potent modulator of microglial gene expression and migration. *J. Neuroinflammation* **2011**, *8*, 1–12. [CrossRef]
43. Tizabi, Y.; Hurley, L.L.; Qualls, Z.; Akinfiresoye, L. Relevance of the anti-inflammatory properties of curcumin in neurodegenerative diseases and depression. *Molecules* **2014**, *19*, 20864–20879. [CrossRef]
44. Yin, H.; Guo, Q.; Li, X.; Tang, T.; Li, C.; Wang, H.; Sun, Y.; Feng, Q.; Ma, C.; Gao, C.; et al. Curcumin Suppresses IL-1β Secretion and Prevents Inflammation through Inhibition of the NLRP3 Inflammasome. *J. Immunol.* **2018**, *200*, 2835–2846. [CrossRef]
45. Jurrmann, N.; Brigelius-Flohe, R.; Bol, G.F. Curcumin blocks interleukin-1 (IL-1) signaling by inhibiting the recruitment of the IL-1 receptor-associated kinase IRAK in murine thymoma EL-4 cells. *J. Nutr.* **2005**, *135*, 1859–1864. [CrossRef]
46. Devi, Y.S.; DeVine, M.; DeKuiper, J.; Ferguson, S.; Fazleabas, A.T. Inhibition of IL-6 signaling pathway by curcumin in uterine decidual cells. *PLoS ONE* **2015**, *10*, e0125627. [CrossRef] [PubMed]
47. Sahebkar, A.; Cicero, A.F.G.; Simental-Mendía, L.E.; Aggarwal, B.B.; Gupta, S.C. Curcumin downregulates human tumor necrosis factor-α levels: A systematic review and meta-analysis ofrandomized controlled trials. *Pharmacol. Res.* **2016**, *107*, 234–242. [CrossRef] [PubMed]
48. Singh, S.; Aggarwal, B.B. Activation of transcription factor NF-κ B is suppressed by curcumin (diferuloylmethane). *J. Biol. Chem.* **1995**, *270*, 24995–25000. [CrossRef] [PubMed]
49. Aggarwal, B.B.; Gupta, S.C.; Sung, B. Curcumin: An orally bioavailable blocker of TNF and other pro-inflammatory biomarkers. *Br. J. Pharmacol.* **2013**, *169*, 1672–1692. [PubMed]
50. Howe, C.L.; LaFrance-Corey, R.G.; Goddery, E.N.; Johnson, R.K.; Mirchia, K. Neuronal CCL2 expression drives inflammatory monocyte infiltration into the brain during acute virus infection. *J. Neuroinflamm.* **2017**, *14*, 1–14. [CrossRef] [PubMed]
51. Zhang, Z.-J.; Zhao, L.-X.; Cao, D.-L.; Zhang, X.; Gao, Y.-J.; Xia, C. Curcumin Inhibits LPS-Induced CCL2 Expression via JNK Pathway in C6 Rat Astrocytoma Cells. *Cell. Mol. Neurobiol.* **2012**, *32*, 1003–1010. [CrossRef] [PubMed]
52. Herman, J.G.; Stadelman, H.L.; Roselli, C.E. Curcumin blocks CCL2-induced adhesion, motility and invasion, in part, through down-regulation of CCL2 expression and proteolytic activity. *Int. J. Oncol.* **2009**, *34*, 1319–1327. [PubMed]
53. Midura-Kiela, M.T.; Radhakrishnan, V.; Kiela, P. Curcumin inhibits interferon-γ signaling in colonic epithelial cells. *Am. J. Physiol. Liver Phisiol.* **2012**, *302*, G86–G96. [CrossRef] [PubMed]
54. Ogadimma, I.; Uzairu, A.; Eyije, S.; Ola, S. Evaluation of the antioxidant properties of curcumin derivatives by genetic function algorithm. *J. Adv. Res.* **2018**, *12*, 47–54.
55. Bendary, E.; Francis, R.R.; Ali, H.M.G.; Sarwat, M.I.; Hady, S. El Antioxidant and structure—Activity relationships (SARs) of some phenolic and anilines compounds. *Ann. Agric. Sci.* **2013**, *58*, 173–181.
56. Menon, V.P.; Sudheer, A.R. Antioxidant and anti-inflamatory properties of curcumin. In *The Molecular Targets and Therapeutic Uses of Curcumin in Health and Disease*; Aggarwal, B.B., Surh, Y.-J., Shishodia, S., Eds.; Springer International Publishing: Cham, Switzerland, 2007; pp. 105–126.
57. Chen, Y.; Xiao, H.; Zheng, J.; Liang, G. Structure-Thermodynamics-Antioxidant Activity Relationships of Selected Natural Phenolic Acids and Derivatives: An Experimental and Theoretical Evaluation. *PLoS ONE* **2015**, *10*, e0121276. [CrossRef] [PubMed]
58. Zbarsky, V.; Datla, K.P.; Parkar, S.; Rai, D.K.; Okezie, I.; Dexter, D.T. Neuroprotective properties of the natural phenolic antioxidants curcumin and naringenin but not quercetin and fisetin in a 6-OHDA model of Parkinson's disease. *Free Radic. Res.* **2009**, *39*, 1119–1125. [CrossRef]
59. Maiti, P.; Dunbar, G.L. Use of curcumin, a natural polyphenol for targeting molecular pathways in treating age-related neurodegenerative diseases. *Int. J. Mol. Sci.* **2018**, *19*, 1637. [CrossRef]
60. Barzegar, A.; Moosavi-movahedi, A.A. Intracellular ROS Protection Efficiency and Free Radical- Scavenging Activity of Curcumin. *PLoS ONE* **2011**, *6*, e26012. [CrossRef]

61. González-Reyes, S.; Guzmán-Beltrán, S.; Medina-Campos, O.N.; Pedraza-Chaverri, J. Curcumin Pretreatment Induces Nrf2 and an Antioxidant Response and Prevents Hemin-Induced Toxicity in Primary Cultures of Cerebellar Granule Neurons of Rats. *Oxid. Med. Cell. Longev.* **2013**, *2013*, 1–14. [CrossRef] [PubMed]
62. Haryuna, T.; Munir, D.; Maria, A.; Bashiruddin, J. The Antioxidant Effect of Curcumin on Cochlear Fibroblasts in Rat Models of Diabetes Mellitus. *Iran J. Otorhinolaryngol.* **2017**, *29*, 197–202. [PubMed]
63. Wahlang, B.; Pawar, Y.B.; Bansal, A.K. Identification of permeability-related hurdles in oral delivery of curcumin using the Caco-2 cell model. *Eur. J. Pharm. Biopharm.* **2011**, *77*, 275–282. [CrossRef]
64. Holder, G.M.; Plummer, J.L.; Ryan, A.J. The metabolism and excretion of curcumin (1,7-bis-(4-hydroxy-3-methoxyphenyl)-1,6-heptadiene-3,5-dione) in the rat. *Xenobiotica* **1978**, *8*, 761–768. [CrossRef]
65. Sharma, R.A. Phase I Clinical Trial of Oral Curcumin: Biomarkers of Systemic Activity and Compliance. *Clin. Cancer Res.* **2004**, *10*, 6847–6854. [CrossRef]
66. Gangurde, A.B.; Kundaikar, H.S.; Javeer, S.D.; Jaiswar, D.R.; Degani, M.S.; Amin, P.D. Enhanced solubility and dissolution of curcumin by a hydrophilic polymer solid dispersion and its in silico molecular modeling studies. *J. Drug Deliv. Sci. Technol.* **2015**, *29*, 226–237. [CrossRef]
67. Chuah, A.M.; Jacob, B.; Jie, Z.; Ramesh, S.; Mandal, S.; Puthan, J.K.; Deshpande, P.; Vaidyanathan, V.V.; Gelling, R.W.; Patel, G.; et al. Enhanced bioavailability and bioefficacy of an amorphous solid dispersion of curcumin. *Food Chem.* **2014**, *156*, 227–233. [CrossRef] [PubMed]
68. Wang, Y.; Wang, C.; Zhao, J.; Ding, Y.; Li, L. Journal of Colloid and Interface Science A cost-effective method to prepare curcumin nanosuspensions with enhanced oral bioavailability. *J. Colloid Interface Sci.* **2017**, *485*, 91–98. [CrossRef] [PubMed]
69. Li, X.; Yuan, H.; Zhang, C.; Chen, W.; Cheng, W.; Chen, X.; Ye, X. Preparation and in-vitro/in-vivo evaluation of curcumin nanosuspension with solubility enhancement. *J. Pharm. Pharmacol.* **2016**, *68*, 980–988. [CrossRef] [PubMed]
70. Dokania, S.; Joshi, A.K. Self-microemulsifying drug delivery system (SMEDDS)—Challenges and road ahead. *Drug Deliv.* **2015**, *22*, 675–690. [CrossRef] [PubMed]
71. Wu, X.; Xu, J.; Huang, X.; Wen, C. Self-microemulsifying drug delivery system improves curcumin dissolution and bioavailability. *Drug Dev. Ind. Pharm.* **2011**, *37*, 15–23. [CrossRef] [PubMed]
72. Jaisamut, P.; Wiwattanawongsa, K.; Graidist, P.; Sangsen, Y.; Wiwattanapatapee, R. Enhanced Oral Bioavailability of Curcumin Using a Supersaturatable Self-Microemulsifying System Incorporating a Hydrophilic Polymer; In Vitro and In Vivo Investigations. *AAPS PharmSciTech* **2018**, *19*, 730–740. [CrossRef]
73. Bele, M.H.; Shaikh, A.A.; Paralkar, S.G. To enhance the solubility of curcumin by solid self-microemulsifying drug delivery system (SMEDDS). *Indo Am. J. Pharm. Res.* **2017**, *7*, 8587–8607.
74. Cui, J.; Yu, B.; Zhao, Y.; Zhu, W.; Li, H.; Lou, H.; Zhai, G. Enhancement of oral absorption of curcumin by self-microemulsifying drug delivery systems. *Int. J. Pharm.* **2009**, *371*, 148–155. [CrossRef]
75. Yallapu, M.M.; Jaggi, M.; Chauhan, S.C. Curcumin nanoformulations: A future nanomedicine for cancer. *Drug Discov. Today* **2012**, *17*, 71–80. [CrossRef]
76. Sun, M.; Su, X.; Ding, B.; He, X.; Liu, X.; Yu, A.; Lou, H.; Zhai, G. Advances in nanotechnology-based delivery systems for curcumin. *Nanomedicine* **2012**, *7*, 1085–1100. [CrossRef]
77. Kreuter, J. Nanoparticles-a historical perspective. *Int. J. Pharm.* **2007**, *331*, 1–10. [CrossRef] [PubMed]
78. Leson, A. There is plenty of room at the bottom. *Vak. Forsch. und Prax.* **2005**, *17*, 123. [CrossRef]
79. Khanna, S.C.; Soliva, M.; Speiser, P. Epoxy resin beads as a pharmaceutical dosage form II: Dissolution studies of epoxy-amine beads and release of drug. *J. Pharm. Sci.* **1969**, *58*, 1385–1388. [CrossRef] [PubMed]
80. Kreuter, J.; Alyautdin, R.N.; Kharkevich, D.A.; Ivanov, A.A. Passage of peptides through the blood-brain barrier with colloidal polymer particles (nanoparticles). *Brain Res.* **1995**, *674*, 171–174. [CrossRef]
81. Müller, R.H.; Maaßen, S.; Weyhers, H.; Mehnert, W. Phagocytic uptake and cytotoxicity of solid lipid nanoparticles (SLN) sterically stabilized with poloxamine 908 and poloxamer 407. *J. Drug Target.* **1996**, *4*, 161–170. [CrossRef] [PubMed]
82. Xu, Y.; Kim, C.S.; Saylor, D.M.; Koo, D. Polymer degradation and drug delivery in PLGA-based drug–polymer applications: A review of experiments and theories. *J. Biomed. Mater. Res. Part B Appl. Biomater.* **2017**, *105*, 1692–1716. [CrossRef] [PubMed]
83. Barenholz, Y. Doxil—The first FDA-approved nano-drug: Lessons learned. *J. Control. Release* **2012**, *160*, 117–134. [CrossRef]

84. Jansook, P.; Ogawa, N.; Loftsson, T. Cyclodextrins: Structure, physicochemical properties and pharmaceutical applications. *Int. J. Pharm.* **2018**, *535*, 272–284. [CrossRef]
85. He, X.; Zhu, Y.; Wang, M.; Jing, G.; Zhu, R.; Wang, S. Antidepressant effects of curcumin and HU-211 coencapsulated solid lipid nanoparticles against corticosterone-induced cellular and animal models of major depression. *Int. J. Nanomed.* **2016**, *11*, 4975–4990. [CrossRef]
86. Kakkar, V.; Muppu, S.K.; Chopra, K.; Kaur, I.P. Curcumin loaded solid lipid nanoparticles: An efficient formulation approach for cerebral ischemic reperfusion injury in rats. *Eur. J. Pharm. Biopharm.* **2013**, *85*, 339–345. [CrossRef]
87. Sandhir, R.; Yadav, A.; Mehrotra, A.; Sunkaria, A.; Singh, A.; Sharma, S. Curcumin nanoparticles attenuate neurochemical and neurobehavioral deficits in experimental model of Huntington's disease. *Neuromol. Med.* **2014**, *16*, 106–118. [CrossRef] [PubMed]
88. Kundu, P.; Das, M.; Tripathy, K.; Sahoo, S.K. Delivery of Dual Drug Loaded Lipid Based Nanoparticles across the Blood-Brain Barrier Impart Enhanced Neuroprotection in a Rotenone Induced Mouse Model of Parkinson's Disease. *ACS Chem. Neurosci.* **2016**, *7*, 1658–1670. [CrossRef] [PubMed]
89. Ramalingam, P.; Ko, Y.T. Enhanced oral delivery of curcumin from N-trimethyl chitosan surface-modified solid lipid nanoparticles: Pharmacokinetic and brain distribution evaluations. *Pharm. Res.* **2015**, *32*, 389–402. [CrossRef] [PubMed]
90. Kakkar, V.; Kaur, I.P. Evaluating potential of curcumin loaded solid lipid nanoparticles in aluminium induced behavioural, biochemical and histopathological alterations in mice brain. *Food Chem. Toxicol.* **2011**, *49*, 2906–2913. [CrossRef] [PubMed]
91. Sadegh, M.S.; Azadi, A.; Izadi, Z.; Kurd, M.; Dara, T.; Dibaei, M.; Sharif Zadeh, M.; Akbari Javar, H.; Hamidi, M. Brain Delivery of Curcumin Using Solid Lipid Nanoparticles and Nanostructured Lipid Carriers: Preparation, Optimization, and Pharmacokinetic Evaluation. *ACS Chem. Neurosci.* **2018**, *10*, 728–739. [CrossRef] [PubMed]
92. Madane, R.G.; Mahajan, H.S. Curcumin-loaded nanostructured lipid carriers (NLCs) for nasal administration: Design, characterization, and in vivo study. *Drug Deliv.* **2016**, *23*, 1326–1334. [PubMed]
93. Fang, M.; Jin, Y.; Bao, W.; Gao, H.; Xu, M.; Wang, D.; Wang, X.; Yao, P.; Liu, L. In vitro characterization and in vivo evaluation of nanostructured lipid curcumin carriers for intragastric administration. *Int. J. Nanomed.* **2012**, *7*, 5395–5404. [CrossRef]
94. Meng, F.; Asghar, S.; Gao, S.; Su, Z.; Song, J.; Huo, M.; Meng, W.; Ping, Q.; Xiao, Y. A novel LDL-mimic nanocarrier for the targeted delivery of curcumin into the brain to treat Alzheimer's disease. *Colloids Surfaces B Biointerfaces* **2015**, *134*, 88–97. [CrossRef]
95. Meng, F.; Asghar, S.; Xu, Y.; Wang, J.; Jin, X.; Wang, Z.; Wang, J.; Ping, Q.; Zhou, J.; Xiao, Y. Design and evaluation of lipoprotein resembling curcumin-encapsulated protein-free nanostructured lipid carrier for brain targeting. *Int. J. Pharm.* **2016**, *506*, 46–56. [CrossRef]
96. Ameruoso, A.; Palomba, R.; Palange, A.L.; Cervadoro, A.; Lee, A.; Di Mascolo, D.; Decuzzi, P. Ameliorating amyloid-β fibrils triggered inflammation via curcumin-loaded polymeric nanoconstructs. *Front. Immunol.* **2017**, *8*, 1411. [CrossRef]
97. Mulik, R.S.; Mönkkönen, J.; Juvonen, R.O.; Mahadik, K.R.; Paradkar, A.R. ApoE3 Mediated Poly(butyl) Cyanoacrylate Nanoparticles Containing Curcumin: Study of Enhanced Activity of Curcumin against Beta Amyloid Induced Cytotoxicity Using In Vitro Cell Culture Model. *Mol. Pharm.* **2010**, *7*, 815–825. [CrossRef] [PubMed]
98. Mulik, R.S.; Mönkkönen, J.; Juvonen, R.O.; Mahadik, K.R.; Paradkar, A.R. ApoE3 mediated polymeric nanoparticles containing curcumin: Apoptosis induced in vitro anticancer activity against neuroblastoma cells. *Int. J. Pharm.* **2012**, *437*, 29–41. [CrossRef]
99. Szymusiak, M.; Hu, X.; Leon Plata, P.A.; Ciupinski, P.; Wang, Z.J.; Liu, Y. Bioavailability of curcumin and curcumin glucuronide in the central nervous system of mice after oral delivery of nano-curcumin. *Int. J. Pharm.* **2016**, *511*, 415–423. [CrossRef]
100. Tsai, Y.M.; Chien, C.F.; Lin, L.C.; Tsai, T.H. Curcumin and its nano-formulation: The kinetics of tissue distribution and blood-brain barrier penetration. *Int. J. Pharm.* **2011**, *416*, 331–338. [CrossRef] [PubMed]
101. Hu, X.; Huang, F.; Szymusiak, M.; Liu, Y.; Wang, Z.J. Curcumin Attenuates Opioid Tolerance and Dependence by Inhibiting Ca^{2+}/Calmodulin-Dependent Protein Kinase II α Activity. *J. Pharmacol. Exp. Ther.* **2015**, *352*, 420–428. [CrossRef] [PubMed]

102. Yadav, A.; Lomash, V.; Samim, M.; Flora, S.J.S. Curcumin encapsulated in chitosan nanoparticles: A novel strategy for the treatment of arsenic toxicity. *Chem. Biol. Interact.* **2012**, *199*, 49–61. [CrossRef] [PubMed]
103. Hashemian, M.; Anisian, D.; Ghasemi-Kasman, M.; Akbari, A.; Khalili-Fomeshi, M.; Ghasemi, S.; Ahmadi, F.; Moghadamnia, A.A.; Ebrahimpour, A. Curcumin-loaded chitosan-alginate-STPP nanoparticles ameliorate memory deficits and reduce glial activation in pentylenetetrazol-induced kindling model of epilepsy. *Prog. Neuro-Psychopharmacol. Biol. Psychiatry* **2017**, *79*, 462–471. [CrossRef]
104. Yang, R.; Zheng, Y.; Wang, Q.; Zhao, L. Curcumin-loaded chitosan–bovine serum albumin nanoparticles potentially enhanced Aβ 42 phagocytosis and modulated macrophage polarization in Alzheimer's disease. *Nanoscale Res. Lett.* **2018**, *13*, 1–9. [CrossRef]
105. Tiwari, S.K.; Agarwal, S.; Seth, B.; Yadav, A.; Nair, S.; Bhatnagar, P.; Karmakar, M.; Kumari, M.; Chauhan, L.K.S.; Patel, D.K.; et al. Curcumin-loaded nanoparticles potently induce adult neurogenesis and reverse cognitive deficits in Alzheimer's disease model via canonical Wnt/β-catenin pathway. *ACS Nano* **2014**, *8*, 76–103. [CrossRef]
106. Pieretti, S.; Ranjan, A.P.; Di Giannuario, A.; Mukerjee, A.; Marzoli, F.; Di Giovannandrea, R.; Vishwanatha, J.K. Curcumin-loaded Poly (D, L-lactide-co-glycolide) nanovesicles induce antinociceptive effects and reduce pronociceptive cytokine and BDNF release in spinal cord after acute administration in mice. *Colloids Surf. B Biointerfaces* **2017**, *158*, 379–386. [CrossRef]
107. Mathew, A.; Fukuda, T.; Nagaoka, Y.; Hasumura, T.; Morimoto, H.; Yoshida, Y.; Maekawa, T.; Venugopal, K.; Kumar, D.S. Curcumin loaded-PLGA nanoparticles conjugated with Tet-1 peptide for potential use in Alzheimer's disease. *PLoS ONE* **2012**, *7*, e32616. [CrossRef] [PubMed]
108. Fan, S.; Zheng, Y.; Liu, X.; Fang, W.; Chen, X.; Liao, W.; Jing, X.; Lei, M.; Tao, E.; Ma, Q.; et al. Curcumin-loaded PLGA-PEG nanoparticles conjugated with B6 peptide for potential use in Alzheimer's disease. *Drug Deliv.* **2018**, *25*, 1091–1102. [CrossRef] [PubMed]
109. Zhang, X.; Li, X.; Hua, H.; Wang, A.; Liu, W.; Li, Y.; Fu, F.; Shi, Y.; Sun, K. Cyclic hexapeptide-conjugated nanoparticles enhance curcumin delivery to glioma tumor cells and tissue. *Int. J. Nanomed.* **2017**, *12*, 5717–5732. [CrossRef] [PubMed]
110. Cui, Y.; Zhang, M.; Zeng, F.; Jin, H.; Xu, Q.; Huang, Y. Dual-Targeting Magnetic PLGA Nanoparticles for Codelivery of Paclitaxel and Curcumin for Brain Tumor Therapy. *ACS Appl. Mater. Interfaces* **2016**, *8*, 32159–32169. [CrossRef] [PubMed]
111. Orunoğlu, M.; Kaffashi, A.; Pehlivan, S.B.; Şahin, S.; Söylemezoğlu, F.; Karlı-Oğuz, K.; Mut, M. Effects of curcumin-loaded PLGA nanoparticles on the RG2 rat glioma model. *Mater. Sci. Eng. C* **2017**, *78*, 32–38. [CrossRef] [PubMed]
112. Zhang, Z.Y.; Jiang, M.; Fang, J.; Yang, M.F.; Zhang, S.; Yin, Y.X.; Li, D.W.; Mao, L.L.; Fu, X.Y.; Hou, Y.; et al. Enhanced Therapeutic Potential of Nano-Curcumin Against Subarachnoid Hemorrhage-Induced Blood–Brain Barrier Disruption Through Inhibition of Inflammatory Response and Oxidative Stress. *Mol. Neurobiol.* **2017**, *54*, 1–14. [CrossRef] [PubMed]
113. Cheng, K.K.; Yeung, C.F.; Ho, S.W.; Chow, S.F.; Chow, A.H.L.; Baum, L. Highly Stabilized Curcumin Nanoparticles Tested in an In Vitro Blood–Brain Barrier Model and in Alzheimer's Disease Tg2576 Mice. *AAPS J.* **2013**, *15*, 324–336. [CrossRef]
114. Yang, L.; Gao, S.; Asghar, S.; Liu, G.; Song, J.; Wang, X.; Ping, Q.; Zhang, C.; Xiao, Y. Hyaluronic acid/chitosan nanoparticles for delivery of curcuminoid and its in vitro evaluation in glioma cells. *Int. J. Biol. Macromol.* **2015**, *72*, 1391–1401. [CrossRef]
115. Mirgani, M.T.; Isacchi, B.; Sadeghizadeh, M.; Marra, F.; Bilia, A.R.; Mowla, S.J.; Najafi, F.; Babaei, E. Dendrosomal curcumin nanoformulation downregulates pluripotency genes via miR-145 activation in U87MG glioblastoma cells. *Int. J. Nanomed.* **2014**, *9*, 403–417.
116. Kumar, A.; Ahuja, A.; Ali, J.; Baboota, S. Curcumin-loaded lipid nanocarrier for improving bioavailability, stability and cytotoxicity against malignant glioma cells. *Drug Deliv.* **2016**, *23*, 214–229. [CrossRef]
117. Nasr, M. Development of an optimized hyaluronic acid-based lipidic nanoemulsion co-encapsulating two polyphenols for nose to brain delivery. *Drug Deliv.* **2016**, *23*, 1444–1452. [CrossRef] [PubMed]
118. Vaz, G.R.; Hädrich, G.; Bidone, J.; Rodrigues, J.L.; Falkembach, M.C.; Putaux, J.L.; Hort, M.A.; Monserrat, J.M.; Varela Junior, A.S.; Teixeira, H.F.; et al. Development of Nasal Lipid Nanocarriers Containing Curcumin for Brain Targeting. *J. Alzheimer's Dis.* **2017**, *59*, 961–974. [CrossRef] [PubMed]

119. Singh, A.K.; Jiang, Y.; Gupta, S.; Younus, M.; Ramzan, M. Anti-Inflammatory Potency of Nano-Formulated Puerarin and Curcumin in Rats Subjected to the Lipopolysaccharide-Induced Inflammation. *J. Med. Food* **2013**, *16*, 899–911. [CrossRef] [PubMed]
120. Cheng, K.K.; Chan, P.S.; Fan, S.; Kwan, S.M.; Yeung, K.L.; Wáng, Y.X.J.; Chow, A.H.L.; Wu, E.X.; Baum, L. Curcumin-conjugated magnetic nanoparticles for detecting amyloid plaques in Alzheimer's disease mice using magnetic resonance imaging (MRI). *Biomaterials* **2015**, *44*, 155–172. [CrossRef] [PubMed]
121. Ghorbani, M.; Bigdeli, B.; Jalili-baleh, L.; Baharifar, H.; Akrami, M.; Dehghani, S.; Goliaei, B.; Amani, A.; Lotfabadi, A.; Rashedi, H.; et al. Curcumin-lipoic acid conjugate as a promising anticancer agent on the surface of gold-iron oxide nanocomposites: A pH-sensitive targeted drug delivery system for brain cancer theranostics. *Eur. J. Pharm. Sci.* **2018**, *114*, 175–188. [CrossRef] [PubMed]
122. Naserzadeh, P.; Hafez, A.A.; Abdorahim, M.; Abdollahifar, M.A.; Shabani, R.; Peirovi, H.; Simchi, A.; Ashtari, K. Curcumin loading potentiates the neuroprotective efficacy of Fe_3O_4 magnetic nanoparticles in cerebellum cells of schizophrenic rats. *Biomed. Pharmacother.* **2018**, *108*, 1244–1252. [CrossRef] [PubMed]
123. Fang, J.H.; Chiu, T.L.; Huang, W.C.; Lai, Y.H.; Hu, S.H.; Chen, Y.Y.; Chen, S.Y. Dual-Targeting Lactoferrin-Conjugated Polymerized Magnetic Polydiacetylene-Assembled Nanocarriers with Self-Responsive Fluorescence/Magnetic Resonance Imaging for in vivo Brain Tumor Therapy. *Adv. Healthc. Mater.* **2016**, *5*, 688–695. [CrossRef]
124. Lazar, A.N.; Mourtas, S.; Youssef, I.; Parizot, C.; Dauphin, A.; Delatour, B.; Antimisiaris, S.G.; Duyckaerts, C. Curcumin-conjugated nanoliposomes with high affinity for Aβ deposits: Possible applications to Alzheimer disease. *Nanomed. Nanotechnol. Biol. Med.* **2013**, *9*, 712–721. [CrossRef]
125. Li, W.; Zhou, M.; Xu, N.; Hu, Y.; Wang, C.; Li, D.; Liu, L.; Li, D. Comparative analysis of protective effects of curcumin, curcumin-β-cyclodextrin nanoparticle and nanoliposomal curcumin on unsymmetrical dimethyl hydrazine poisoning in mice. *Bioengineered* **2016**, *7*, 334–341. [CrossRef]
126. Citron, M. Alzheimer's disease: Strategies for disease modification. *Nat. Rev. Drug Discov.* **2010**, *9*, 387–398. [CrossRef]
127. Ballatore, C.; Lee, V.M.-Y.; Trojanowski, J.Q. Tau-mediated neurodegeneration in Alzheimer's disease and related disorders. *Nat. Rev. Neurosci.* **2007**, *8*, 663–672. [CrossRef] [PubMed]
128. Djiokeng Paka, G.; Doggui, S.; Zaghmi, A.; Safar, R.; Dao, L.; Reisch, A.; Klymchenko, A.; Roullin, V.G.; Joubert, O.; Ramassamy, C. Neuronal Uptake and Neuroprotective Properties of Curcumin-Loaded Nanoparticles on SK-N-SH Cell Line: Role of Poly(lactide-co-glycolide) Polymeric Matrix Composition. *Mol. Pharm.* **2016**, *13*, 391–403. [CrossRef] [PubMed]
129. Barbara, R.; Belletti, D.; Pederzoli, F.; Masoni, M.; Keller, J.; Ballestrazzi, A.; Vandelli, M.A.; Tosi, G.; Grabrucker, A.M. Novel Curcumin loaded nanoparticles engineered for Blood-Brain Barrier crossing and able to disrupt Aβ aggregates. *Int. J. Pharm.* **2017**, *526*, 413–424. [CrossRef] [PubMed]
130. Huang, N.; Lu, S.; Liu, X.-G.; Zhu, J.; Wang, Y.-J.; Liu, R.-T. PLGA nanoparticles modified with a BBB-penetrating peptide co-delivering Aβ generation inhibitor and curcumin attenuate memory deficits and neuropathology in Alzheimer's disease mice. *Oncotarget* **2017**, *8*, 81001–81013. [PubMed]
131. Siddique, Y.H.; Khan, W.; Singh, B.R.; Naqvi, A.H. Synthesis of Alginate-Curcumin Nanocomposite and Its Protective Role in Transgenic *Drosophila* Model of Parkinson's Disease. *ISRN Pharmacol.* **2013**, *2013*, 794582. [CrossRef] [PubMed]
132. Bollimpelli, V.S.; Kumar, P.; Kumari, S.; Kondapi, A.K. Neuroprotective effect of curcumin-loaded lactoferrin nano particles against rotenone induced neurotoxicity. *Neurochem. Int.* **2016**, *95*, 37–45. [CrossRef] [PubMed]
133. Zhang, N.; Yan, F.; Liang, X.; Wu, M.; Shen, Y.; Chen, M.; Xu, Y.; Zou, G.; Jiang, P.; Tang, C.; et al. Localized delivery of curcumin into brain with polysorbate 80-modified cerasomes by ultrasound-targeted microbubble destruction for improved Parkinson's disease therapy. *Theranostics* **2018**, *8*, 2264–2277. [CrossRef] [PubMed]

5

Ethanolic Extract of Folium Sennae Mediates the Glucose Uptake of L6 Cells by GLUT4 and Ca^{2+}

Ping Zhao [1,2,*], Qian Ming [1], Junying Qiu [1], Di Tian [1], Jia Liu [1], Jinhua Shen [1], Qing-Hua Liu [1] and Xinzhou Yang [2,3,*]

1 Institute for Medical Biology & Hubei Provincial Key Laboratory for Protection and Application of Special Plants in the Wuling Area of China, College of Life Sciences, South-Central University for Nationalities, Wuhan 430074, China; 18062196191@163.com (Q.M.); qiu927633@163.com (J.Q.); tiandi_2983@126.com (D.T.); 13512566172@163.com (J.L.); shenjinhua2013@163.com (J.S.); qinghualiu95@163.com (Q.-H.L.)

2 National Demonstration Center for Experimental Ethnopharmacology Education, South-Central University for Nationalities, Wuhan 430074, China

3 School of Pharmaceutical Sciences, South-Central University for Nationalities, 182 Min-Zu Road, Wuhan 430074, China

* Correspondence: p.zhao@scuec.edu.cn (P.Z.); xzyang@mail.scuec.edu.cn (X.Y.);

Academic Editor: Pinarosa Avato

Abstract: In today's world, diabetes mellitus (DM) is on the rise, especially type 2 diabetes mellitus (T2DM), which is characterized by insulin resistance. T2DM has high morbidity, and therapies with natural products have attracted much attention in the recent past. In this paper, we aimed to study the hypoglycemic effect and the mechanism of an ethanolic extract of Folium Sennae (FSE) on L6 cells. The glucose uptake of L6 cells was investigated using a glucose assay kit. We studied glucose transporter 4 (GLUT4) expression and AMP-activated protein kinase (AMPK), protein kinase B (PKB/Akt), and protein kinase C (PKC) phosphorylation levels using western blot analysis. GLUT4 trafficking and intracellular Ca^{2+} levels were monitored by laser confocal microscopy in L6 cells stably expressing IRAP-mOrange. GLUT4 fusion with plasma membrane (PM) was observed by myc-GLUT4-mOrange. FSE stimulated glucose uptake; GLUT4 expression and translocation; PM fusion; intracellular Ca^{2+} elevation; and the phosphorylation of AMPK, Akt, and PKC in L6 cells. GLUT4 translocation was weakened by the AMPK inhibitor compound C, PI3K inhibitor Wortmannin, PKC inhibitor Gö6983, G protein inhibitor PTX/Gallein, and PLC inhibitor U73122. Similarly, in addition to PTX/Gallein and U73122, the IP3R inhibitor 2-APB and a 0 mM Ca^{2+}-EGTA solution partially inhibited the elevation of intracellular Ca^{2+} levels. BAPTA-AM had a significant inhibitory effect on FSE-mediated GLUT4 activities. In summary, FSE regulates GLUT4 expression and translocation by activating the AMPK, PI3K/Akt, and G protein–PLC–PKC pathways. FSE causes increasing Ca^{2+} concentration to complete the fusion of GLUT4 vesicles with PM, allowing glucose uptake. Therefore, FSE may be a potential drug for improving T2DM.

Keywords: FSE; T2DM; GLUT4; Ca^{2+}; L6 cell

---

1. Introduction

Diabetes mellitus (DM) is a chronic metabolic disorder resulting from insufficient insulin secretion or insulin dysfunction. It may lead to a series of complications such as renal failure, cardiovascular disease, blindness, hypertension, non-alcoholic fatty liver disease (NAFLD), and obesity [1,2]. The global prevalence of DM is on the rise, especially in developing countries [3]. T2DM is the most prevalent form of DM and accounts for more than 90% of the cases of DM [4]. Insulin resistance is the typical feature of T2DM, which causes cells to stop responding adequately to the standard role of insulin. While the body continues to produce insulin, the cells in the body become resistant to its effects. Therefore, cells cannot effectively process insulin, resulting in hyperglycemia [5–7].

Blood glucose influx into cells requires glucose transporter family proteins (GLUTs) [1]. With the onset of hyperglycemia, the glucose uptake in the adipose tissue and muscles is mostly mediated by GLUT4, an isoform of a family of sugar transporter proteins (encoded on the SLC2A4 gene) containing 12 transmembrane domains. GLUT4 continuously recycles between intracellular vessels and the plasma membrane (PM) [8,9]. After insulin stimulation, GLUT4 proteins are mobilized to PM immediately, which enhances the rate of exocytosis and their fusion with PM (this process is synonymous with GLUT4 translocation). The increase in PM GLUT4 leads to glucose uptake [10]. Previous studies have reported that defective GLUT4 translocation is a feature of insulin resistance and an essential precursor of T2DM [4,7,11]. Thus, GLUT4 as a key regulatory target for glucose homeostasis is widely used in antidiabetic drug research.

Intracellular cytosolic free Ca^{2+} comes from both extracellular Ca^{2+} influx and Ca^{2+} release from intracellular stores (including sarcoplasmic reticulum, lysosomes, and mitochondria). As an important second messenger, it participates in many physiological activities of cells. Numerous studies have highlighted the role of cytosolic Ca^{2+} in GLUT4 synthesis, GLUT4 traffic (endocytosis and exocytosis), and glucose uptake. Wright reported that the treatment of L6 muscle cells with agents that increase Ca^{2+} leads to an increase in the GLUT4 protein content [12]. Li et al. found that Ca^{2+} signals promote GLUT4 exocytosis and reduce its endocytosis in muscle cells [13]. Johanna et al. described the role of Ca^{2+} influx for insulin-mediated glucose uptake in skeletal muscles [14]. Contreras-Ferrat et al. clearly showed that an inositol 1,4,5-triphosphate (IP3)-dependent Ca^{2+} release pathway is required for insulin-stimulated GLUT4 translocation and glucose uptake in cardiomyocytes [15]. Similarly, it has been reported that the AMPK, PKC, and insulin-dependent pathways were relatively independent of Ca^{2+}-regulated GLUT4 traffic [16–19]. Furthermore, increases in intracellular Ca^{2+} levels, even at concentrations too low to induce contractions, provide the signal to activate GLUT4 translocation in skeletal muscles [17].

Because of serious economic burdens and side effects of chemical agent-based DM treatment strategies [7,20,21], natural drug products are gaining popularity because of their various advantages, such as fewer side effects, better patient tolerance, relatively lower cost, and acceptance due to the long history of use. An important cause of these products' efficacy is that, unlike a single chemical entity aimed at a specific single target, many Chinese herbal medicines (such as the multi-flavonoid-rich plant extracts) are thought to alleviate the disorder of diabetes mellitus through an integrated effect upon multitarget sites [22,23]. Current studies have shown that phytochemicals, polysaccharides, flavonoids, terpenoids, tannins, steroids, and other chemicals naturally found in plants possess antidiabetic activity [8,24,25]. The two main antidiabetic agents represented by metformin and flavonoids were derived from medicinal plants. Folium Sennae, also called the senna leaf, is derived from the dried leaflets of *Cassia angustifolia Vahl* or *Cassia acutifolia Delile*, and belongs to the dicotyledonous leguminous family. It is native to India and Egypt, and is widely distributed in the Taiwan, Guangdong, Guangxi, and Yunnan provinces of China [26]. The Chinese Pharmacopoeia (2010) and Chinese Materia Medica state that senna leaves contain four sennosides (A, B, C, and D), rhein, emodin, chrysophanol, aloe-emodin, physcion, tinnevellin glucoside, kaempferol, phytosterol and its glycosides, pine camphor, salicylic acid, and several other ingredients. In addition to being well known as a natural laxative [27], the senna leaf has been found to exhibit antioxidant [28], antibacterial [29], anti-inflammatory [30], antitumor [31], analgesic [32], antimalarial [33], and antidiabetic [34] activities. Ayinla et al. reported that the ethanolic leaf extract of Senna fistula improved hematologic parameters, lipid profiles, and oxidative stress in alloxan-induced diabetic rats [35]. Thilagam et al. discovered that the ethanolic leaf extract of Senna surattensis inhibited the carbohydrate digestive enzymes and increased the peripheral glucose uptake in the isolated rat hemidiaphragm model [34]. Malematja et al. showed that Senna italica leaf acetone extract promoted glucose uptake and anti-obesity through the PI3K-dependent pathway [36]. However, only a few studies have assessed the possible hypoglycemic properties and hypoglycemic mechanisms of Folium Sennae (FSE).

In the present study, we observed that FSE displayed a strong effect in promoting glucose uptake, GLUT4 expression and translocation, and cytosolic Ca^{2+} levels in L6 rat skeletal muscle cells. We observed that FSE induced GLUT4 expression and translocation through the AMPK, PI3K/Akt, and PKC signaling pathways. FSE also increased cytosolic Ca^{2+} concentration by extracellular Ca^{2+} influx or/and intracellular Ca^{2+} release of G protein-IP3-IP3R signals, which assisted GLUT4 movement and stimulated glucose uptake. We elucidated the mechanism of action and validated the beneficial effects of FSE as an antidiabetic agent.

2. Results

2.1. FSE Increases GLUT4 Expression Levels and Glucose Uptake in L6 Cells

To confirm the possible hypoglycemic activity of FSE, we first studied its glucose uptake effect. As shown in Figure 1A, L6 cells were serum-deprived and then incubated with 100 nM insulin or different concentrations of FSE for 1 h. When compared with the control group, insulin (positive control) and 30, 60, and 120 μg/mL of FSE significantly promoted the glucose uptake of cells by 2.04-fold, 1.87-fold, 1.95-fold, and 1.68-fold, respectively. This result was based on the corresponding MTT assay after drug treatment. MTT results showed that neither FSE nor insulin caused toxicity to L6 cells (Figure S1). In the next step, we chose 60 μg/mL as the best concentration of FSE. To understand whether FSE affected the expression of the glucose regulator GLUT4, the total protein and mRNA of GLUT4 and the mRNA of IRAP in L6 cells were extracted after stimulation with insulin or FSE. The results showed that 100 nM insulin and 60 μg/mL FSE increased the protein expression of GLUT4 by 2.13-fold and 1.89-fold, respectively (Figure 1B). The fold increases of GLUT4 mRNA levels were even more prominent, at 4.13-fold with insulin and 2.8-fold with FSE (Figure 1C). In addition, as a resident protein of GLUT4 storage vesicles, insulin-regulated aminopeptidase (IRAP) also changed at the mRNA level, with 1.46-fold from insulin treatment and 1.70-fold from FSE treatment (Figure 1D).

2.2. FSE Stimulates GLUT4 Translocation and Increases Intracellular Ca^{2+} Levels

Since intracellular GLUT4 translocation to the cell surface can exert glucose uptake function, we further analyzed GLUT4 translocation in L6 cells under FSE treatment. L6 cells stably expressing IRAP-mOrange (L6-mOrange-IRAP) were transfected with red fluorescent protein (mOrange)-tagged IRAP. IRAP was initially found in specialized vesicles containing GLUT4, which immediately migrated to the cell surface along with GLUT4 after receiving insulin [37]. Some evidences proved that IRAP was highly co-localized with GLUT4 [38,39]. We used Fluo-4 AM fluorescent dyes during loading of cells with Ca^{2+} and monitored the translocation of GLUT4 and intracellular Ca^{2+} changes in live cells by real-time fluorescence microscopy. As a comparative insulin treatment, the image showed that the intracellular IRAP-mOrange signal was enhanced and signal accumulation appeared in adjacent PM region. Green fluorescence was significantly brightened after 100 nM insulin treatment in intracellular Ca^{2+} detection (Figure S2). Similarly, the IRAP fluorescence intensity in cytoplasm was obviously raised after the addition of 60 μg/mL FSE, and a substantial amount of red fluorescence accumulated at the cell periphery as revealed by IRAP-mOrange signals. Meanwhile, the green fluorescence of Ca^{2+} was densely distributed in the cells (Figure 2A). The fold growth curve increased with IRAP level at the PM region or with intracellular Ca^{2+}, and it increased in a time-dependent manner (Figure 2B). Our studies suggested that FSE promoted glucose uptake not only by stimulating GLUT4 expression and translocation but also by increasing intracellular Ca^{2+} levels.

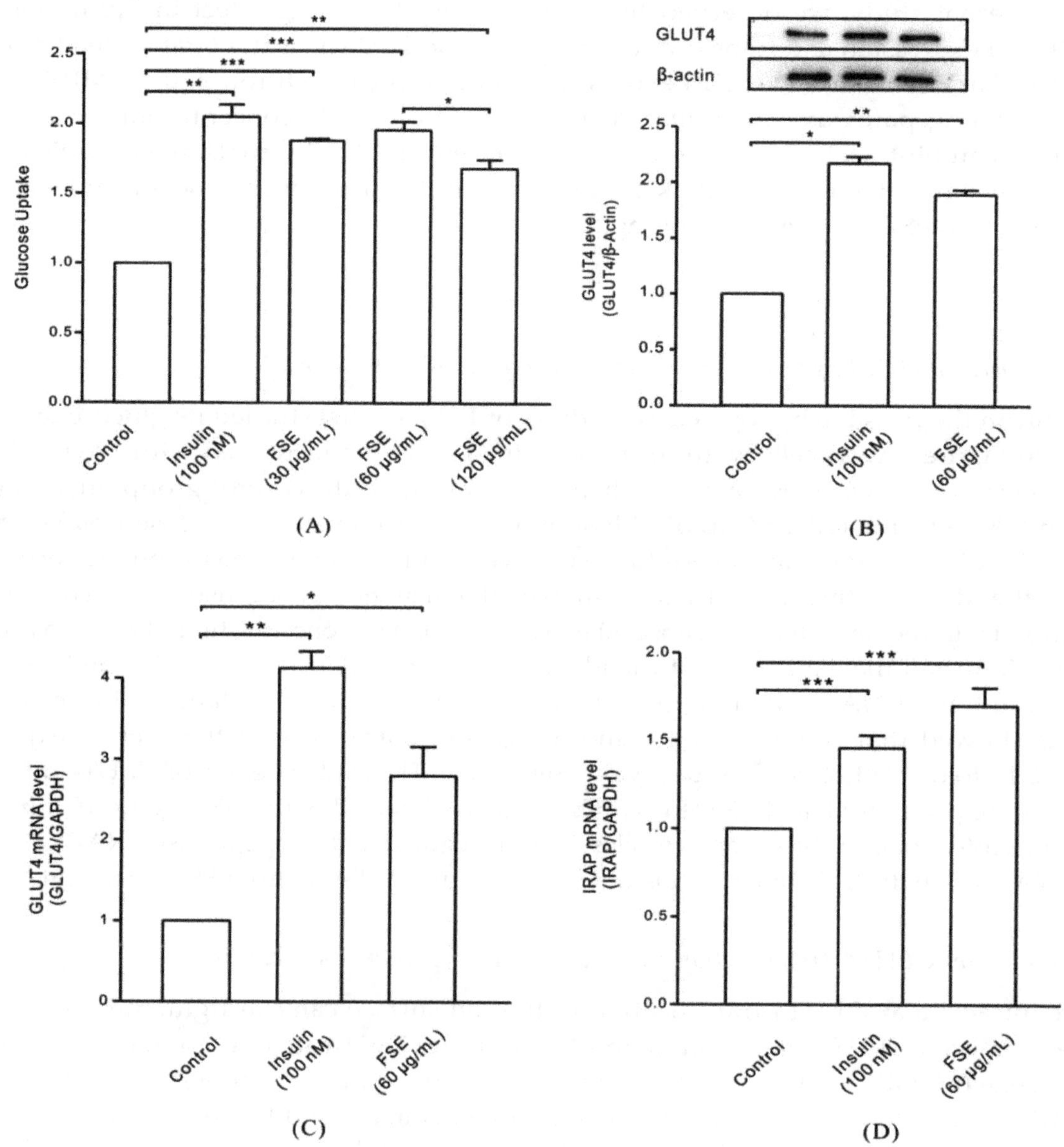

Figure 1. Enhancing the effects of Folium Sennae (FSE) on glucose uptake and GLUT4 expression in L6 cells. Insulin as a positive control. (**A**) Cells were incubated with 100 nM insulin or 30, 60, and 120 μg/mL FSE for 1 h, and glucose uptake was measured using a glucose assay kit. (**B**) Cells were stimulated with 100 nM insulin or 60 μg/mL FSE for 30 min. Whole cell lysates were subjected to western blot analysis for GLUT4, and the protein expression level was normalized against β-actin. (**C**) Cells were treated with 100 nM insulin or 60 μg/mL FSE for 30 min. GAPDH was used to normalize the mRNA level, and the relative expression of GLUT4 mRNA was investigated by real-time PCR. (**D**) Cells were treated with 100 nM insulin or 60 μg/mL FSE for 30 min. GAPDH was used to normalize the mRNA level, and the relative expression of IRAP mRNA was investigated by real-time PCR. The data were obtained from three independent repeated experiments. Significance analysis: * $p < 0.05$; ** $p < 0.01$; *** $p < 0.001$.

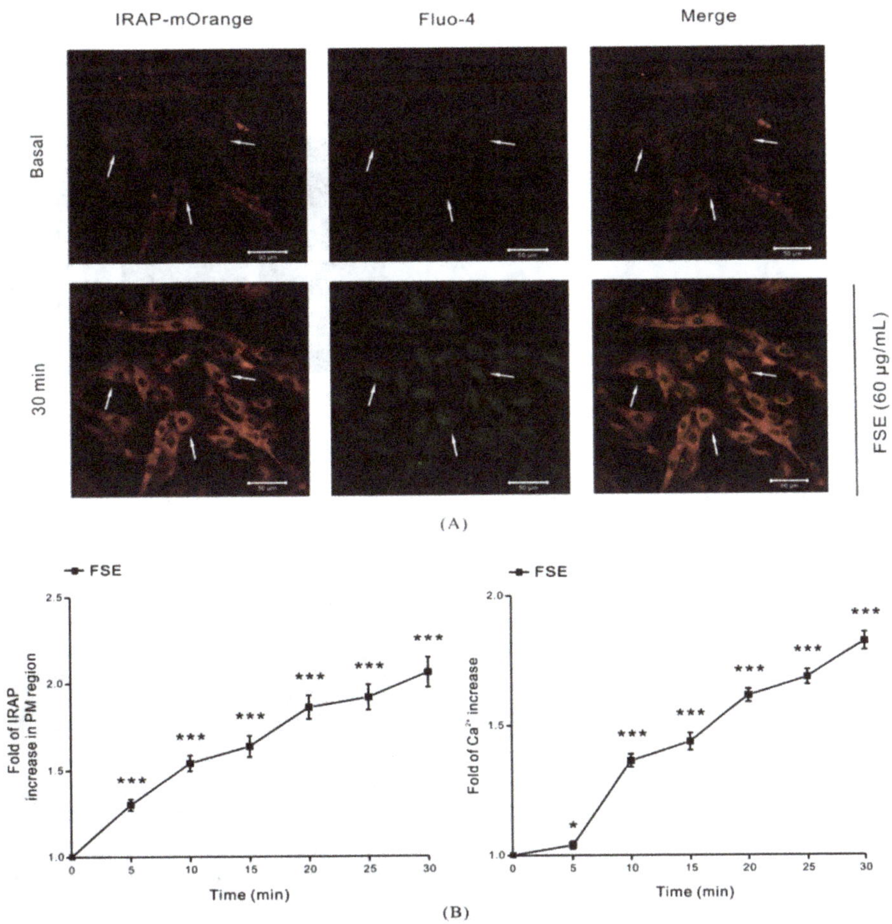

Figure 2. Stimulating effects of FSE on GLUT4 translocation and intracellular Ca^{2+} level. The red fluorescence of IRAP-mOrange stably expressed in L6 cells and the green fluorescence of Ca^{2+} were simultaneously observed by confocal microscope. Scale bar = 50 μm. (**A**) Intracellular Ca^{2+} was stained with Flou-4 AM for 20 min, followed by stimulation with 60 μg/mL FSE for 30 min. IRAP-mOrange fluorescence intensity and intracellular Ca^{2+} fluorescence concentration were detected at excitation wavelengths of 555 nm and 488 nm, respectively, and fluorescence superposition displayed specific positioning. (**B**) The cell images were recorded over 30 min, and the red fluorescence from the outside edges of cells and the green fluorescence of the whole cells were collected. Fluorescence quantization was done with Zeiss 2010 software. Significance analysis: * $p < 0.05$; *** $p < 0.001$.

2.3. *The Role of Cytosolic Ca^{2+} in FSE-Mediated GLUT4 Translocation*

In order to determine whether the increase of intracellular Ca^{2+} concentration after FSE stimulation was related to GLUT4 translocation, we blocked the different sources of intracellular Ca^{2+} before treatment with 60 μg/mL FSE to observe the GLUT4 translocation. FSE-induced increase of intracellular Ca^{2+} was partially inhibited with the removal of extracellular Ca^{2+}, but the FSE-mediated increase of IRAP fluorescence in the PM region remained unchanged (Figure 3A). This phenomenon can be explained by the observation that for FSE to evoke the rise of intracellular Ca^{2+}, it needs at least to mobilize extracellular Ca^{2+} influx. In addition, when 0 mM extracellular Ca^{2+}+BAPTA-AM was used to chelate cytosolic Ca^{2+}, the FSE-induced increase of intracellular Ca^{2+} was completely inhibited, and the increase of IRAP fluorescence in the PM region was also obviously blocked (Figure 3B). These findings supported the idea that cytosolic Ca^{2+} plays an important role in the process of FSE-induced GLUT4 translocation to the PM.

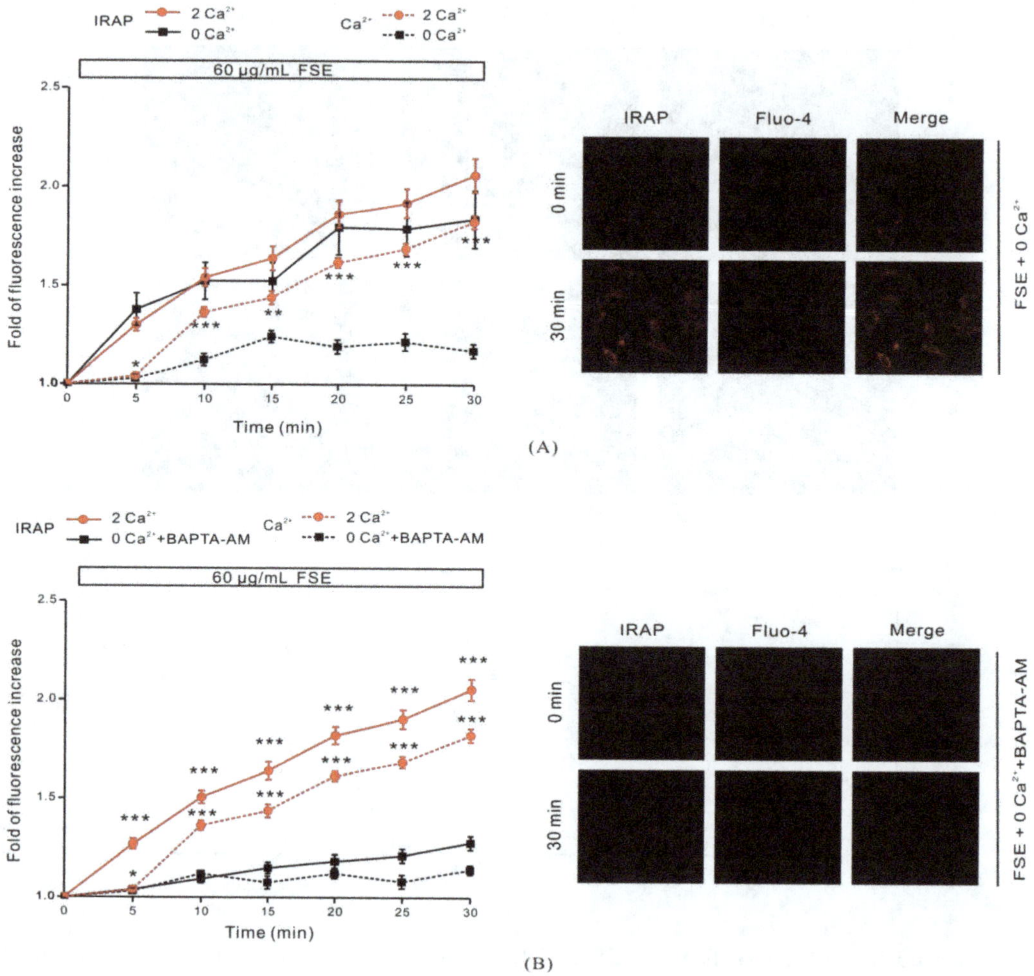

Figure 3. Role of intracellular Ca^{2+} on FSE-induced GLUT4 translocation. (**A**) After intracellular Ca^{2+} was loaded with Fluo-4 AM, cells were treated with 60 μg/mL FSE for 30 min under 0 mM extracellular Ca^{2+} conditions. * $p < 0.05$; ** $p < 0.01$; *** $p < 0.001$. (**B**) Cells were incubated for 30 min under the condition of 0 mM extracellular Ca^{2+} + 10 μM BAPTA-AM chelated intracellular Ca^{2+}, followed by stimulation with 60 μg/mL FSE for 30 min to quantify IRAP-mOrange fluorescence in the PM region and intracellular Ca^{2+} levels. Significance analysis: * $p < 0.05$; ** $p < 0.01$; *** $p < 0.001$.

2.4. FSE Enhances GLUT4 Translocation and Expression through the AMPK, PI3K/Akt, and PKC Pathways

Next, we attempted to shed light on some of the signaling pathways involved in GLUT4 translocation and expression. After treatment with AMPK inhibitor Compound C (10 μM, 30 min), PI3K inhibitor Wortmannin (100 nM, 30 min), or PKC inhibitor Gö6983 (10 μM, 30 min), the increase of IRAP fluorescence in the PM region induced by 60 μg/mL FSE was inhibited (Figure 4A), and the inhibition from compound C (Figure 4A, left) and Gö6983 (Figure 4A, right) was stronger than that from Wortmannin (Figure 4A, middle). This indicated that AMPK, PI3K/Akt, and PKC may be involved in FSE-mediated GLUT4 expression and translocation. Following this, we used western blot analysis to verify our conjecture. Compared with the control group, the expression levels of GLUT4 protein in L6 cells were increased by 1.87-fold (FSE), 1.33-fold (FSE+Compound C), 1.63-fold (FSE+Wortmannin), and 1.35-fold (FSE+Gö6983) after treatment with FSE and/or these different inhibitors (Figure 4B). Consistent with Figure 4, the three inhibitors also exhibited their inhibitory effects on FSE-mediated GLUT4 protein expression (vs. FSE). Western blotting of the signaling pathway-related proteins revealed that the phosphorylation levels of AMPK, Akt, and PKC in L6 cells after treatment with 60 μg/mL FSE were upregulated by 1.36-fold, 1.72-fold, and 1.92-fold, respectively. Also, FSE's effects were slightly lower than 1.54-fold of what was seen with 100 μg/mL metformin, 1.94-fold of what was seen with 100 nM insulin, and 2.74-fold of what was seen with 200 nM phorbol ester (PMA) in the positive control groups (Figure 4C–E). The above results showed that the increase in FSE-induced GLUT4 expression was dependent on AMPK, Akt, and PKC activities, and the FSE-promoted GLUT4 translocation also occurred through the AMPK, PI3K/Akt, and PKC pathways.

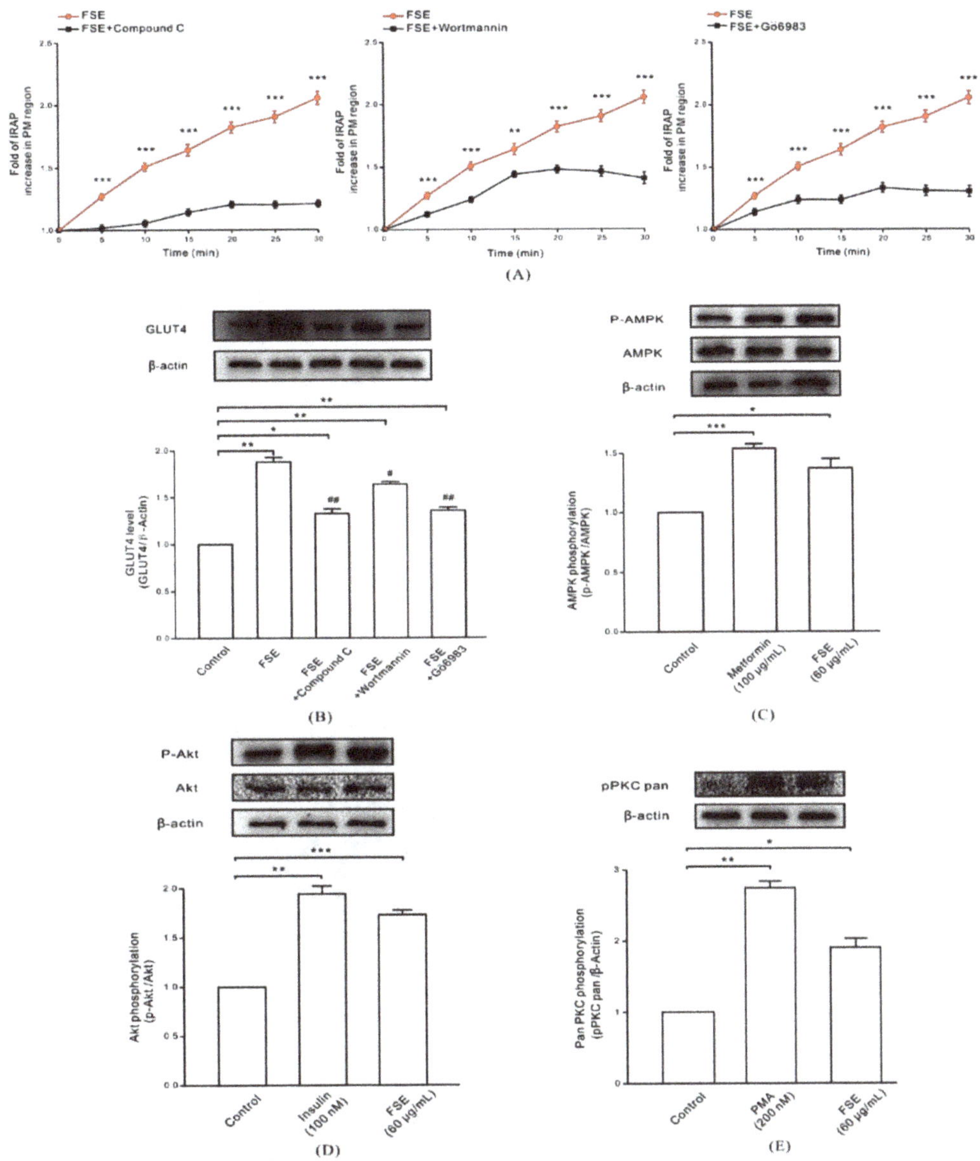

Figure 4. Effect of FSE on the AMPK, PI3K/Akt, and PKC signaling pathways and related proteins. (**A**) Cells were incubated with 10 μM compound C (AMPK inhibitor), 100 nM Wortmannin (PI3K inhibitor), or 10 μM Gö6983 (PKC inhibitor) for 30 min, and then treated with 60 μg/mL FSE. We calculated the fold of IRAP fluorescence increases in the PM region. * $p < 0.05$; ** $p < 0.01$; *** $p < 0.001$. (**B**) Cells were incubated with 10 μM compound C, 100 nM Wortmannin, or 10 μM Gö6983 inhibitor for 30 min and then were stimulated with 60 μg/mL FSE for 30 min. Whole cell lysates were subjected to western blot analysis for GLUT4 protein expression levels. * $p < 0.05$; ** $p < 0.01$, vs control group; # $p < 0.05$; ## $p < 0.01$, vs. FSE group. (**C**) L6 cells were treated with 100 μg/mL metformin (overnight) or 60 μg/mL FSE (30 min) and then analyzed for phosphorylated-AMPK, total AMPK, and β-actin protein level by western blot analysis. * $p < 0.05$; *** $p < 0.001$. (**D**) Cells were treated with 100 nM insulin or 60 μg/mL FSE for 30 min, followed by western blot analysis of phosphorylated Akt, total Akt, and β-actin. ** $p < 0.01$; *** $p < 0.001$. (**E**) Cells were treated with 200 nM PMA (4 h) or 60 μg/mL FSE (30 min), and western blot was used to analyze the phosphorylated protein level of PKC in L6 cells. Data were from three independent repeated experiments. * $p < 0.05$; ** $p < 0.01$.

2.5. G Protein and PLC Regulate FSE-Mediated Intracellular Ca^{2+} Increases and GLUT4 Translocation

G protein and PLC are upstream of the PKC pathway, and IP3R is one of the major receptors that trigger intracellular Ca^{2+} release. We investigated how G protein and PLC regulate FSE-induced Ca^{2+} increase and GLUT4 translocation. Cells treated with the Gβγ protein inhibitor 100 μM Gallein or Gα protein inhibitor 100 μM PTX for 6–8 h, or PLC inhibitor 2 μM U73122 for 30 min, significantly inhibited FSE-induced IRAP fluorescence intensity and intracellular Ca^{2+} elevation (Figure 5A–C). The results implied that FSE enhanced GLUT4 translocation via the G protein-PLC-PKC signaling pathway.

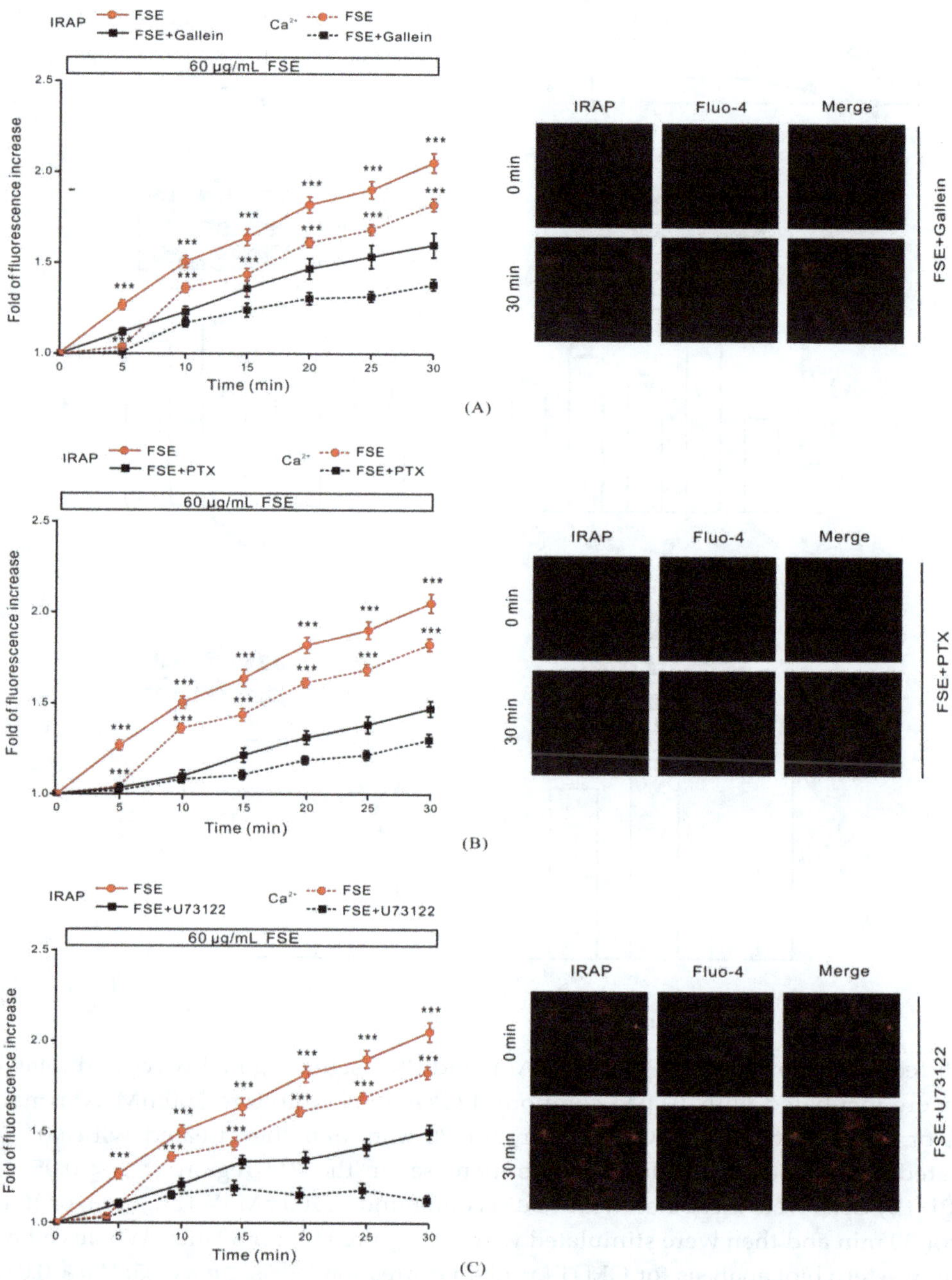

Figure 5. G protein-PLC signaling regulated FSE-mediated GLUT4 translocation and intracellular Ca^{2+} increase. (**A**) Cells were incubated for 6–8 h with 100 μM Gallein (Gβγ protein inhibitor) and then treated with 60 μg/mL FSE. * $p < 0.05$; *** $p < 0.001$. (**B**) Cells were incubated for 6–8 h with 100 μM PTX (Gα protein inhibitor), followed by the addition of 60 μg/mL FSE. *** $p < 0.001$. (**C**) Cells were treated with 2 μM U73122 (PLC inhibitor) for 30 min and were then stimulated by 60 μg/mL FSE. The IRAP-mOrange fluorescence in the PM region and the intracellular Ca^{2+} levels were quantified by Zeiss 2010 software. Significance analysis: * $p < 0.05$; *** $p < 0.001$.

2.6. IP3R Is Involved in FSE-Triggered Intracellular Ca^{2+} Release

The result shown in Figure 3 suggested the potential impact of intracellular Ca^{2+} release in the process of FSE-mediated GLUT4 translocation and the increase in intracellular Ca^{2+} levels. To support this hypothesis, we used 100 μM 2-APB to block IP3R-regulated intracellular Ca^{2+} release. We found that 2-APB had no effect on FSE-mediated GLUT4 translocation under 2 mM extracellular Ca^{2+}, but it evidently inhibited FSE-triggered Ca^{2+} release (Figure 6A). The ryanodine receptor (RyR), another channel that releases Ca^{2+} in the sarcoplasmic reticulum (SR)/endoplasmic reticulum (ER) [40], has attracted much attention due to its manipulation of intracellular Ca^{2+} output. Inhibition of RyR with 30 μM ryanodine had no effect on either GLUT4 translocation or intracellular Ca^{2+} increase mediated by FSE (Figure 6B). These findings indicated that IP3R, rather than RyR, was involved in the FSE-triggered increases of intracellular Ca^{2+}.

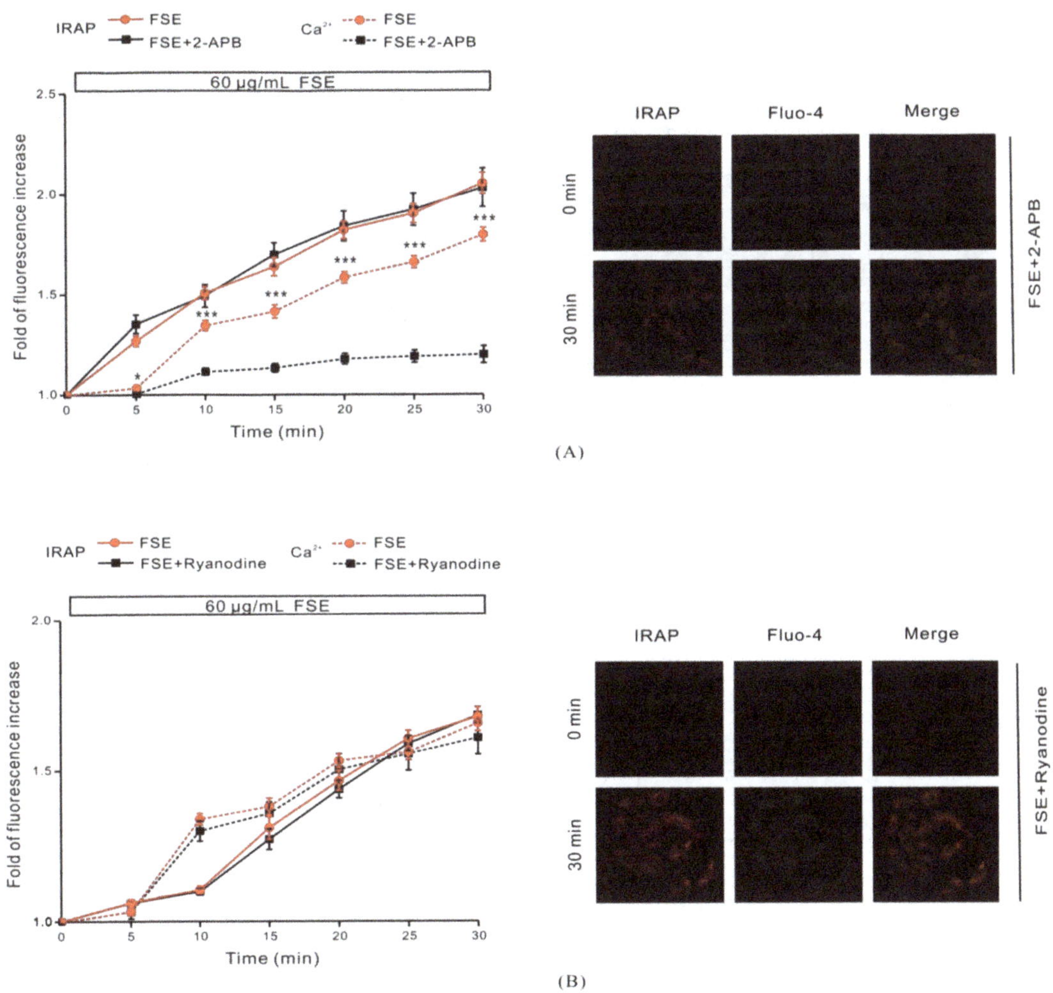

Figure 6. The IP3R receptor is involved in FSE-stimulated intracellular Ca^{2+} release. (**A**) Under extracellular 2 mM Ca^{2+}, cells were treated with 100 μM 2-APB (IP3RS blocker) for 30 min and then treated with 60 μg/mL FSE. (**B**) Under extracellular 2 mM Ca^{2+}, cells were incubated with 30 μM Ryanodine (RyR blocker) for 30 min, and the changes of IRAP-mOrange in the PM area and intracellular Ca^{2+} were measured after stimulation with 60 μg/mL FSE. Significance analysis: * $p < 0.05$; ** $p < 0.01$; *** $p < 0.001$.

2.7. Ca^{2+} Is Required for GLUT4 Insertion into the PM

Some studies have shown that Ca^{2+}-assisted binding of GLUT4 to the PM is involved in preparation for glucose uptake by cells [41,42]. In our study, myc-labeled GLUT4 was used to observe the fusion of GLUT4 vesicles with the PM in L6 cells stably expressing myc-GLUT4-mOrange. Fluorescence imaging revealed that FITC labeling for anti-myc antibody was not detected on the cell surface in the absence of drug stimulation. When we treated the cells for 30 min with 100 nM insulin and 60 μg/mL FSE, we observed significant increases of FITC fluorescence signals on the cell surfaces (Figure 7A). However, the FSE-induced FITC fluorescence signal on the cell surface was seriously suppressed under the condition of 0 mM extracellular Ca^{2+}/0 mM extracellular Ca^{2+} + 10 μM BAPTA-AM. On the other hand, the proportion of FITC-positive cells in the total number of mOrange cells showed (Figure 7B) that 0 mM Ca^{2+} + 10 μM BAPTA-AM had stronger inhibitory effects on FSE-mediated GLUT4 fusion with PM than the 0 mM Ca^{2+} group.

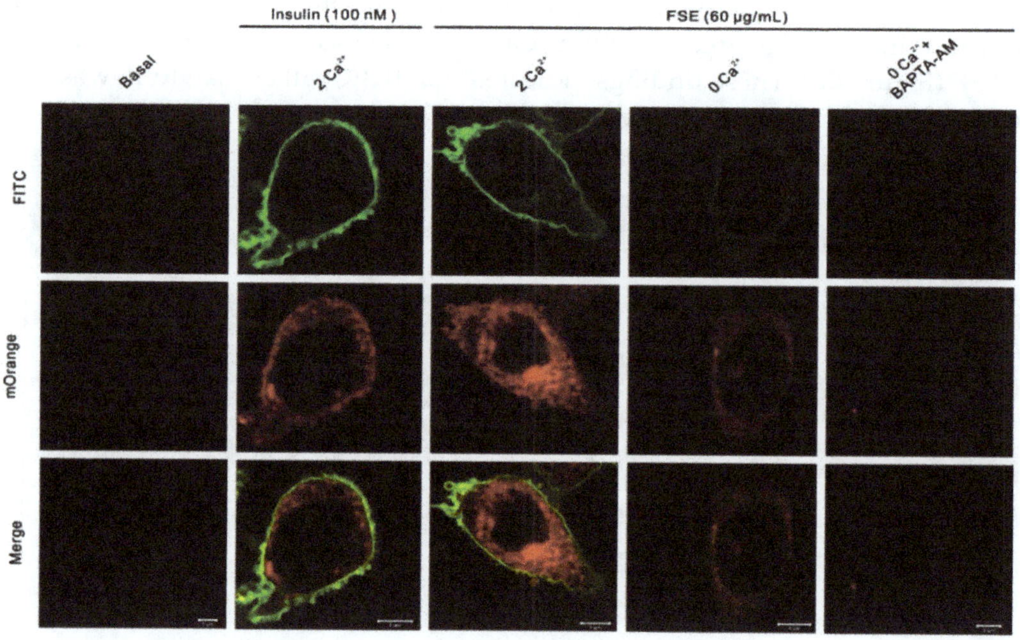

(A)

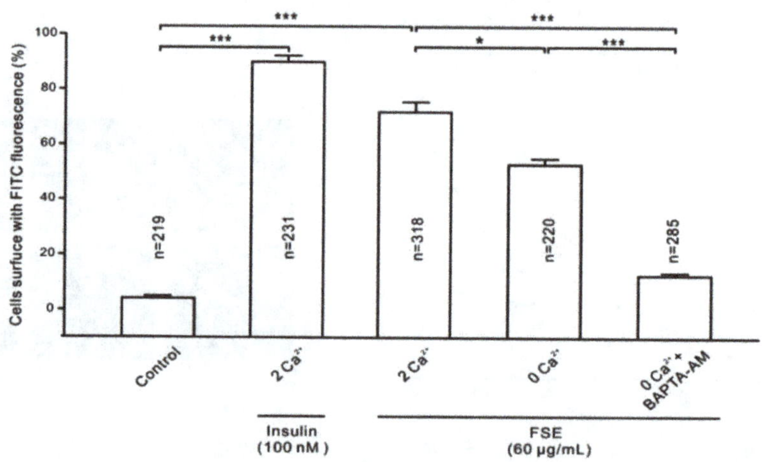

(B)

Figure 7. Involvement of Ca^{2+} in the fusion of GLUT4 and PM induced by FSE. (**A**) L6 cells transfected with plasmid GV348-myc-GLUT4-mOrange encoding an mOrange fusion protein with myc epitope-tagged GLUT4 (myc-GLUT4-FITC). Cells were stimulated with 100 nM insulin or 60 μg/mL FSE under 2 mM extracellular Ca^{2+}, 0 mM Ca^{2+}, and 0 mM Ca^{2+}+BAPTA-AM conditions. Then, cells were fixed and subjected to specific immunofluorescence antibody staining. The mOrange red fluorescence and FITC green fluorescence were detected by confocal microscopy at 555 nm and 488 nm excitation wavelengths, respectively. Scale bar = 5 μm. (**B**) The percentage of FITC-positive cells in the total mOrange cell population was counted. The results shown were from three independent replicate experiments. Significance analysis: * $p < 0.05$; ** $p < 0.01$; *** $p < 0.001$.

2.8. FSE-Induced Ca^{2+} Increases Improve Glucose Uptake in L6 Cells

To clarify the relationship between FSE-mediated glucose uptake and Ca^{2+}, a glucose uptake experiment was performed under various Ca^{2+} conditions. Results demonstrated that there was no significant difference in the glucose uptake between the groups in the absence of FSE or in the insulin-positive control group, whereas glucose uptake by cells was remarkably increased by 1.58-fold after the addition of FSE for 1 h in the culture medium with 2 mM extracellular Ca^{2+}. Similarly, insulin treatment showed a 1.68-fold increase in glucose uptake. To a certain extent, 0 mM extracellular Ca^{2+} inhibited the effect of FSE by 1.3-fold or the effect of insulin by 1.28-fold. Meanwhile, insulin or FSE-mediated glucose uptake was completely blocked under 0 mM Ca^{2+}+BAPTA-AM, which indicated that Ca^{2+} plays a crucial role in the FSE-induced glucose uptake process (Figure 8).

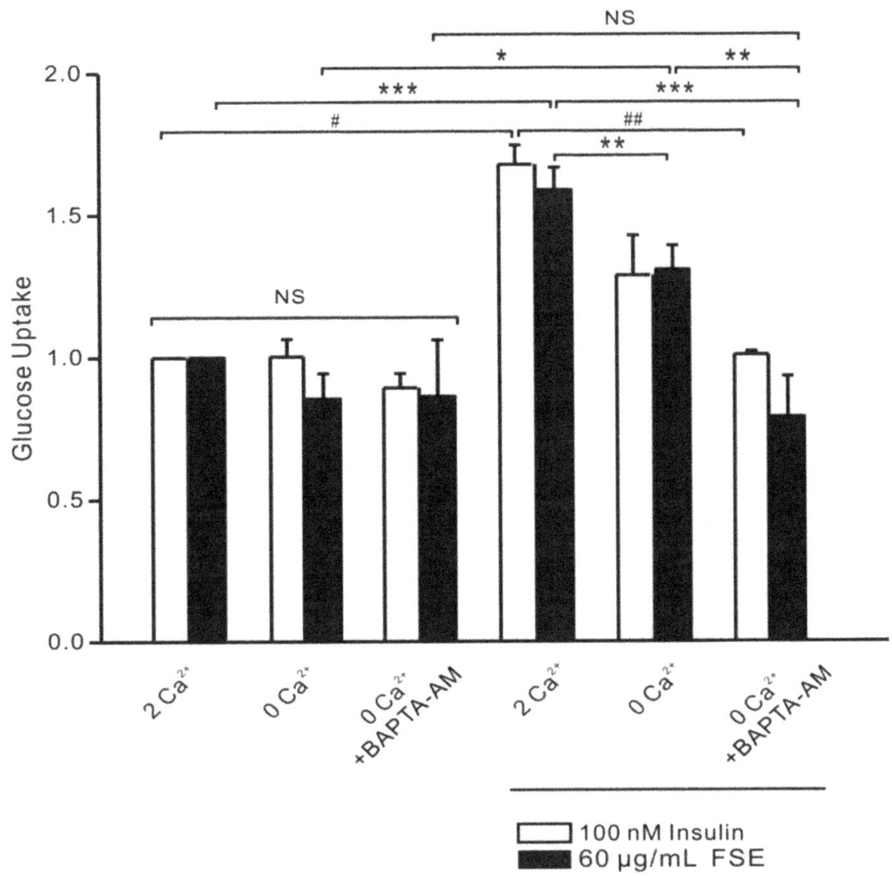

Figure 8. Increased effect of FSE on glucose uptake via Ca^{2+} signaling. Glucose uptake was measured using a glucose assay kit. L6 cells were serum-deprived for 2 h and incubated in 2 mM extracellular Ca^{2+}, 0 mM extracellular Ca^{2+}, or 0 mM extracellular Ca^{2+} + 10 μM BAPTA-AM chelated intracellular Ca^{2+} conditions. Cells were stimulated with vehicle, 60 μg/mL FSE, or 100 nM insulin for 1 h, and then the glucose uptake was measured. The experimental data are from six independent repeated experiments. Significant analysis: FSE group, * $p < 0.05$; ** $p < 0.01$; *** $p < 0.001$. Insulin group, # $p < 0.05$; ## $p < 0.01$.

3. Discussion

Diabetes has long been a global health problem. In particular, the high proportion of T2DM characterized by insulin resistance in DM has become the focus of DM research [43]. Skeletal muscle is the primary tissue for insulin-stimulated glucose uptake in the body. It consumes glucose and is responsible for approximately 80% of the postprandial glucose intake and consumption, and is therefore recognized as an important therapeutic target tissue for insulin resistance [11,44]. GLUT4 plays a crucial role in maintaining systemic glucose homeostasis. It is mostly intracellular in the unstimulated state but is acutely redistributed to the PM in response to insulin, contraction, and other stimuli [9]. The amount of glucose uptake is determined by the number of GLUT4 molecules on the muscle cell membranes [36,45]. Relevant studies reported that GLUT4 translocation and fusion with PM were the main rate-limiting steps for glucose disposal [46,47]. The existing synthetic antidiabetic drugs often exhibit side effects or resistance that pose a huge challenge to managing diabetes [43]. It is, therefore, necessary to find better medicines from herbs or natural products. Consequently, we extracted the effective products from the natural medicinal plant Folium Sennae. We investigated the potential activity of FSE on glucose uptake in L6 rat skeletal muscle cells in regard to GLUT4 expression, translocation, and fusion with PM and the participation of Ca^{2+} in this process.

It has been reported that an ethanolic extract of the leaves of *Senna surattensis* increased glucose uptake in an isolated rat hemidiaphragm model [34]. However, little is known about how FSE exerts its hypoglycemic mechanism in vivo. In this study, we first investigated the effect of FSE on the glucose uptake of L6 cells. Consistent with the reported results, FSE significantly increased glucose uptake in L6 cells. We also discovered that FSE upregulated GLUT4 mRNA and protein expression in GLUT4 molecular assays. The results suggested that there was some connection between FSE-induced glucose uptake and intracellular GLUT4 and IRAP motion (Figure 1).

Next, in order to observe the translocation of GLUT4 caused by FSE, we studied L6-IRAP-mOrange cells under confocal microscopy. Due to the high colocalization of intracellular IRAP and GLUT4 [48], IRAP was used as a reporter molecule to track and quantify dynamic information about GLUT4 in real time. Our results showed that FSE promoted the increase in IRAP expression in cytosol. By collecting red fluorescence in the periphery of the cells, we found marked increases in IRAP in the PM region, which indicated that FSE promoted GLUT4 translocation (Figure 2A,B). In this way, FSE-mediated increases in GLUT4 transcription and translation are able to provide more GLUT4 traffic to the PM, triggering glucose uptake in L6 cells. Previous studies have shown that increasing intracellular cytosolic Ca^{2+} concentration increases cell surface GLUT4 levels [19]. We observed that upon intracellular Ca^{2+} loading, the fluorescent indicator also increased almost synchronously with GLUT4. This phenomenon implied that FSE-enhanced GLUT4 translocation may mobilize intracellular Ca^{2+}.

We then sought to search for the signal transduction pathways by which FSE stimulates GLUT4 expression and translocation. There are various signaling pathways which are involved in GLUT4 translocation and/or expression, such as the AMPK pathway, the PI3K/Akt pathway, and the PKC pathway. AMPK, a key signaling molecule stimulated by muscle contraction, activates to cause GLUT4 translocation [45]. GLUT4 is a member of the glycolytic enzyme genes. Its expression was activated under the effect of the AMPK agonist AICAR [49]. PI3K can catalyze the phosphorylation of phosphatidylinositol 4,5-diphosphate (PIP2) to PIP3, activating the downstream signaling factor Akt by phosphorylation, thereby promoting GLUT4 translocation to the PM to absorb glucose into the muscle [44,50]. The PKCα inhibitor dioleoyl phosphoethanolamine retained cell surface GLUT4 by inhibiting PKCα-driven internalization in adipocytes. PKC β and λ were involved in the insulin signaling cascade causing PKC-meditated GLUT4 traffic in skeletal muscle cells [19,51]. When we studied which of the three signaling pathways was/were involved in FSE-mediated glucose uptake, we found that both Compound C and Gö6983 remarkably inhibited the promotion by FSE of GLUT4 translocation and expression, but the inhibition effect of Wortmannin was relatively weak (Figure 4A,B). This suggested that the PI3K/Akt pathway was not dominant in the process of FSE-mediated GLUT4 translocation. Furthermore, the observation that FSE increased the phosphorylation of AMPK, Akt, and PKC proteins in L6 cells further conjectured that FSE-induced glucose uptake was associated with the AMPK, Akt, and PKC signaling pathways (Figure 4C–E).

To study the relationship between FSE-mediated GLUT4 translocation and Ca^{2+}, we partially removed Ca^{2+} and found that 0 mM extracellular Ca^{2+} partially inhibited FSE-induced Ca^{2+} elevation but did not affect GLUT4 translocation (Figure 3A). While the intracellular and extracellular Ca^{2+} were all chelated, the FSE-induced Ca^{2+} increase was almost completely blocked and the GLUT4 translocation was also severely inhibited (Figure 3B), and it was certified that cytosolic Ca^{2+}

participated in FSE-induced GLUT4 translocation. In order to examine the source of cytosolic Ca^{2+}, internal Ca^{2+} release was also studied, in addition to external Ca^{2+} influx. IP3R and RyR are two important barriers to the release of Ca^{2+} from intracellular Ca^{2+} stores, controlling the output of internal Ca^{2+} [18]. Similar to 0 mM Ca^{2+}, FSE-mediated Ca^{2+} increase was obviously inhibited after 2-APB blocking IP3R. Nevertheless, GLUT4 translocation was not altered (Figure 6A). However, the inhibition of RyR did not have any impact on FSE-triggered Ca^{2+} elevation or GLUT4 translocation. These results showed that FSE-induced Ca^{2+} elevation may be related to IP3R (Figure 6B). To explain why simply blocking the external or internal Ca^{2+} source to reduce cytosolic Ca^{2+} concentration does not inhibit GLUT4 translocation of FSE, we propose that the lower Ca^{2+} concentration can cause the GLUT4 translocation process via FSE while Ca^{2+} can be obtained from another source, even if one of the sources was blocked.

G protein and PLC are upstream of the PKC signaling pathway and IP3R [52]. This provides a potential breakthrough point for simultaneously refining the pathway of FSE-regulated intracellular Ca^{2+} release and GLUT4 translocation. We found that G protein and PLC inhibitors disrupted the FSE-induced Ca^{2+} increase and displayed varying degrees of suppression efficacy. This was demonstrated by the observation that FSE induced intracellular Ca^{2+} release through the G protein-PLC-IP3-IP3R pathway. Regarding the partial inhibition of G protein and PLC inhibitors of GLUT4 translocation, we concluded that FSE-regulated GLUT4 translocation not only depends on one pathway, but may involve two or more signaling pathways (Figure 5A–C).

In addition, our studies testified that FSE increases Ca^{2+} to enhance GLUT4 insertion into the PM and increases glucose uptake. GLUT4 fusion is the last step in glucose uptake and several studies have reported a key role for Ca^{2+}/calmodulin in the late stages of GLUT4 vesicle docking/fusion [53,54]. As shown in Figures 7 and 8, both FSE-mediated GLUT4-PM fusion and glucose uptake were somewhat attenuated under conditions of abolishment of extracellular Ca^{2+}. When free Ca^{2+} ions were fully chelated by EGTA and BAPTA-AM, FSE-induced membrane fusion and especially glucose uptake were also seriously diminished. It can be seen that FSE-mediated membrane fusion and glucose uptake require Ca^{2+}, which makes Ca^{2+} indispensable in these steps.

Throughout the course of this research, the signaling pathways induced by FSE-mediated glucose uptake were found to be quite diverse. This diversity may be attributed to the differences in the active ingredients of FSE. Based on the components of FSE as described above, many interesting results have been found. For example, through inhibiting mitochondrial complex I activity, emodin increases cellular ROS and Ca^{2+} influx to activate AMPK, causing GLUT4 translocation and glucose uptake [55]. Emodin significantly improved the blood glucose of diabetic rats by activating the PI3K/Akt/GSK-3β signaling pathway [56]. Isolated chrysophanol from rhubarb rhizome increased tyrosine phosphorylation of the insulin receptor (IR) and accelerated GLUT4 mRNA expression [57]. Aloe-emodin glycosides stimulated glucose transport and glycogen storage through PI3K-dependent mechanisms in L6 myotubes [58]. Long-term dietary supplementation of kaempferol promoted the expression of AMPK and GLUT4 in skeletal muscles, thereby preventing hyperglycemia in middle-aged obese mice [59]. These statements implied that the FSE-regulated glucose pathway is a complex and vast network. Our study shows for the first time that FSE regulates glucose metabolism through the PKC pathway, but it is not clear which active ingredient plays a role in it and is worth further exploration. Besides, this research on FSE is limited to the cellular level; hence the hypoglycemic effect at the animal level remains to be explored.

In conclusion, FSE promoted GLUT4 expression and translocation through the AMPK, Akt, and G protein-PLC-PKC pathways. FSE increased Ca^{2+} concentration by external Ca^{2+} influx and internal Ca^{2+} release of G protein-PLC-IP3-IP3R signals to assist GLUT4 traffic and PM fusion, ultimately leading to glucose uptake (Figure 9). Therefore, FSE is expected to become an effective drug for the treatment of insulin resistance.

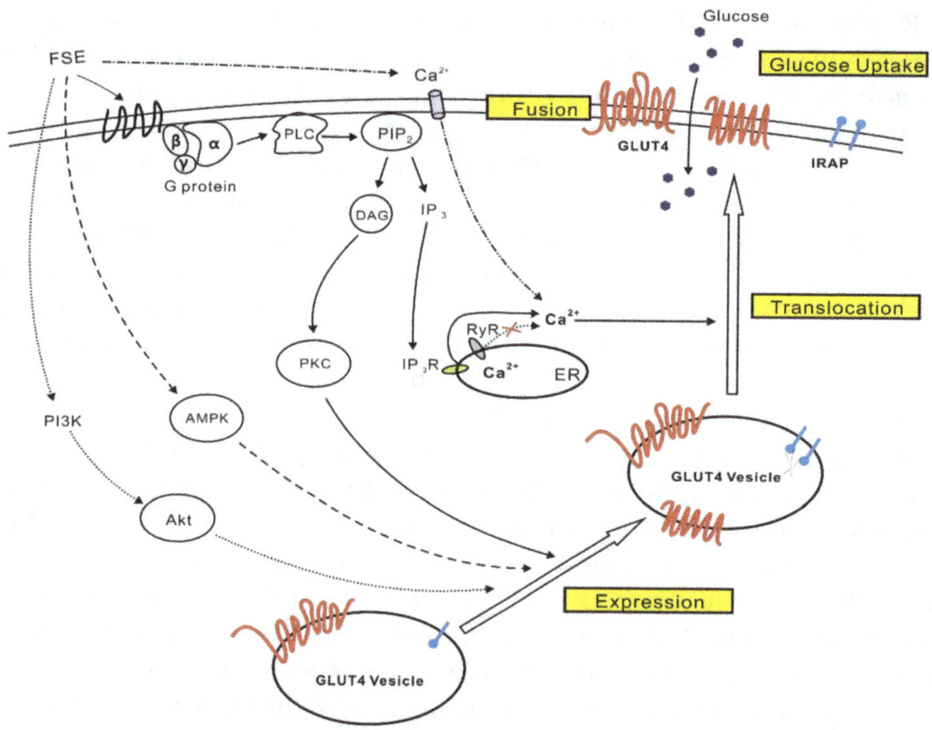

Figure 9. Proposed mechanism of FSE for the enhancement of glucose uptake in L6 cells. FSE promotes GLUT4 expression and translocation via the activation the AMPK, IP3K/Akt, and G protein-PLC-PKC pathways. Moreover, the increase in cytosolic Ca^{2+} induced by the G-protein-PLC-IP3-IP3R-Ca^{2+} pathway or/and by extracellular Ca^{2+} influx assists GLUT4 trafficking and fusion to PM, ultimately triggering glucose uptake.

4. Materials and methods

4.1. Reagents and Solutions

Alpha-MEM (α-MEM) and penicillin streptomycin solution were purchased from Gibco (Gran Island, NY, USA). Fetal bovine serum (FBS) was purchased from Hyclone (Logan, UT, USA). The glucose assay kit was purchased from Cayman Chemical Company (Ann Arbor, MI, USA). Fluo-4 AM was obtained from Invitrogen (Camarillo, CA, USA). Compound C was purchased from Selleckchem (Houston, TX, USA). Wortmannin, BAPTA-AM, U73122, Ryanodine, and 2-APB were purchased from Sigma (St. Louis, MO, USA). Gallein and PTX were purchased from Tocris Bioscience (Bristol, UK). Gö6983 was from EMD Millipore (Billerica, MA, USA). GLUT4 antibody, β-actin antibody, phospho-AMPKα (Thr172) antibody, AMPK antibody, phospho-Akt (Ser473) antibody, Anti-Akt antibody, and phospho-PKC pan (Thr410) antibody were from Cell Signaling Technology (Beverly, MA, USA). HRP goat anti-mouse and goat anti-rabbit IgG antibody were from CWBIO (Beijing, China), anti-c-myc mouse monoclonal antibody and FITC antibody were purchased from TransGen Biotech (Beijing, China), Phorbol 12-myristate 13-acetate (PMA) was purchased from Ascent Scientific (Cambridge, MA), metformin and insulin were obtained from Yuanye biological (shanghai, China). 2 mM Ca^{2+} (pss): 135 NaCl, 5 KCl, 1 $MgCl_2$, 2 $CaCl_2$, 10 HEPES, and 10 glucose (pH 7.4). 0 mM Ca^{2+}-EGTA: 135 NaCl, 5 KCl, 1 $MgCl_2$, 0.5 EGTA, 10 HEPES, and 10 glucose (pH 7.4). PBS buffer: 137 NaCl, 2.7 KCl, 10 Na_2HPO_4, 2 KH_2PO_4, and the volume is adjusted to 1 L with ultrapure water (PH 7.4).

4.2. Plant Collection and Preparation

Dried plant material was ground into a fine powder using a commercial electric blender and stored in air-tight containers. Fifty grams of leaf material was soaked in 500 mL of 70% industrial ethanol for 30 h, and then refluxed in a 60 °C water bath. The extraction procedure was repeated three times in order to extract as much of the components as possible. The extract was filtered using Whatman no. 1 filter paper and dried under a stream of cold air. The ethanolic extract of Folium Sennae (FSE) was dissolved in 3% dimethylsulfoxide (DMSO) for biological detection.

4.3. L6 Cell Culture and Treatment

L6 myoblasts were grown in α-MEM containing 10% (*v*/*v*) FBS, 100 units/mL penicillin, and 100 μg/mL streptomycin in 5% CO_2 at 37 °C. L6 cells were harvested after about 80% confluent and used in all experiments. Prior to any treatment, the cells were serum-deprived for 2 h. After treatment, the cells were divided into different drug treatment groups.

4.4. Amount of Glucose Uptake into Cells

The glucose uptake stimulatory effect of FSE was determined in L6 cells by a previously reported method [60] with slight modifications [61,62]. Briefly, L6 cells were grown in 96-well culture plates at 37 °C under 5% CO_2 and cultured for 3–4 days until the cells were confluent. Next, cells were starved for 2 h with 100 μL serum-free α-MEM medium and then treated with 60 μg/mL FSE or 100 nM insulin or vehicle control dissolved in 100 μL serum-free α-MEM medium for 1 h. Insulin was used as positive control. The concentration of glucose remaining in the media was determined according to the glucose assay kit manufacturer's instructions using an Infinite M200 Pro microplate reader (Tecan, Croedig, Austria) with a 505 nm wavelength. Meanwhile, cell numbers from each group were analyzed using tetrazolium salt (3-(4,5-dimethylthiazol-2-yl)-2,5-diphenyltetrazolium) bromide (MTT). For analysis, 20 μL of MTT substrate was added to each well and the plates were incubated for an additional 4 h at 37 °C with 5% CO_2. The medium was removed, and the cells were solubilized in 150 μL DMSO. The colorimetric analysis was performed at a wavelength of 492 nm. The amount of glucose uptake in each group was calculated by using the amount of glucose uptake for the corresponding cell counts. Three independent experiments were conducted, comparing the control group (control), the insulin group (insulin), and the added drug group (FSE).

4.5. Western Blotting Analyses

L6 cells were serum-deprived for 2 h, then treated with FSE (60 μg/mL for 30 min), insulin (100 nM for 30 min), PMA (200 nM for 4 h) or metformin (100 μg/mL overnight), Wortmannin (100 nM for 30 min), Gö6983 (10 μM for 30 min), Compound C (10 μM for 30 min). Next, the cells were placed on ice, washed three times with cold PBS, and treated with a protease inhibitor cocktail (Roche, Basel, Switzerland) and phosphatase inhibitor cocktail (Selleckchem, Houston, TX, USA) at 4 °C. Cells were then lysed as described previously [60]. After cell debris was removed, supernatants containing proteins were collected. Equal amounts of protein were separated by 10% (*v*/*v*) SDS-PAGE and transferred to polyvinylidene difluoride (PVDF) membranes. Blots were incubated with 5% BSA blocking solution at 4 °C, overnight with a primary antibody (1:1000), and then incubated with corresponding horseradish peroxidase-conjugated secondary antibody (1:10,000) for 1 h at room temperature. The intensity of protein bands was quantitated using a ChemiDoc XRS system (Bio-Rad, Hercules, CA, USA).

4.6. RT-PCR

The L6 cells were subjected to the same western blotting operation described above and divided into control, insulin, and FSE groups. Total RNA was extracted using TRIzol reagent (Invitrogen) including chloroform extraction and isopropanol precipitation. The RNA initial extract of each sample was washed and dried with 75% ethanol and then dissolved in 50 μL DEPC water. The quality of each RNA extraction was confirmed by electrophoresis on a 1% agarose gel. Next, 2 μg of total RNA from each sample was reverse-transcribed using the RevertAid First Strand cDNA Synthesis Kit (Thermo Scientific, Wilmington, DE, USA) in a 20 μL reaction according to the manufacturer's protocol. The PCR conditions were set as follows: initial activation of Taq polymerase at 95 °C for 10 min, 35 cycles of PCR amplification at 95 °C for 15 s, and annealing/elongation at 60 °C for 1 min. cDNA products were diluted with RNAse-free water, and then real-time PCR was performed using the FastStart Universal SYBR Green PCR Master ROX (Roche) system on the 7500 Fast Real-Time PCR System instrument (Applied Biosystems, Foster City, CA, USA). Primer sequences were as follows: rat GAPDH (NCBI RefSeq NM_017008.4), F: 5′-TACAGCAACAGGGTGGTGGAC-3′, R: 5′-GGGATGGAATTGTGAGGGAGA-3′; rat GLUT4 (NCBI RefSeq NM_012751.1), F: 5′-CTTCCTTCTATTTGCCGTCCTC-3′, R: 5′-GCTGCTGTTTCCTTCATCCTG-3′; rat IRAP (NCBI Refseq NM_001113403.2), F: 5′-GTGGGGACTAAGGGCGAAAA- 3′ R:5′-CATACATCCGGACCTCCACG-3′. Relative quantification results obtained for the target genes were normalized using the $2^{-\Delta\Delta CT}$ method.

4.7. Fluorescence Microscopy for Detection of IRAP Translocation and Ca^{2+}

L6 cells were transfected with pIRAP-mOrange cDNAs (presented by Professor Xu Tao, Chinese Academy of Sciences) using Lipofectamine 2000 as per the manufacturer's protocol [2]. Stably expressing IRAP-mOrange of L6 cells (L6 IRAP-mOrange) were seeded into a glass slide and incubated overnight until differentiated and confluent over the slides. Cells were starved in serum-free α-MEM for 2 h. For loading the dye, cells were incubated in 2 μM fluo4-AM (Invitrogen, Carlsbad, CA, USA) for 20 min at 37 °C, followed by a wash with PSS, and then treated with 60 μg/mL FSE or other related signaling pathway protein inhibitors. Red fluorescence (555 nm) and green fluorescence (488 nm) images of cells were simultaneously taken with the LSM700 laser scanning confocal microscope (Carl Zeiss, Jena, Germany). The IRAP-mOrange translocation and intracellular Ca^{2+} levels were monitored as spatial and temporal changes in the fluorescence intensity of the indicator mOrange and dye Fluo4, respectively. In the absence of stimulation, GLUT4 and IRAP are present in intracellular GLUT storage vesicles (GSVs). Many studies have reported that GLUT4 and IRAP displayed a high co-localization relationship [63], thus, detecting the IRAP can indirectly reflect the localization of GLUT4. The images were captured with 555 nm or 488 nm excitation laser every 10 s in the first 5 min and then every 5 min over 25 min.

4.8. Immunofluorescence of GLUT4 Fusion with PM

L6 cells were transfected by lentivirus with GV348 plasmid DNA encoding myc, GLUT4, and mOrange constructs of the myc-GLUT4-mOrange fusion protein. GLUT4myc cDNA was constructed by inserting the human c-myc epitope (14 amino acids) into the first ectodomain of GLUT4, as described [64]. Live cell imaging was performed to measure membrane fusion and GLUT4 trafficking with myc and mOrange as molecular probes, respectively [42]. A single clone containing the highest fluorescence intensity was selected and used for the following experiments. The GV348-myc-GLUT4-mOrange of L6 cells were seeded onto the glass slide, incubated until they reached 80% confluence, and then serum-deprived for 2 h. In addition to the control group and the 100 nM insulin-positive control group of 2 mM Ca^{2+}, the cells were treated with 60 μg/mL FSE under the conditions of 2 mM Ca^{2+}, 0 mM Ca^{2+}, and 0 mM Ca^{2+}+BAPTA-AM, respectively. After 30 min of stimulation, the cells were fixed with 4% paraformaldehyde. Then, 50 mM glycine was used to remove impurities which would cause background signals. Then samples were blocked with PBS containing with 2% FBS for 1 h. Afterward, cells were labeled with anti-c-myc mouse monoclonal antibody (1:200) and goat anti-mouse IgG (H+L) FITC-conjugated secondary antibody (1:200). Cell images of green fluorescent protein (FITC) and mOrange fluorescence were measured by the LSM700 microscope (Carl Zeiss).

4.9. Statistical Analysis

Data are presented as the mean ± SEM of at least three independent experiments. All statistical analyses were performed using OriginPro 8 (OriginLab, Northampton, MA, USA). Multigroup comparisons were conducted by one-way analysis of variance and differences between two group means were compared by Student's t-test. p values < 0.05 were considered to represent statistical significance. The n values represent the number of cells.

5. Conclusions

The present study showed that FSE promoted GLUT4 expression and translocation in L6 cells via the AMPK, PI3K/Akt, and G protein-PLC-PKC signaling pathways. It also increased Ca^{2+} concentration in the form of external Ca^{2+} influx and Ca^{2+} pool release, assisting GLUT4-PM fusion to enhance glucose uptake. These results suggested the possibility of FSE being used as a novel hypoglycemic agent for the treatment of T2DM.

Author Contributions: P.Z. and Q.M. contributed equally to this study. P.Z. contributed to study design and guidance. Q.M. conducted the experiments and wrote the manuscript. J.Q. provided the raw materials for FSE. D.T. and J.L. participated in data interpretation. J.S., Q.-H.L., P.Z., and X.Y. supervised this study and edited the manuscript.

Acknowledgments: Authors are thankful to Tao Xu for providing the IRAP-mOrange L6 cell lines. We are also deeply grateful to Pingsheng Liu for providing L6 cells.

References

1. Kang, O.H.; Shon, M.Y.; Kong, R.; Seo, Y.S.; Zhou, T.; Kim, D.Y.; Kim, Y.S.; Kwon, D.Y. Anti-diabetic effect of black ginseng extract by augmentation of AMPK protein activity and upregulation of GLUT2 and GLUT4 expression in db/db mice. *BMC Complement. Altern. Med.* **2017**, *17*, 341. [CrossRef] [PubMed]
2. Yang, J.; Zhao, P.; Wan, D.; Zhou, Q.; Wang, C.; Shu, G.; Mei, Z.; Yang, X. Antidiabetic Effect of Methanolic Extract from Berberis julianae Schneid. via Activation of AMP-Activated Protein Kinase in Type 2 Diabetic Mice. *Evid. Based Complement. Altern. Med.* **2014**, *2014*, 106206. [CrossRef] [PubMed]
3. Zhang, M.; Li, X.; Liang, H.; Cai, H.; Hu, X.; Bian, Y.; Dong, L.; Ding, L.; Wang, L.; Yu, B.; et al. Semen Cassiae Extract Improves Glucose Metabolism by Promoting GlUT4 Translocation in the Skeletal Muscle of Diabetic Rats. *Front. Pharmacol.* **2018**, *9*, 235. [CrossRef] [PubMed]
4. Huang, Y.; Hao, J.; Tian, D.; Wen, Y.; Zhao, P.; Chen, H.; Lv, Y.; Yang, X. Antidiabetic Activity of a Flavonoid-Rich Extract From Sophora davidii (Franch.) Skeels in KK-Ay Mice via Activation of AMP-Activated Protein Kinase. *Front. Pharmacol.* **2018**, *9*, 760. [CrossRef] [PubMed]
5. Cai, Y.; Wang, Y.; Zhi, F.; Xing, Q.C.; Chen, Y.Z. The Effect of Sanggua Drink Extract on Insulin Resistance through the PI3K/AKT Signaling Pathway. *Evid. Based Complement. Altern. Med.* **2018**, *2018*, 9407945.
6. Kamakura, R.; Son, M.J.; de Beer, D.; Joubert, E.; Miura, Y.; Yagasaki, K. Antidiabetic effect of green rooibos (Aspalathus linearis) extract in cultured cells and type 2 diabetic model KK-A(y) mice. *Cytotechnology* **2015**, *67*, 699–710. [CrossRef] [PubMed]
7. Choi, J.; Kim, K.J.; Koh, E.J.; Lee, B.Y. Gelidium elegans Extract Ameliorates Type 2 Diabetes via Regulation of MAPK and PI3K/Akt Signaling. *Nutrients* **2018**, *10*, 51. [CrossRef] [PubMed]
8. Kadan, S.; Sasson, Y.; Saad, B.; Zaid, H. Gundelia tournefortii Antidiabetic Efficacy: Chemical Composition and GLUT4 Translocation. *Evid. Based Complement. Altern. Med.* **2018**, *2018*, 8294320. [CrossRef] [PubMed]
9. Chanda, D.; Luiken, J.J.; Glatz, J.F. Signaling pathways involved in cardiac energy metabolism. *FEBS Lett.* **2016**, *590*, 2364–2374. [CrossRef] [PubMed]
10. Zaid, H.; Antonescu, C.N.; Randhawa, V.K.; Klip, A. Insulin action on glucose transporters through molecular switches, tracks and tethers. *Biochem. J.* **2008**, *413*, 201–215. [CrossRef] [PubMed]
11. Vlavcheski, F.; Baron, D.; Vlachogiannis, I.A.; MacPherson, R.E.K.; Tsiani, E. Carnosol Increases Skeletal Muscle Cell Glucose Uptake via AMPK-Dependent GLUT4 Glucose Transporter Translocation. *Int. J. Mol. Sci.* **2018**, *19*, 1321. [CrossRef] [PubMed]

12. Wright, D.C. Mechanisms of calcium-induced mitochondrial biogenesis and GLUT4 synthesis. *Appl. Physiol. Nutr. Metab.* **2007**, *32*, 840–845. [CrossRef] [PubMed]
13. Li, Q.; Zhu, X.; Ishikura, S.; Zhang, D.; Gao, J.; Sun, Y.; Contreras-Ferrat, A.; Foley, K.P.; Lavandero, S.; Yao, Z.; et al. Ca^{2+} signals promote GLUT4 exocytosis and reduce its endocytosis in muscle cells. *Am. J. Physiol. Endocrinol. Metab.* **2014**, *307*, E209–E224. [CrossRef] [PubMed]
14. Lanner, J.T.; Katz, A.; Tavi, P.; Sandstrom, M.E.; Zhang, S.J.; Wretman, C.; James, S.; Fauconnier, J.; Lannergren, J.; Bruton, J.D.; et al. The role of Ca^{2+} influx for insulin-mediated glucose uptake in skeletal muscle. *Diabetes* **2006**, *55*, 2077–2083. [CrossRef] [PubMed]
15. Contreras-Ferrat, A.E.; Toro, B.; Bravo, R.; Parra, V.; Vasquez, C.; Ibarra, C.; Mears, D.; Chiong, M.; Jaimovich, E.; Klip, A.; et al. An inositol 1,4,5-triphosphate (IP3)-IP3 receptor pathway is required for insulin-stimulated glucose transporter 4 translocation and glucose uptake in cardiomyocytes. *Endocrinology* **2010**, *151*, 4665–4677. [CrossRef] [PubMed]
16. Wijesekara, N.; Tung, A.; Thong, F.; Klip, A. Muscle cell depolarization induces a gain in surface GLUT4 via reduced endocytosis independently of AMPK. *Am. J. Physiol. Endocrinol. Metab.* **2006**, *290*, E1276–E1286. [CrossRef] [PubMed]
17. Waller, A.P.; Kalyanasundaram, A.; Hayes, S.; Periasamy, M.; Lacombe, V.A. Sarcoplasmic reticulum Ca^{2+} ATPase pump is a major regulator of glucose transport in the healthy and diabetic heart. *Biochim. Biophys. Acta* **2015**, *1852*, 873–881. [CrossRef] [PubMed]
18. Contreras-Ferrat, A.; Llanos, P.; Vasquez, C.; Espinosa, A.; Osorio-Fuentealba, C.; Arias-Calderon, M.; Lavandero, S.; Klip, A.; Hidalgo, C.; Jaimovich, E. Insulin elicits a ROS-activated and an IP(3)-dependent Ca(2)(+) release, which both impinge on GLUT4 translocation. *J. Cell Sci.* **2014**, *127*, 1911–1923. [CrossRef] [PubMed]
19. Deng, B.; Zhu, X.; Zhao, Y.; Zhang, D.; Pannu, A.; Chen, L.; Niu, W. PKC and Rab13 mediate Ca^{2+} signal-regulated GLUT4 traffic. *Biochem. Biophys. Res. Commun.* **2018**, *495*, 1956–1963. [CrossRef] [PubMed]
20. Singh, S.; Loke, Y.K.; Furberg, C.D. Long-term risk of cardiovascular events with rosiglitazone: A meta-analysis. *JAMA* **2007**, *298*, 1189–1195. [CrossRef] [PubMed]
21. Schuster, D.P.; Duvuuri, V. Diabetes mellitus. *Clin. Podiatr. Med. Surg.* **2002**, *19*, 79–107. [CrossRef]
22. Li, W.L.; Zheng, H.C.; Bukuru, J.; De Kimpe, N. Natural medicines used in the traditional Chinese medical system for therapy of diabetes mellitus. *J. Ethnopharmacol.* **2004**, *92*, 1–21. [CrossRef] [PubMed]
23. Chen, J.; Mangelinckx, S.; Adams, A.; Wang, Z.T.; Li, W.L.; De Kimpe, N. Natural flavonoids as potential herbal medication for the treatment of diabetes mellitus and its complications. *Nat. Prod. Commun.* **2015**, *10*, 187–200. [PubMed]
24. Zaid, H.; Mahdi, A.A.; Tamrakar, A.K. Natural Active Ingredients for Diabetes and Metabolism Disorders Treatment. *Evid. Based Complement. Altern. Med.* **2016**, *2016*, 2965214. [CrossRef] [PubMed]
25. Testa, R.; Bonfigli, A.R.; Genovese, S.; De Nigris, V.; Ceriello, A. The Possible Role of Flavonoids in the Prevention of Diabetic Complications. *Nutrients* **2016**, *8*, 310. [CrossRef] [PubMed]
26. Kundu, S.; Roy, S.; Nandi, S.; Ukil, B.; Lyndem, L.M. Senna alexandrina Mill. induced ultrastructural changes on Hymenolepis diminuta. *J. Parasit. Dis.* **2017**, *41*, 147–154. [CrossRef] [PubMed]
27. Rama Reddy, N.R.; Mehta, R.H.; Soni, P.H.; Makasana, J.; Gajbhiye, N.A.; Ponnuchamy, M.; Kumar, J. Next Generation Sequencing and Transcriptome Analysis Predicts Biosynthetic Pathway of Sennosides from Senna (*Cassia angustifolia* Vahl.), a Non-Model Plant with Potent Laxative Properties. *PLoS ONE* **2015**, *10*, e0129422. [CrossRef] [PubMed]
28. Muanda, F.N.; Bouayed, J.; Djilani, A.; Yao, C.; Soulimani, R.; Dicko, A. Chemical Composition and, Cellular Evaluation of the Antioxidant Activity of Desmodium adscendens Leaves. *Evid. Based Complement. Altern. Med.* **2011**, *2011*, 620862. [CrossRef] [PubMed]
29. Elansary, H.O.; Szopa, A.; Kubica, P.; Ekiert, H.; Ali, H.M. Bioactivities of Traditional Medicinal Plants in Alexandria. *Evid. Based Complement. Altern. Med.* **2018**, *2018*, 1463579. [CrossRef] [PubMed]
30. Susunaga-Notario Adel, C.; Perez-Gutierrez, S.; Zavala-Sanchez, M.A.; Almanza-Perez, J.C.; Gutierrez-Carrillo, A.; Arrieta-Baez, D.; Lopez-Lopez, A.L.; Roman-Ramos, R.; Flores-Saenz, J.L.; Alarcon-Aguilar, F.J. Bioassay-guided chemical study of the anti-inflammatory effect of Senna villosa (Miller) H.S. Irwin & Barneby (Leguminosae) in TPA-induced ear edema. *Molecules* **2014**, *19*, 10261–10278. [PubMed]

31. Pereira, R.M.; Ferreira-Silva, G.A.; Pivatto, M.; Santos Lde, A.; Bolzani Vda, S.; Chagas de Paula, D.A.; Oliveira, J.C.; Viegas Junior, C.; Ionta, M. Alkaloids derived from flowers of Senna spectabilis, (-)-cassine and (-)-spectaline, have antiproliferative activity on HepG2 cells for inducing cell cycle arrest in G1/S transition through ERK inactivation and downregulation of cyclin D1 expression. *Toxicol. In Vitro* **2016**, *31*, 86–92. [CrossRef] [PubMed]
32. Hishe, H.Z.; Ambech, T.A.; Hiben, M.G.; Fanta, B.S. Anti-nociceptive effect of methanol extract of leaves of Senna singueana in mice. *J. Ethnopharmacol.* **2018**, *217*, 49–53. [CrossRef] [PubMed]
33. Hiben, M.G.; Sibhat, G.G.; Fanta, B.S.; Gebrezgi, H.D.; Tesema, S.B. Evaluation of Senna singueana leaf extract as an alternative or adjuvant therapy for malaria. *J. Tradit. Complement. Med.* **2016**, *6*, 112–117. [CrossRef] [PubMed]
34. Thilagam, E.; Parimaladevi, B.; Kumarappan, C.; Mandal, S.C. Alpha-Glucosidase and alpha-amylase inhibitory activity of Senna surattensis. *J. Acupunct. Meridian. Stud.* **2013**, *6*, 24–30. [CrossRef] [PubMed]
35. Ayinla, T.M.; Owoyele, V.B.; Yakubu, T.M. Effect of Ethanolic Leaf Extract of Senna Fistula on some Haematological Parameters, Lipid Profile and Oxidative Stress in Alloxan-induced Diabetic Rats. *Niger. J. Physiol. Sci.* **2015**, *30*, 87–93. [PubMed]
36. Malematja, R.O.; Bagla, V.P. Potential Hypoglycaemic and Antiobesity Effects of Senna italica Leaf Acetone Extract. *Evid. Based Complement. Altern. Med.* **2018**, *2018*, 5101656. [CrossRef] [PubMed]
37. Ismail, M.A.; Mateos, L.; Maioli, S.; Merino-Serrais, P. 27-Hydroxycholesterol impairs neuronal glucose uptake through an IRAP/GLUT4 system dysregulation. *J. Exp. Med.* **2017**, *214*, 699–717. [CrossRef] [PubMed]
38. Li, Y.; Zheng, L.; Wang, D.; Zhang, X.; Li, J.; Ali, S.; Lu, J.; Zong, H.; Xu, X. Staurosporine as an agonist for induction of GLUT4 translocation, identified by a pH-sensitive fluorescent IRAP-mOrange2 probe. *Biochem. Biophys. Res. Commun.* **2016**, *480*, 534–538. [CrossRef] [PubMed]
39. Jiang, L.; Fan, J.; Bai, L.; Wang, Y.; Chen, Y.; Yang, L.; Chen, L.; Xu, T. Direct quantification of fusion rate reveals a distal role for AS160 in insulin-stimulated fusion of GLUT4 storage vesicles. *J. Biol. Chem.* **2008**, *283*, 8508–8516. [CrossRef] [PubMed]
40. Zeng, B.; Chen, G.L.; Daskoulidou, N.; Xu, S.Z. The ryanodine receptor agonist 4-chloro-3-ethylphenol blocks ORAI store-operated channels. *Br. J. Pharmacol.* **2014**, *171*, 1250–1259. [CrossRef] [PubMed]
41. Yu, H.; Rathore, S.S.; Davis, E.M.; Ouyang, Y.; Shen, J. Doc2b promotes GLUT4 exocytosis by activating the SNARE-mediated fusion reaction in a calcium- and membrane bending-dependent manner. *Mol. Biol. Cell* **2013**, *24*, 1176–1184. [CrossRef] [PubMed]
42. Xie, X.; Gong, Z.; Mansuy-Aubert, V.; Zhou, Q.L.; Tatulian, S.A.; Sehrt, D.; Gnad, F.; Brill, L.M.; Motamedchaboki, K.; Chen, Y.; et al. C2 domain-containing phosphoprotein CDP138 regulates GLUT4 insertion into the plasma membrane. *Cell Metab.* **2011**, *14*, 378–389. [CrossRef] [PubMed]
43. Xing, Q.; Chen, Y. Antidiabetic Effects of a Chinese Herbal Medicinal Compound Sangguayin Preparation via PI3K/Akt Signaling Pathway in db/db Mice. *Evid. Based Complement. Altern. Med.* **2018**, *2018*, 2010423. [CrossRef] [PubMed]
44. Tian, C.; Chang, H. Wushenziye Formula Improves Skeletal Muscle Insulin Resistance in Type 2 Diabetes Mellitus via PTP1B-IRS1-Akt-GLUT4 Signaling Pathway. *Evid. Based Complement. Altern. Med.* **2017**, *2017*, 4393529. [CrossRef] [PubMed]
45. Zhang, C.; Jiang, Y.; Liu, J.; Jin, M.; Qin, N.; Chen, Y.; Niu, W.; Duan, H. AMPK/AS160 mediates tiliroside derivatives-stimulated GLUT4 translocation in muscle cells. *Drug Des. Dev. Ther.* **2018**, *12*, 1581–1587. [CrossRef] [PubMed]
46. Beaton, N.; Rudigier, C.; Moest, H.; Muller, S.; Mrosek, N.; Roder, E.; Rudofsky, G.; Rulicke, T.; Ukropec, J.; Ukropcova, B.; et al. TUSC5 regulates insulin-mediated adipose tissue glucose uptake by modulation of GLUT4 recycling. *Mol. Metab.* **2015**, *4*, 795–810. [CrossRef] [PubMed]
47. Waller, A.P.; Burns, T.A.; Mudge, M.C.; Belknap, J.K.; Lacombe, V.A. Insulin resistance selectively alters cell-surface glucose transporters but not their total protein expression in equine skeletal muscle. *J. Vet. Intern. Med.* **2011**, *25*, 315–321. [CrossRef] [PubMed]
48. Werno, M.W.; Chamberlain, L.H. S-acylation of the Insulin-Responsive Aminopeptidase (IRAP): Quantitative analysis and Identification of Modified Cysteines. *Sci. Rep.* **2015**, *5*, 12413. [CrossRef] [PubMed]

49. Grigorash, B.B.; Suvorova, I.I.; Pospelov, V.A. AICAR-Dependent Activation of AMPK Kinase Is Not Accompanied by G1/S Block in Mouse Embryonic Stem Cells. *Mol. Biol. (Mosk)* **2018**, *52*, 489–500. [CrossRef] [PubMed]
50. Wang, C.; Deng, Y.; Yue, Y.; Chen, W.; Zhang, Y.; Shi, G.; Wu, Z. Glutamine Enhances the Hypoglycemic Effect of Insulin in L6 Cells via Phosphatidylinositol-3-Kinase (PI3K)/Protein Kinase B (AKT)/Glucose Transporter 4 (GLUT4) Signaling Pathway. *Med. Sci. Monit.* **2018**, *24*, 1241–1250. [CrossRef] [PubMed]
51. Nishizaki, T. Dioleoylphosphoethanolamine Retains Cell Surface GLUT4 by Inhibiting PKCalpha-Driven Internalization. *Cell. Physiol. Biochem.* **2018**, *46*, 1985–1998. [CrossRef] [PubMed]
52. Litosch, I. Regulating G protein activity by lipase-independent functions of phospholipase C. *Life Sci.* **2015**, *137*, 116–124. [CrossRef] [PubMed]
53. Whitehead, J.P.; Molero, J.C.; Clark, S.; Martin, S.; Meneilly, G.; James, D.E. The role of Ca^{2+} in insulin-stimulated glucose transport in 3T3-L1 cells. *J. Biol. Chem.* **2001**, *276*, 27816–27824. [CrossRef] [PubMed]
54. Klip, A. The many ways to regulate glucose transporter 4. *Appl. Physiol. Nutr. Metab.* **2009**, *34*, 481–487. [CrossRef] [PubMed]
55. Song, P.; Kim, J.H.; Ghim, J.; Yoon, J.H.; Lee, A.; Kwon, Y.; Hyun, H.; Moon, H.Y.; Choi, H.S.; Berggren, P.O.; et al. Emodin regulates glucose utilization by activating AMP-activated protein kinase. *J. Biol. Chem.* **2013**, *288*, 5732–5742. [CrossRef] [PubMed]
56. Jing, D.; Bai, H.; Yin, S. Renoprotective effects of emodin against diabetic nephropathy in rat models are mediated via PI3K/Akt/GSK-3beta and Bax/caspase-3 signaling pathways. *Exp. Ther. Med.* **2017**, *14*, 5163–5169. [PubMed]
57. Lee, M.S.; Sohn, C.B. Anti-diabetic properties of chrysophanol and its glucoside from rhubarb rhizome. *Biol. Pharm. Bull.* **2008**, *31*, 2154–2157. [CrossRef] [PubMed]
58. Anand, S.; Muthusamy, V.S.; Sujatha, S.; Sangeetha, K.N.; Bharathi Raja, R.; Sudhagar, S.; Poornima Devi, N.; Lakshmi, B.S. Aloe emodin glycosides stimulates glucose transport and glycogen storage through PI3K dependent mechanism in L6 myotubes and inhibits adipocyte differentiation in 3T3L1 adipocytes. *FEBS Lett.* **2010**, *584*, 3170–3178. [CrossRef] [PubMed]
59. Alkhalidy, H.; Moore, W.; Zhang, Y.; McMillan, R. Small Molecule Kaempferol Promotes Insulin Sensitivity and Preserved Pancreatic beta-Cell Mass in Middle-Aged Obese Diabetic Mice. *J. Diabetes Res.* **2015**, *2015*, 532984. [CrossRef] [PubMed]
60. Zhou, Q.; Yang, X.; Xiong, M.; Xu, X.; Zhen, L.; Chen, W.; Wang, Y.; Shen, J.; Zhao, P.; Liu, Q.H. Chloroquine Increases Glucose Uptake via Enhancing GLUT4 Translocation and Fusion with the Plasma Membrane in L6 Cells. *Cell. Physiol. Biochem.* **2016**, *38*, 2030–2040. [CrossRef] [PubMed]
61. Zhou, F.; Furuhashi, K.; Son, M.J.; Toyozaki, M.; Yoshizawa, F.; Miura, Y.; Yagasaki, K. Antidiabetic effect of enterolactone in cultured muscle cells and in type 2 diabetic model db/db mice. *Cytotechnology* **2017**, *69*, 493–502. [CrossRef] [PubMed]
62. Zhao, Y.; He, J.; Yang, L.; Luo, Q.; Liu, Z. Histone Deacetylase-3 Modification of MicroRNA-31 Promotes Cell Proliferation and Aerobic Glycolysis in Breast Cancer and Is Predictive of Poor Prognosis. *J. Breast Cancer* **2018**, *21*, 112–123. [CrossRef] [PubMed]
63. Huang, M.; Deng, S.; Han, Q.; Zhao, P.; Zhou, Q.; Zheng, S.; Ma, X.; Xu, C.; Yang, J.; Yang, X. Hypoglycemic Activity and the Potential Mechanism of the Flavonoid Rich Extract from Sophora tonkinensis Gagnep. in KK-Ay Mice. *Front. Pharmacol.* **2016**, *7*, 288. [CrossRef] [PubMed]
64. Wang, Q.; Khayat, Z.; Kishi, K.; Ebina, Y.; Klip, A. GLUT4 translocation by insulin in intact muscle cells: Detection by a fast and quantitative assay. *FEBS Lett.* **1998**, *427*, 193–197. [CrossRef]

6

Cytotoxicity-Guided Isolation of Two New Phenolic Derivatives from *Dryopteris fragrans* (L.) Schott

Tong Zhang [1], Li Wang [2], De-Hua Duan [1], Yi-Hao Zhang [1], Sheng-Xiong Huang [2,*] and Ying Chang [1,*]

1 College of Life Science, Northeast Agricultural University, Harbin 150030, China; shmzhyzt@163.com (T.Z.); myrddh@163.com (D.-H.D.); yhzneau@163.com (Y.-H.Z.)
2 State Key Laboratory of Phytochemistry and Plant Resources in West China, Kunming Institute of Botany, Chinese Academy of Sciences, Kunming 650201, China; jasminewangli@126.com
* Correspondence: sxhuang@mail.kib.ac.cn (S.-X.H.); changying@neau.edu.cn (Y.C.);

Academic Editor: Pinarosa Avato

Abstract: *Dryopteris fragrans* is a valuable medicinal plant resource with extensive biological activities including anti-cancer, anti-oxidation, and anti-inflammation activities. This work aims to study further the cytotoxic constituents from *Dryopteris fragrans*. In this work, two new phenolic derivatives known as dryofragone (**1**) and dryofracoumarin B (**2**) with six known compounds (**3–8**) were isolated from the petroleum ether fraction of the methanol extract of the aerial parts of *Dryopteris fragrans* (L.) Schott by two round cytotoxicity-guided tracking with the 3-(4,5-dimethyl-2-thiazolyl)-2,5-diphenyl-2-*H*-tetrazolium bromide (MTT) assay and cell counting kit-8 (CCK-8) assay. Their structures were elucidated by the extensive spectroscopic analysis (^{1}H-NMR, ^{13}C-NMR, and two dimensions NMR), chemical derivatization, and comparison with data reported in the literature. All the isolates were evaluated for their cytotoxicity against nine cancer cell lines as well as their in vitro immunomodulatory activity. The results showed that compounds have a modest cytotoxicity toward human HeLa cell line with IC_{50} value below 30 μM and compounds **4** and **5** may modulate immunity to affect the growth of tumor cells.

Keywords: cytotoxicity-guided; phenolic derivatives; *Dryopteris fragrans*; chemical derivatization; immuno-regulation activity

---

1. Introduction

Dryopteris fragrans (L.) Schott (Figure 1) belonging to the genus Dryopteris is a perennial herb with aroma widely distributed throughout the world and is mostly distributed in the alpine and volcanic regions of Northeast China [1,2]. *D. fragrans* has been used as folk medicine for treating arthritis and skin diseases such as psoriasis, dermatophytosis, and more [3]. Previous phytochemical investigations on this plant have led to the identification of terpenoids [4], phloroglucinols [5], glucosides [6], and other phenolic derivatives such as coumarin [3]. The earlier biological studies have shown that *D. fragrans* was a valuable medicinal plant resource with extensive biological activities including anti-cancer, anti-oxidation, insect repellent, anti-microbial, and anti-inflammation activities [3–7].

Of its various biological effects, the mechanism of anti-cancer effects has been studied most. Dryofragin, which is a derivative of phloroglucinol, was found to activate the endogenous pathway of apoptosis by affecting the changes of ROS in mitochondria and inducing changes in mitochondria in breast cancer cell MCF-7 and to cause tumor cell apoptosis by the apoptosis-related protein Bcl-2, Bax, Caspase-9, Caspase-3, and PARP [8]. It has also been reported to be an inhibitor of migration and invasion of the human osteosarcoma cell line U2OS through the PI3K/Akt and MAPK energy pathway involving MMP-2/9 and TIMP-1/2 proteins [9]. Aspidin PB, which is another phloroglucinol derivative from *D. fragrans*, has been recorded as a tumor cell-inhibiting agent for its impact on cyclin p53/p21 and mitochondrial changes in human osteosarcoma cells Saos-2, U2OS, and HOS [10]. In addition, there have been many other reports on compounds from *D. fragrans* with cytotoxicity [11–13]. To further study cytotoxic constituents from *D. fragrans*, a cytotoxicity-guided isolation of the extract of *D. fragrans* was designed. The isolation of two new phenolic derivatives and six known compounds by cytotoxicity-guided tracking as well as their cytotoxicity and immunomodulatory activity detection is described in this paper.

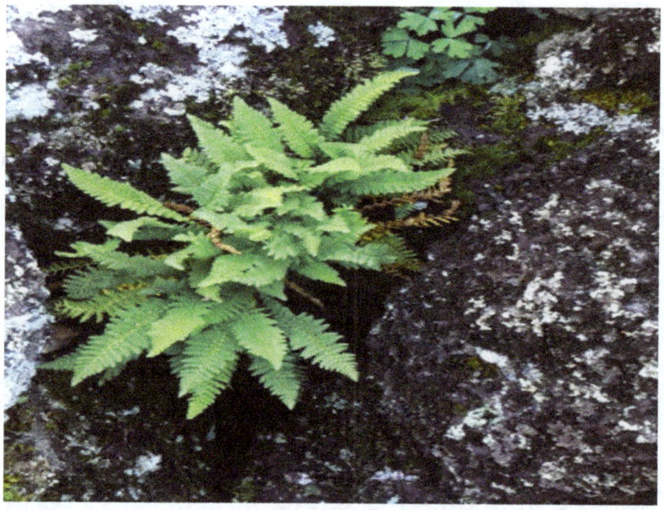

Figure 1. *Dryopteris fragrans* plant.

2. Results and Discussion

2.1. Determination of Isolated Compounds

After two round cytotoxicity screening by MTT [14] and CCK-8 [15] assay, Fractions SG1-SG7 from the petroleum ether-soluble part with prominent cytotoxic activities were selected as the bioactive sites (Figures S1 and S2). Two new phenolic derivatives known as dryofragone (**1**) and dryofracoumarin B (**2**) (Figure 2) along with six known compounds (**3–8**) (Figure 2), were isolated from the above seven bioactive fractions by using extensive chromatographic methods like silica gel, MCI gel, Sephadex LH-20, and HPLC. The known compounds were identified as dryofracoumarin A (**3**) [3], vitamin E quinone (**4**) [16], albicanol (**5**) [5], 2′,4′-dihydroxy-6′-methoxy-3′,5′-dimethylchalcone (**6**) [17], norflavesone (**7**) [18], and aspidinol (**8**) [19] by comparing their ^{1}H- and ^{13}C-NMR data with that reported in the literature.

Compound **1** was obtained as yellow powder from $CHCl_3$. The HR-ESI-MS data (*m/z* 239.0926 $[M - H]^-$, calcd for 239.0925) of **1** showed the molecular formula $C_{12}H_{16}O_5$, which correspond to five degrees of unsaturation. The IR spectrum of **1** displayed hydroxyls (3321 cm^{-1}), carbonyl groups (1714 cm^{-1}), and double bonds (1607 cm^{-1}) absorptions. The red shifted hydroxyl signal (3321 cm^{-1}) also showed that some hydroxyls in **1** were involved in the hydrogen bonding interaction. The ^{1}H-NMR spectrum of **1** (Table 1) showed one 3H-singlet at δ_H 1.54 for a tertiary methyl group, one 3H-singlet at δ_H 3.91 for a methoxy group, one 3H-triplet at δ_H 1.01 for a primary methyl group, and an olefinic proton at δ_H 5.37. The ^{13}C-NMR spectrum of **1** revealed 12 resonance signals including two ketone carbons at δ_C 196.3 (conjugated) and 203.7, two pair of olefinic carbons (δ_C 189.4, 176.0, 104.5 and 94.5) with two oxygenated sites (δ_C 189.4 and 176.0), an oxygenated tertiary carbon (δ_C 75.4), a methoxy carbon (δ_C 57.4), two aliphatic methylene carbon (δ_C 41.0 and 18.7), and two methyl carbons (δ_C 30.2 and 14.1). The above evidence indicated that compound **1** presumably possessed an oxygenated phloroglucinol core [20]. This inference was further confirmed by the 2D-NMR spectra

(Figure 3). The long-range HMBC couplings—H-4/C-2, C-3, C-5, and C-6 as well as Me-11/C-1, C-2, and C-3 demonstrated the presence of a cyclohexadiene moiety with two oxygen-bearing carbon at C-2 and C-5. The HMBC correlation from a methoxy at δ_H 3.91 (Me-12) to a quaternary olefinic carbon at δ_C 176.0 (C-3) revealed that a methoxy was located at C-3. Furthermore, a butyryl was linked to C-6, which was supported by the HMBC correlations from protons at C-8 (δ_H 2.99 and 2.92) to carbons at δ_C 104.5 (C-6), 203.7 (C-7), 18.7 (C-9), and 14.1 (C-10), respectively. The CD experiment towards compound **1** was performed. However, the CD spectrum (Figure S9) of **1** showed no characteristic cotton effect. Compound **1** was considered to be a pair of enantiomers.

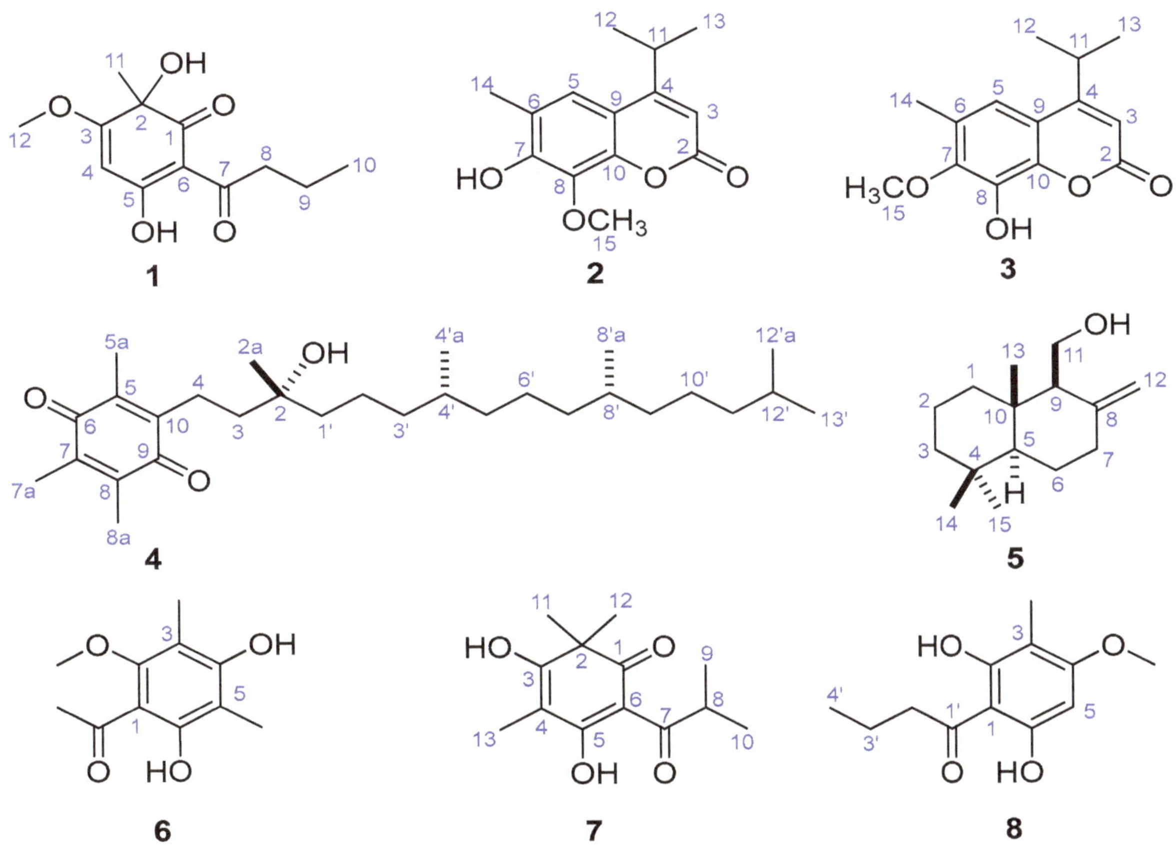

Figure 2. Structures of compounds **1–8**.

Table 1. NMR data for Compound **1** (TMS as the internal standard, δ in ppm, J in Hz) [a].

No.	δ_H	δ_C	No.	δ_H	δ_C
1		196.32 (C)	8a	2.99 (1H, m)	41.04 (CH_2)
2		75.37 (C)	8b	2.92 (1H, m)	
3		176.04 (C)	9	1.69 (2H, m)	18.71 (CH_2)
4	5.37 (1H, s)	94.49 (CH)	10	1.01 (3H, t, J = 7.4)	14.07 (CH_3)
5		189.34 (C)	11	1.54 (3H, s)	30.20 (CH_3)
6		104.49 (C)	12	3.91 (3H, s)	57.35 (CH_3)
7		203.65 (C)			

[a] ^{1}H-NMR and ^{13}C-NMR data were recorded in $CDCl_3$ at 600 MHz and 150 MHz, respectively.

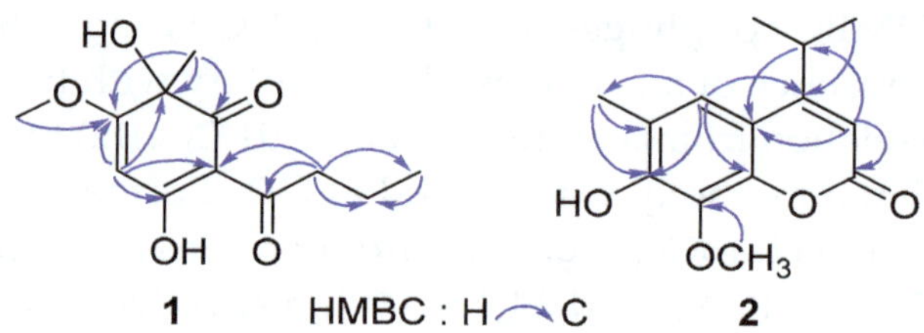

Figure 3. Key HMBC correlations of **1** and **2**.

Therefore, the structure of **1** was concluded to be a new acylphloroglucinol, 6-isobutyryl-2, 5-dihydroxy-2-methyl-3-methoxy-cyclohexa-3,5-dien-1-one, and was named dryofragone.

Compound **2** was obtained as a mixture with compound **3** initially. The ^{13}C-NMR spectrum of the mixture revealed 28 resonance signals (Figure S12) in which half were consistent with the data reported for a coumarin and dryofracoumarin A (**3**) [3]. However, the ESI-MS data (*m/z* 249[M + H]$^+$, 271[M + Na]$^+$, 287[M + K]$^+$) of the mixture showed only one molecular weight (248 Da), which aligned with that of **3**. Consequently, the other half of carbon resonance signals in the ^{13}C-NMR for the mixture, which were highly similar with that of **3**, were supposed to be of an isomer of **3** featuring exchanged positions of hydroxyl and methoxy groups in the coumarin core. Based on the large space size of tert-butyl dimethyl silicyl group, which can strike the balance of molecular polarity for compounds **2** and **3** and the high yield of the desilication step, a silicon etherification-desilication procedure was designed for the isolation of the mixture (See Section 3.5 and Figure 4). NMR data of compounds **2** and **3** are shown in Table 2. After the chemical derivatization, compound **2** was afforded as a simplex. The IR spectrum of **2** exhibited a signal of hydroxyl with no hydrogen bonds (3548 cm^{-1}), a strong band at 1668 cm^{-1} for the lactone subunit in coumarin core, and absorptions (1636, 1602, 1572 cm^{-1}) of benzene ring moiety in coumarin. The HR-ESI-MS data (*m/z* 247.0975 [M − H]$^-$, calcd for 247.0976) indicated a molecular formula $C_{14}H_{16}O_4$ with seven degrees of unsaturation for **2**. The HMBC correlations (Figure 3) from Me-12 and -13 (δ_H 1.30 × 2) to C-4 (δ_C 163.0) as well as the correlations from H-11(δ_H 3.25) to C-3 (δ_C 107.8), C-4 (δ_C 163.0), and C-9 (δ_C 112.2), which suggests that an isopropyl was fused to C-4. Another HMBC correlation Me-15/C-8 verified that a methoxyl group was linked to C-8. In addition, the HMBC correlations from an isolated methyl (δ_H 2.31) to C-5 (δ_C 120.0), C-6 (δ_C 121.1), and C-7 (δ_C 150.0) inferred a methyl at C-6 in **2**. The above analyses disclosed our former hypothesis. As a result, the structure of **2** was determined to be 7-hydroxy-6-methyl-8-methoxy-4-isopropyl-2H-chromen-2-one, which was given the trivial name of dryofracoumarin B.

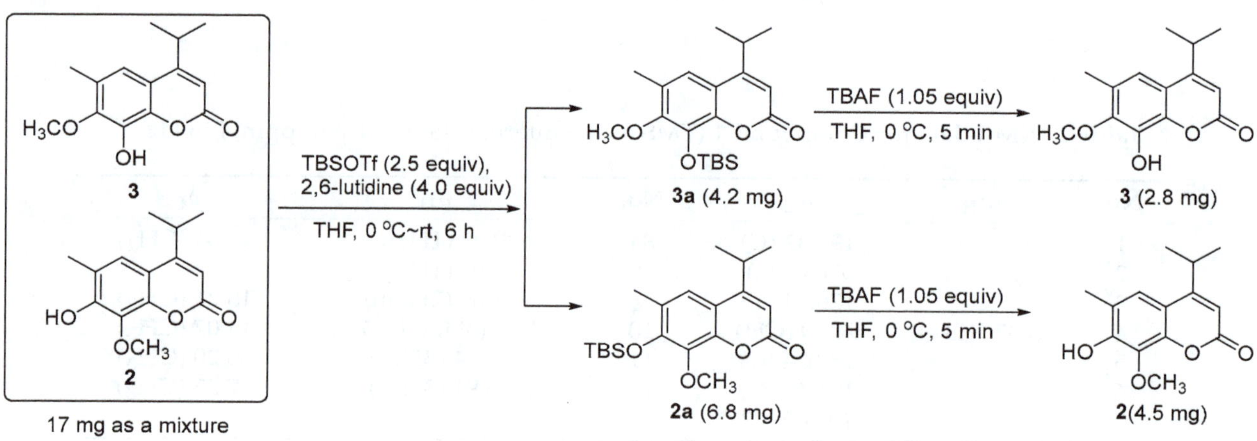

Figure 4. Silicon etherification involved the isolation of **2** and **3**.

Table 2. NMR data for compound **2** and **3** (TMS as the internal standard, δ in ppm, J in Hz) [a].

No.	2		3	
	δ_H	δ_C	δ_H	δ_C
1				
2		161.5 (C)		161.1 (C)
3	6.16 (1H, s)	107.8 (CH)	6.22 (1H, s)	109.2 (CH)
4		163.0 (C)		163.0 (C)
5	7.17 (1H, s)	120.0 (CH)	7.01 (1H, s)	115.5 (CH)
6		121.1 (C)		127.5 (C)
7		150.0 (C)		147.8 (C)
8		133.6 (C)		136.7 (C)
9		112.2 (C)		114.5 (C)
10		145.5 (C)		141.3 (C)
11	3.25 (1H, m)	28.7 (CH)	3.25 (1H, m)	28.7 (CH)
12	1.30 (3H, d, J = 6.8)	22.1 (CH_3)	1.31 (3H, d, J = 6.8)	21.9 (CH_3)
13	1.30 (3H, d, J = 6.8)	22.1 (CH_3)	1.31 (3H, d, J = 6.8)	21.9 (CH_3)
14	2.31 (3H, s)	15.9 (CH_3)	2.32 (3H, s)	16.3 (CH_3)
15	4.08 (3H, s)	61.9 (OCH_3)	3.95 (3H, s)	60.5 (OCH_3)

[a] ^{1}H-NMR and ^{13}C-NMR data were recorded in $CDCl_3$ at 600 MHz and 150 MHz, respectively.

2.2. *In Vitro Cytotoxicity and Immunomodulatory Activity Detection*

For all the isolates, their cytotoxicities against nine human cancer cell lines known as HepG2, A549, HeLa, U251, HOS, MG63, U2OS, MB231, and SKBR-3 as well as their immuno-regulation activities were evaluated. The cytotoxicities were screened using the CCK-8 assay [15]. The IC_{50} values of cytotoxicities for the eight compounds are shown in Table 3. For compounds isolated by cytotoxicity-guided tracking, they exhibited moderate activities to the HeLa cell line and weak activities to glioma, liver cancer, and lung cancer cell lines. However, they were not very sensitive to osteosarcoma and breast cancer cell lines when compared to the crude extract. For their immuno-regulation activities, LPS stimulated THP-1 cells were used as the in vitro model for the detection [21]. Fenofibrate (Feno) pre-treatment (20 μM) was used as a positive control [21]. The results for immuno-regulation activities are shown in Figure 5. Only compounds **4** and **5** could enhance the secretion of the factors *TNF-α* and *IL-1β*. The results showed that compounds **4** and **5** may activate the LPS signaling pathway, which may modulate immunity to affect the growth of tumor cells.

Table 3. IC_{50} values (μM) of cytotoxicity for eight compounds against nine human cancer cell lines.

Compound	HepG2	A549	HeLa	U251	HOS	MG63	U2OS	MB231	SKBR-3
1	-	45.86 ± 1.64	25.37 ± 2.62	46.13 ± 1.90	-	-	-	-	-
2	45.52 ± 3.21	47.70 ± 2.43	15.12 ± 4.01	46.14 ± 2.40	-	-	-	25.59 ± 2.30	-
3	48.39 ± 2.15	38.01 ± 3.56	-	-	-	-	-	38.09 ± 2.40	-
4	38.13 ± 1.03	37.41 ± 1.24	1.24 ± 0.08	-	-	-	47.56 ± 2.23	41.95 ± 2.35	-
5	-	49.74 ± 3.35	-	-	-	-	-	-	-
6	-	47.42 ± 2.25	-	-	-		-	-	-
7	-	40.03 ± 0.98	-	-	-	-	-	-	
8	18.02 ± 0.89	-	17.76 ± 3.43	41.21 ± 1.35	43.67 ± 2.52	22.76 ± 2.65	36.36 ± 1.32	39.61 ± 1.50	33.40 ± 1.50
Taxol [a]	5.32 ± 0.12	3.46 ± 0.23	0.17 ± 0.02	5.02 ± 0.21	3.71 ± 0.33	5.86 ± 0.24	1.01 ± 0.03	6.23 ± 0.36	3.12 ± 0.25

Note: IC_{50} values represented the means ± SD of six independent experiments and "-" means the IC_{50} value is above 50 μM. [a] Taxol was used as a positive control.

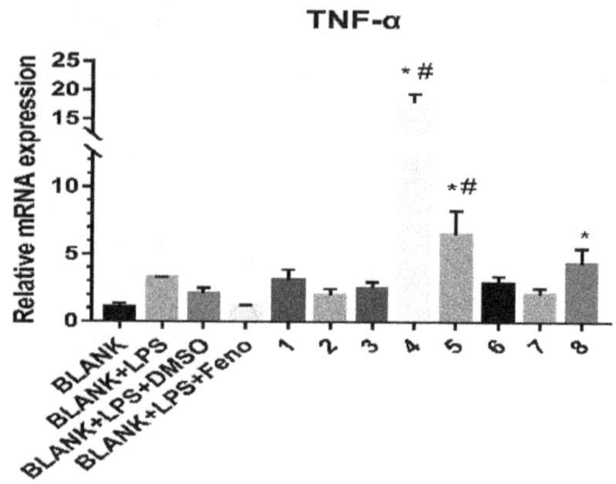

(A)

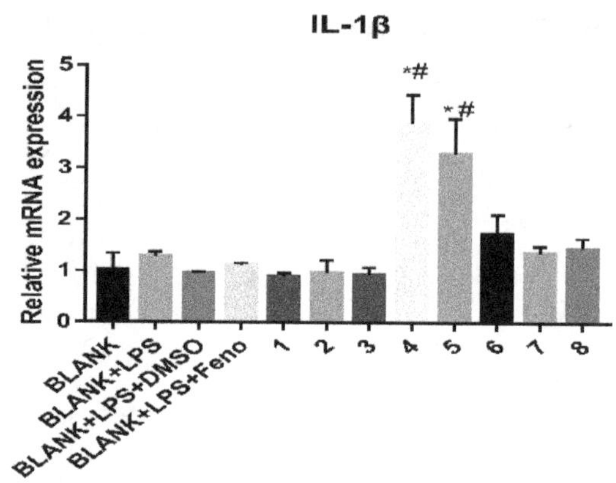

(B)

Figure 5. The influence of eight compounds on immuno-regulation factors over a period of 24 h. (**A**) for the factor *TNF-α* and (**B**) for the factor *IL-1β*. The "*" indicates that there were significant differences ($p < 0.05$) between other compounds and the BLANK group amd the "#" indicates that there were significant differences ($p < 0.05$) between other compounds and the BLANK + LPS group. Each value represented the means ± SD of three independent experiments.

3. Materials and Methods

3.1. General Experimental Procedures

Optical rotations were recorded in MeOH using a JASCO P-1020 Polarimeter (Jasco Corp., Tokyo, Japan). UV spectra were acquired in MeOH with a Shimadzu UV-2401PC UV-VIS spectrophotometer (Shimadzu Corp., Kyoto, Japan). IR spectra were measured on a Bruker Tensor 27 FTIR Spectrometer with KBr disks (Bruker Corp., Karlsruhe, Germany). ^{1}H-NMR, ^{13}C-NMR, and 2D NMR spectra were recorded in $CDCl_3$ using a Bruker AVANCE III-600 spectrometer or a Bruker DRX-400 spectrometer (Bruker Corp., St. Gallen, Switzerland). TMS was used as the internal standard. ESI-MS spectra were recorded using a Waters Xevo TQ-S Ultra High Pressure Liquid Chromatography Triple Quadrupole Mass Spectrometer (Waters Corp., Manchester, UK). HR-ESI-MS data were obtained using an Agilent G6230 Q-TOF mass instrument (Agilent Corp., Santa Clara, CA, USA). Column chromatography (CC) was performed using a silica gel (200–300 mesh, Qingdao Marine Chemical Inc., Qingdao, China), MCI gel CHP 20P (75–150 μm, Mitsubishi Corp., Tokyo, Japan), and Sephadex LH-20 (25–100 mm, Pharmacia Biotech Ltd., Uppsala, Sweden). Thin-layer chromatography (TLC) was performed using pre-coated silica gel GF254 plates (0.25 mm in thickness for analysis and 0.60 mm thickness for preparation, Qingdao Marine Chemical Inc., Qingdao, China) with various solvent systems. Spots were visualized under UV light (254 nm) and colored by iodine and by spraying silica gel plates with 10% H_2SO_4 in MeOH followed by heating. Preparative HPLC separations were performed on a CXTH system equipped with a UV3000 detector (Beijing Chuangxintongheng Instruments Co. Ltd., Beijing, China), and a Kromasil C_{18} column (250 mm × 20 mm i.d., 5 mm, EKA Chemicals Corp., Bohus, Sweden) using a flow rate of 8.0 mL/min at a column temperature of 25 °C. Semi-preparative HPLC was conducted on a HITACHI Chromaster system (Hitachi Ltd., Tokyo, Japan) equipped with an Agilent ZORBAXSB-C_{18} column (150 mm × 9.4 mm i.d., 5 mm, Agilent Corp., Santa Clara, CA, USA) using a flow rate of 3.0 mL/min at a column temperature of 25 °C. The detection was performed with a DAD detector.

3.2. Plant Material

The aerial parts of *Dryopteris fragrans* (L.) Schott were collected in June 2016 from the Wudalianchi scenic area, Heihe City, Helongjiang Province, China and identified by Prof. Baodong Liu from the

Harbin Normal University. A voucher specimen (No. df-20070702-9) was deposited in the Plant Herbarium of Northeast Agricultural University in Harbin, China.

3.3. Determination of Anti-Tumor Fraction of *Dryopteris fragrans*

After methanol extraction, the crude extract was then partitioned with petroleum ether (rt), dichloromethane (DCM) (rt), EtOAc (rt), and n-BuOH (rt) in sequence. The crude extract was divided into six parts (the whole extracts, petroleum ether layer, DCM layer, EtOAc layer, n-BuOH layer, and water phase). Each fraction was dissolved in DMSO and the final concentration of DMSO in the cell culture medium was no more than 0.1%. The osteosarcoma cell lines HOS and MG63 were used as the first round screening target in MTT [14] for the above six parts of the crude extracts. As shown in Figure S1, petroleum ether fraction of crude extracts had the most obvious cytotoxic effects at the point of 48 h. The petroleum ether fraction was then divided into 14 sub-fractions (Fr SG1-SG14) by using silica gel column chromatography. The above 14 fractions were then subjected to MTT or CCK-8 assay [15] against HepG2, MB231, and MG63 cell lines, respectively. As shown in Figure S2, Fractions SG1–SG7 from the petroleum ether-soluble part exhibited prominent cytotoxic activities.

3.4. Extraction and Isolation

The air-dried aerial parts of *Dryopteris fragrans* (L.) Schott powder (2 kg) were extracted with 100% methanol (20 L × 2 d × 3) and ultrasonized (40 Hz) for 4 h at each time. After filtration, the filtrate was concentrated to yield the crude extract. The crude extract was then suspended in water (1.5 L) and partitioned with petroleum ether (3 × 1.5 L), DCM (3 × 1.5 L), EtOAc (3 × 1.5 L), and n-BuOH (3 × 1.5 L) sequentially. Guided by the first round cytotoxicity screening, the petroleum ether fraction (54 g) was chosen for further isolation. The petroleum ether-soluble part was then subjected to silica gel CC and eluted with petroleum ether–EtOAc (1:0–0:1) to create 14 fractions (SG1–SG14). According to the second round cytotoxicity screening, Fractions SG1–SG7 were selected as the isolation targets for the next step. Fractions SG1 and SG2 were not actually involved in the next step because their low polarities made an effective separation on column chromatography difficult.

Fraction SG3 (5.93 g) was submitted to the silica gel CC (petroleum ether–EtOAc 1:0–0:1) and Sephadex LH-20 CC (MeOH–$CHCl_3$ 1:1) and followed by preparative TLC (petroleum ether–EtOAc 11:2, Rf = 0.53) to afford compound **4** (14.4 mg). Compound **5** (103.2 mg) was isolated from Fraction SG4 (5.01 g) by undergoing a protocol of repeated silica gel CC (petroleum ether–EtOAc 1:0–10:1), Sephadex LH-20 CC (MeOH–CHCl3 1:1), and preparative TLC (petroleum ether–EtOAc 8:1, Rf = 0.40). Fraction SG6 (3.54 g) was chromatographed on MCI CC (MeOH–H_2O 40:60 to 100:0) to yield 16 sub-fractions (Fr M1–M16). Further purification of Fr. M6 by semi-preparative HPLC (MeOH: H_2O 53:47) resulted in the isolation of compounds **6** (15.8 mg) and **7** (10.0 mg). Fraction SG7 (2.49 g) was further separated by MCI CC (MeOH–H_2O 20:80 to 100:0) to yield 11 fractions (Fr. M_21–M_211). Compound **1** (4.5 mg) was purified from Fraction M_24 using semi-preparative HPLC (MeOH:H_2O 58:42). In the same way, compound **8** (2.0 mg) was obtained from Fraction M_27. Compounds **2** and **3** were obtained as a mixture (17.0 mg) from Fraction M_26 by semi-preparative HPLC (MeOH:H_2O 77:23). They were separated by a silicon etherification-desilication procedure (See Section 3.5).

Dryofragone (**1**): yellow powder ($CHCl_3$). $[\alpha]_D^{23.7}$ −20.3 (*c* 0.10, MeOH); UV (MeOH) λ_{max} (log ε): 198 (3.17) nm, 241 (3.38) nm, 276 (3.20) nm, 320 (3.14) nm, IR (KBr) ν_{max} IR (KBr) ν_{max} 3321, 2929, 1714, 1607, 1533, 1442, 1231, 1104; ^{1}H-NMR (600 MHz, $CDCl_3$): δ_H 5.37 (1H, s, H-4), 3.91 (3H, s, Me-12), 2.99 (1H, m, H-8a), 2.92 (1H ,m, H-8b), 1.69 (2H, m, H-9), 1.54 (3H, s, Me-11), 1.01 (3H, t, *J* = 7.4 Hz, Me-10); 203.7 (C-7), 196.3 (C-1), 189.4 (C-5), 176.0 (C-3), 104.5 (C-6), 94.5 (C-4), 75.4 (C-2), 57.4 (C-12), 41.0 (C-8), 30.2 (C-11), 18.7 (C-9),14.1 (C-10), ESI-MS *m/z* 239 $[M-H]^-$, and HR-ESI-MS *m/z* 239.0926 $[M-H]^-$ (calcd for $C_{12}H_{15}O_5$, 239.0925).

3.5. Silicon Etherification Involved Isolation of 2 and 3

3.5.1. Silicon Etherification of the Mixture of Compounds **2** and **3**

With regard to the solution of the mixture of Compounds **2** and **3** (17 mg, 0.068 mmol) in dry DCM (0.5 mL), 2,6-luditine (30 µL, 0.27 mmol, 4.0 equiv) was added at 0 °C, which is followed by the addition of TBSOTf (35 µL, 0.17 mmol, 2.5 equiv). The resulting mixture was warmed to room temperature (rt) naturally, stirred for 6 h, and then quenched with water (2.0 mL). The mixture was then stirred for 10 min, followed by an extraction with EtOAc (10.0 mL) three times, and the EtOAc layer was dried over anhydrous Na_2SO_4 and subsequently concentrated. The residue was further purified by semi-preparative HPLC (85% MeOH in H_2O, 3 mL/min, a HITACHI Chromaster system equipped with a DAD detector, an Agilent ZORBAX SB-C_{18} column, 150 mm × 9.4 mm i.d., 5 µm) to yield compound **2a** (6.8 mg, t_R = 19.8 min) and **3a** (4.2 mg, t_R = 15.8 min) as white solids. Compound **2a**: ^{1}H-NMR (400 MHz, $CDCl_3$): δ_H 7.17 (1H, s, H-5), 6.18 (1H, s, H-3), 3.91 (3H, s, Me-15), 3.24 (1H, m, H-11), 2.29 (3H, s, Me-14), 1.30 (6H, d, J = 6.8 Hz, Me-12, 13), 1.03 (9H, s, Me-19, 20, 21), 0.24 (6H, s, Me-16, 17), ^{13}C-NMR (100 MHz, $CDCl_3$): δ_C 162.5 (C-4), 161.7 (C-2), 150.1 (C-7), 146.9 (C-10), 138.3 (C-8), 126.5 (C-6), 119.5 (C-5), 113.4 (C-9), 108.5 (C-3), 61.1 (C-15), 28.7 (C-11), 26.1 × 3 (C-19, 20, 21), 22.1 × 2 (C-12, 13), 19.0 (C-18), 17.7 (C-14), −4.0 × 2 (C-16, 17). Compound **3a**: ^{1}H-NMR (400 MHz, $CDCl_3$): δ_H 7.07 (1H, s, H-5), 6.21 (1H, s, H-3), 3.82 (3H, s, Me-15), 3.24 (1H, m, H-11), 2.32 (3H, s, Me-14), 1.30 (6H, d, J = 6.8 Hz, Me-12, 13), 1.08 (9H, s, Me-19, 20, 21), 0.25 (6H, s, Me-16, 17), ^{13}C-NMR (100 MHz, $CDCl_3$): δ_C 162.2 (C-4), 161.4 (C-2), 152.5 (C-7), 145.3 (C-10), 137.2 (C-8), 127.8 (C-6), 117.0 (C-5), 115.4 (C-9), 109.8 (C-3), 60.2 (C-15), 28.7 (C-11), 25.9 × 3 (C-19, 20, 21), 22.1 × 2 (C-12, 13), 18.8 (C-18), 16.4 (C-14), −4.2 × 2 (C-16, 17).

3.5.2. Desilication of Compound **2a**

To a solution of compound **2a** (6.8 mg, 0.0188 mmol) in dry THF (0.1 mL), TBAF (1 M in THF, 19 µL, 0.0197 mmol, 1.05 equiv) was added at 0 °C. The resulting mixture was stirred at 0 °C for 5 min and then quenched by adding 1.0 mL of the saturated ammonium chloride aqueous solution. The resulting mixture was then extracted by EtOAc (5.0 mL) three times and the combined organic extracts were dried over anhydrous Na_2SO_4 and were then concentrated. The residue was purified by using flash column chromatography on the silica gel (200–300 mush, 1.0 × 3.0 cm, petroleum ether/EtOAc 4:1), which yielded compound **2** (4.5 mg, 96.6% yield) as a white solid. Compound **2**: UV (MeOH) λ_{max} (log ε): 206 (3.81) nm, 218 (3.52) nm, 250 (2.78) nm, 330 (3.29) nm; IR (KBr) ν_{max} 3548, 3466, 3169, 2942, 1668, 1602, 1460, 1404, 1229, 1094, 1024, 925, 856; ^{1}H-NMR (600 MHz, $CDCl_3$): δ_H 7.17 (1H, s, H-5), 6.16 (1H, s, H-3), 4.08 (3H, s, Me-15), 3.25 (1H, m, H-11), 2.31 (3H, s, Me-14), 1.30 (3H, d, J = 6.8 Hz, Me-12), 1.30 (3H, d, J = 6.8 Hz, Me-13); ^{13}C-NMR (150 MHz, $CDCl_3$): δ_C 163.0 (C-4), 161.5 (C-2), 150.0 (C-7), 145.5 (C-10), 133.6 (C-8), 121.1 (C-6), 120.0 (C-5), 112.2 (C-9), 107.8 (C-3), 61.9 (C-15), 28.7 (C-11), 22.1 (C-12), 22.1 (C-13), 15.9 (C-14), HR-ESI-MS: m/z 247.0975[M − H]$^-$, calcd. 247.0976 for $C_{14}H_{15}O_4$.

3.5.3. Desilication of Compound **3a**

To a solution of compound **3a** (4.2 mg, 0.0116 mmol) in dry THF (0.1 mL), TBAF (1 M in THF, 12 µL, 0.0121 mmol, 1.05 equiv) was added at 0 °C. The resulting mixture was stirred at 0 °C for 5 min and then quenched by adding 1.0 mL of saturated ammonium chloride aqueous solution. The resulting mixture was then extracted by EtOAc (5.0 mL) three times and the combined organic extracts were dried over anhydrous Na_2SO_4 and concentrated. The residue was purified by flash column chromatography on the silica gel (200–300 mush, 1.0 × 3.0 cm, petroleum ether/EtOAc 4:1), which yielded compound **3** (2.8 mg, 97.4% yield) as a white solid. Compound **3**: ^{1}H-NMR (600 MHz, $CDCl_3$): δ_H 7.01 (1H, s, H-5), 6.22 (1H, s, H-3), 3.95 (3H, s, Me-15), 3.25 (1H, m, H-11), 2.32 (3H, s, Me-14), 1.31 (6H, d, J = 6.8 Hz, Me-12, 13); ^{13}C-NMR (150 MHz, $CDCl_3$): δ_C 163.0 (C-4), 161.1 (C-2),

147.8 (C-7), 141.3 (C-10), 136.7 (C-8), 127.5 (C-6), 115.5 (C-5), 114.5 (C-9), 109.2 (C-3), 60.5 (C-15), 28.7 (C-11), 21.9 (C-12 & C-13), and 16.3 (C-14).

3.6. MTT and CCK-8 Assay

Human HepG2, HeLa, U251, HOS, MG63, U2OS, MB231, and SKBR-3 cells were obtained from the Cell Library of Committee on Type Culture Collection of Chinese Academy of Sciences (Shanghai, China). Cells were cultured at 37 °C, 5% CO_2 in the Dulbecco's Modified Eagle's medium (DMEM), Minimum Eagle's medium (MEM), or the Roswell Park Memorial Institute (RPMI) medium containing 10% FBS, 100 U/mL penicillin, and 100 U/mL streptomycin.

Compounds **1–8** were dissolved in DMSO and diluted with DMEM medium (containing 1% FBS and 100 U/mL penicillin/streptomycin) for certain concentrations (1.5625 μM, 3.125 μM, 6.25 μM, 12.5 μM, 25 μM, 50 μM, and 100 μM). The concentration of DMSO in the final solutions was no more than 0.1%. Human HepG2, HeLa, U251, HOS, MG63, U2OS, MB231, and SKBR-3 cells were seeded in 96-well micro-titer plates (100 μL, 1×10^4 cells/well). When the cells grew to certain concentrations (70%–80% of the well), the medium was removed and the diluted compounds (200 μL) were added to each well. Blank (only medium) and control (cells with DMEM medium) group were set to calculate the cell viability and Taxol was used as a positive control. After 48 h, the 96-well micro-titer plates were taken out from the incubator and the medium was removed. When using the MTT assay, DMEM medium (200 μL) should be first added into the well and then followed by MTT (20 μL, 5 mg/mL dissolved in PBS). After culturing for 4 h, the 96-well micro-titer plates were taken out from the incubator and the medium was removed and then 150 μL of DMSO was added into the well. The absorbance was measured by a microplate reader (Bio-Rad, America) at 560 nm. When using CCK-8 assay, DMEM medium (100 μL) should be first added into the well and then CCK-8 (Dojindo, Kumamoto, Japan) followed. After culturing for 2.5 h, the 96-well micro-titer plates were taken out from the incubator and the absorbance was measured by a microplate reader at 450 nm. The cell viability = (Lab group − Blank group)/(Control group − Blank group) and the IC_{50} value was calculated by the software GraphPad Prism 7.0 with the cell viability value.

3.7. Immunoregulation Activity

THP-1 cells were obtained from the Harbin medical university and was cultured in RPMI medium. The cell was seeded in 6-well plate (2 mL, 2×10^6 cell/well) and starved for 12 h. Lipopolysaccharide (LPS, Sigma, St. Louis, MI, USA) (2 mg/mL in PBS) was then added in the well to stimulate the cell. One hour later, each compound was dissolved in DMSO at a concentration of 20 μM. It was added in the well and cultivated for 24 h. The cell was then collected. Following the manufacturer's instructions, the Trizol reagent (Invitrogen, Carlsbad, CA, USA) was used to isolate the total RNA of THP-1 cell. The extracted total RNA was dissolved in RNA enzyme-free water and added into a 100 μL reaction mixture for reverse transcription into complementary DNA (cDNA). The extracted RNA solution contained 8 μg, 8 μL of 50 pmol/μL Oligo d(T)18 and the volume was brought up to 46 μL with RNA enzyme-free water, incubated at 70 °C for 5 min, and then 4 °C for 5 min. Afterward, 20 μL of 2.5 μmol/mL dNTP, 20 μL of 5× RT buffer, 8 μL of dTT, 2 μL of RNA inhibitor, and 4 μL of M-MLV were added and the mixture was incubated at 42 °C for 3 h. The 100 μL mixture was stored at −20 °C for qualitative PCR (qPCR). Detected via qPCR, the gene expression levels were identified with a LightCycler® 480 System (Roche, Basel, Switzerland) using the TransStart® Tip Green qPCR SuperMix (TRANSGEN BIOTECH, Beijing, China). The cDNA was added into a 20 μL reaction mixture: 10 μL of 2× TransStart® Tip Green qPCR SuperMix, 2 μL of cDNA Template (100–200 pg), 0.8 μL of primer mixture (10 μM), 0.4 μL of Passive Reference Dye (50×), and 6.8 μL of ddH_2O. The PCR procedure includes a temperature of 94 °C and a time period of 30 s followed by 40 cycles at 94 °C for 5 s, 57 °C for 15 s, and 72 °C for 10 s. The β-actin gene was used a control to quantify other genes. The results were calculated using $2^{-\Delta\Delta Ct}$ where $\Delta\Delta Ct$ = (Ct Target − Ct β-actin)Lab − (Ct Target − Ct β-actin) Control. Primers of the target gene TNF-α, IL-1β, and β-actin were designed by Primer 5.0 software following the published gene sequence in GenBank: TNF-α Forward: CAGCAAGGGACAGCAGAGG, Reverse: AGTATGTGAGAGGAAGAGAACC; IL-1β Forward: TGATGGCTTATTACAGTGGCAATG, Reverse: TGATGGCTTATTACAGTGGCAATG; β-actin Forward: ATCGGCAATGAGCGGTTCC, Reverse: ATCGGCAATGAGCGGTTCC.

4. Conclusions

In this work, two new phenolic derivatives dryofragone (**1**) and dryofracoumarin B (**2**) were isolated from *Dryopteris fragrans* by cytotoxicity-guided tracking. Two coumarin isomers dryofracoumarin B (**2**) and dryofracoumarin A (**3**) were separated by a silicon etherification-desilication procedure. Compounds (**4**) and (**6**) were first reported in this plant. The cytotoxicity and immuno-regulation activity were examined among the eight compounds and the relationship between cytotoxicity and immuno-regulation activity revealed that compounds may activate the LPS signaling to regulate the growth of tumor cells through immuno-regulation. This relation needs further study.

Author Contributions: S.-X.H. and Y.C. handled the conceptualization. T.Z. managed the data curation. T.Z. performed a formal analysis. S.-X.H. and Y.C. handled the funding acquisition. T.Z., L.W., D.-H.D., and Y.-H.Z. were responsible for the methodology. L.W. handled the software. S.-X.H. and Y.C. supervised the project. T.Z. wrote the original draft. Writing—review & editing, L.W. took part in reviewing and editing the manuscript.

Acknowledgments: This work received no external funding and was financially supported by the National Natural Science Foundation of China (No. 81522044 to S.-X.H.), the Applied Basic Research Foundation of Yunnan Province (No. 2013HA022 to S.-X.H.), Foundation from Chinese Academy of Sciences (QYZDB-SSW-SMC051 to S.-X.H.), and the National Natural Science Foundation of China (No. 31570189 to Y.C.). We appreciate the help of Yunzhou Wu and Wenfei Wang in this work.

References

1. Kuang, H.; Zhang, Y.; Li, G.; Zeng, W.; Wang, H.; Song, Q. A new phenolic glycoside from the aerial parts of *Dryopteris fragrans*. *Fitoterapia* **2008**, *79*, 319–320. [CrossRef] [PubMed]
2. Patama, T.T.; Widen, C.J. Phloroglucinol derivatives from *Dryopteris fuscoatra* and *D. hawaiiensis*. *Phytochemistry* **1991**, *30*, 3305–3310. [CrossRef]
3. Zhao, D.D.; Zhao, Q.S.; Liu, L.; Chen, Z.Q.; Zeng, W.M.; Lei, H.; Zhang, Y.L. Compounds from *Dryopteris fragrans* (L.) Schott with cytotoxic activity. *Molecules* **2014**, *19*, 3345–3355. [CrossRef] [PubMed]
4. Huang, Y.H.; Zeng, W.M.; Li, G.Y.; Liu, G.Q.; Zhao, D.D.; Wang, J.; Zhang, Y.L. Characterization of a new sesquiterpene and antifungal activities of chemical constituents from *Dryopteris fragrans* (L.) Schott. *Molecules* **2013**, *19*, 507–513. [CrossRef] [PubMed]
5. Ito, H.; Muranaka, T.; Mori, K.; Jin, Z.X.; Tokuda, H.; Nishino, H.; Yoshida, T. Ichthyotoxic phloroglucinol derivatives from *Dryopteris fragrans* and their anti-tumor promoting activity. *Chem. Pharm. Bull.* **2000**, *31*, 1190–1195. [CrossRef]
6. Peng, B.; Bai, R.F.; Li, P.; Han, X.Y.; Wang, H.; Zhu, C.C.; Zeng, Z.P.; Chai, X.Y. Two new glycosides from *Dryopteris fragrans* with anti-inflammatory activities. *J. Asian Nat. Prod. Res.* **2016**, *18*, 59–64. [CrossRef] [PubMed]
7. Li, X.J.; Wang, W.; Luo, M.; Li, C.Y.; Zu, Y.G.; Mu, P.S.; Fu, Y.J. Solvent-free microwave extraction of essential oil from *Dryopteris fragrans* and evaluation of antioxidant activity. *Food Chem.* **2012**, *133*, 437–444. [CrossRef] [PubMed]
8. Zhang, Y.; Luo, M.; Zu, Y.; Fu, Y.; Gu, C.; Wang, W.; Yao, L.; Efferth, T. Dryofragin, a phloroglucinol derivative, induces apoptosis in human breast cancer MCF-7 cells through ROS-mediated mitochondrial pathway. *Chem. Biol. Interact.* **2012**, *199*, 129–136. [CrossRef] [PubMed]
9. Wan, D.; Jiang, C.; Hua, X.; Wang, T.; Chai, Y. Cell cycle arrest and apoptosis induced by aspidin PB through the p53/p21 and mitochondria-dependent pathways in human osteosarcoma cells. *Anti Cancer Drugs* **2015**, *26*, 931–941. [CrossRef] [PubMed]

10. Su, Y.; Wan, D.; Song, W. Dryofragin inhibits the migration and invasion of human osteosarcoma U2OS cells by suppressing MMP-2/9 and elevating TIMP-1/2 through PI3K/AKT and p38 MAPK signaling pathways. *Anti Cancer Drugs* **2016**, *27*, 660–668. [CrossRef] [PubMed]
11. Sun, Y.; Gao, C.; Luo, M.; Wang, W.; Gu, C.; Zu, Y.; Li, J.; Efferth, T.; Fu, Y. Aspidin PB, a phloroglucinol derivative, induces apoptosis in human hepatocarcinoma HepG2 cells by modulating PI3K/Akt/GSK3β pathway. *Chem. Biol. Interact.* **2013**, *201*, 1–8. [CrossRef] [PubMed]
12. Sun, Y.; Mu, F.; Li, C.; Wang, W.; Luo, M.; Fu, Y.; Zu, Y. Aspidin BB, a phloroglucinol derivative, induces cell cycle arrest and apoptosis in human ovarian HO-8910 cells. *Chem. Biol. Interact.* **2013**, *204*, 88–97. [CrossRef] [PubMed]
13. Zhong, Z.C.; Zhao, D.D.; Liu, Z.D.; Jiang, S.; Zhang, Y.L. A new human cancer cell proliferation inhibition sesquiterpene, dryofraterpene A, from medicinal plant *Dryopteris fragrans* (L.) Schott. *Molecules* **2017**, *22*, 180. [CrossRef] [PubMed]
14. Elisia, I.; Popovich, D.G.; Hu, C.; Kitts, D.D. Evaluation of viability assays for anthocyanins in cultured cells. *Phytochem. Anal.* **2008**, *19*, 479–486. [CrossRef] [PubMed]
15. Kang, D.; Gong, Y.; Zhu, Y.; Li, A.; Dong, N.; Piao, Y.; Yuan, Y. The biological activity of *H. pylori* SlyD in vitro. *Helicobacter* **2013**, *18*, 347–355. [CrossRef] [PubMed]
16. Cho, J.G.; Lee, D.Y.; Lee, J.W.; Lee, D.G.; Lee, Y.H.; Kim, S.Y.; Kim, S.H. Acyclic diterpenoids from the leaves of *Capsicum annuum*. *J. Korean Soc. Appl. Biol. Chem.* **2009**, *52*, 128–132. [CrossRef]
17. Amzad, H.M. Synthesis of 2′,4′-dihydroxy-6′-methoxy-3′,5′-dimethylchalcone. *Bangladesh J. Sci. Ind. Res.* **2001**, *36*, 50–54.
18. Ayräs, P.; Lötjönen, S.; Widén, C.J. NMR spectroscopy of naturally occurring phloroglucinol derivatives. *Planta Med.* **1981**, *42*, 187–194. [CrossRef] [PubMed]
19. Lobo-Echeverri, T.; Rivero-Cruz, J.F.; Su, B.N.; Chai, H.B.; Cordell, G.A.; Pezzuto, J.M.; Swanson, S.M.; Soejarto, D.D.; Kinghorn, A.D. Constituents of the leaves and twigs of *Calyptranthes pallens* collected from an experimental plot in Southern Florida. *J. Nat. Prod.* **2005**, *68*, 577–580. [CrossRef] [PubMed]
20. Ito, T.; Nisa, K.; Rakainsa, S.K.; Lallo, S.; Morita, H. New phloroglucinol derivatives from Indonesian *Baeckea frutescens*. *Tetrahedron* **2017**, *73*, 1177–1181. [CrossRef]
21. Yang, L.; Guo, H.; Li, Y.; Meng, X.; Yan, L.; Dan, Z.; Wu, S.; Zhou, H.; Peng, L.; Xie, Q.; et al. Oleoylethanolamide exerts anti-inflammatory effects on LPS-induced THP-1 cells by enhancing PPARα signaling and inhibiting the NF-κB and ERK1/2/AP-1/STAT3 pathways. *Sci. Rep.* **2016**, *6*, 34611. [CrossRef] [PubMed]

7

Phenolic Compounds from *Humulus lupulus* as Natural Antimicrobial Products: New Weapons in the Fight against Methicillin Resistant *Staphylococcus aureus*, *Leishmania mexicana* and *Trypanosoma brucei* Strains

Laetitia Bocquet [1], Sevser Sahpaz [1], Natacha Bonneau [1], Claire Beaufay [2], Séverine Mahieux [3], Jennifer Samaillie [1], Vincent Roumy [1], Justine Jacquin [1], Simon Bordage [1], Thierry Hennebelle [1], Feng Chai [4], Joëlle Quetin-Leclercq [2], Christel Neut [3] and Céline Rivière [1,*]

1 EA 7394—ICV, Charles Viollette Research Institute, SFR Condorcet FR CNRS 3417, Univ. Lille, INRA, ISA-Yncréa, Univ. Artois, Univ. Littoral Côte d'Opale, 3 rue du Professeur Laguesse, 59000 Lille, France; laetitia.bocquet1309@gmail.com (L.B.); sevser.sahpaz@univ-lille.fr (S.S.); natacha.bonneau@univ-lille.fr (N.B.); jennifer.samaillie@univ-lille.fr (J.S.); vincent.roumy@univ-lille.fr (V.R.); justine.jacquin@yncrea.fr (J.J.); simon.bordage@univ-lille.fr (S.B.); thierry.hennebelle@univ-lille.fr (T.H.)

2 Pharmacognosy Research group, Louvain Drug Research Institute, Université Catholique de Louvain, 1200 Brussels, Belgium; claire.beaufay@uclouvain.be (C.B.); joelle.leclercq@uclouvain.be (J.Q.-L.)

3 U995—LIRIC, Lille Inflammation Research International Center, Univ. Lille, Inserm, CHU Lille, 59000 Lille, France; severine.mahieux@univ-lille.fr (S.M.); christel.neut@univ-lille.fr (C.N.)

4 U1008—Controlled Drug Delivery Systems and Biomaterials, Univ. Lille, Inserm, CHU Lille, 59000 Lille, France; feng.chai@univ-lille.fr

* Correspondence: celine.riviere@univ-lille.fr;

Academic Editor: Pinarosa Avato

Abstract: New anti-infective agents are urgently needed to fight microbial resistance. Methicillin-resistant *Staphylococcus aureus* (MRSA) strains are particularly responsible for complicated pathologies that are difficult to treat due to their virulence and the formation of persistent biofilms forming a complex protecting shell. Parasitic infections caused by *Trypanosoma brucei* and *Leishmania mexicana* are also of global concern, because of the mortality due to the low number of safe and effective treatments. Female inflorescences of hop produce specialized metabolites known for their antimicrobial effects but underexploited to fight against drug-resistant microorganisms. In this study, we assessed the antimicrobial potential of phenolic compounds against MRSA clinical isolates, *T. brucei* and *L. mexicana*. By fractionation process, we purified the major prenylated chalcones and acylphloroglucinols, which were quantified by UHPLC-UV in different plant parts, showing their higher content in the active flowers extract. Their potent antibacterial action (MIC < 1 μg/mL for the most active compound) was demonstrated against MRSA strains, through kill curves, post-antibiotic effects, anti-biofilm assays and synergy studies with antibiotics. An antiparasitic activity was also shown for some purified compounds, particularly on *T. brucei* (IC_{50} < 1 to 11 μg/mL). Their cytotoxic activity was assessed both on cancer and non-cancer human cell lines.

Keywords: *Humulus lupulus*; prenylated phenolic compounds; antimicrobial agents; methicillin-resistant *Staphylococcus aureus*; *Leishmania mexicana mexicana*; *Trypanosoma brucei brucei*

1. Introduction

Multidrug-resistant microorganisms are rapidly spreading throughout the world leading to treatment failures [1]. Antibacterial resistance in humans is affected by an inappropriate or excessive use of antibiotics in human health but is also partially affected by the use of antibiotics in animal-rearing. Some national action plans, such as restrictive measures of antibiotic use in human and animal health, are now imposed in all parts of the world but the problem of antimicrobial resistance is far from being solved [2,3]. Therefore, the discovery of new antimicrobial compounds is crucial.

Several plant-derived natural products, characterized by a huge structural diversity, including phenolic compounds, are cited as antimicrobial agents and resistance-modifying agents (RMAs) [4]. They could constitute a valuable interim solution, until new classes of antibiotics are discovered [5].

Methicillin-resistant *Staphylococcus aureus* (MRSA) strains are considered as a very urgent health problem because of their propagation in the last 15 years in the elderly and in immunocompromised patients, mainly due to their increasing implication in nosocomial infections and the lack of development of new antimicrobials. In 2016, the percentage of MRSA among all *S. aureus* isolates remained above 25% in several countries in Southern Europe and greater than 15% in France, especially for invasive isolates [6]. MRSA is also one of the principal multi-resistant bacterial pathogen responsible for complicated skin and hospital-acquired infections, associated with high mortality rates [7,8]. Furthermore, these strains are very often involved in infections of diabetic foot ulcers characterized by frequent complications and risks of lower-limb amputations [9]. *S. aureus* has the ability, like most Gram-positive organisms, to acquire resistance to practically all useful antibiotics. Several mechanisms can explain this resistance: modification of target sites, enzymatic degradation or structural modification of antibiotics and, expression of efflux pumps [5,10–12]. These bacteria also produce virulence factors involved in pathogenesis like adhesion and biofilm formation, which enhance bacterial resistance [13,14].

On the other hand, many parasitic infections deserve a special attention due to the lack of effective treatments. *Trypanosoma brucei* is a parasite conveyed by the tsetse fly and responsible for the Human African Trypanosomiasis (HAT) or sleeping sickness. This fatal disease if untreated leads to central nervous system disturbances, including sensory, motor and psychic troubles and neuroendocrine abnormalities [15,16]. Leishmaniasis, caused by different *Leishmania* species, is responsible for chronic skin and visceral diseases transmitted by sand-flies [17].

Hop (*Humulus lupulus* L.) is a climbing dioecious plant belonging to the Cannabaceae family. This species is cultivated worldwide for its female inflorescences (cones), usually called "hops", which are used in the brewing industry. The compounds sought by brewers are prenylated acylphloroglucinol derivatives, also called bitter acids and in particular α-acids (humulone derivatives) which are isomerized into iso-α-acids during the brewing process. These compounds confer some bitterness and antiseptic properties to beer [18]. This plant is also known to have many pharmacological activities, including sedative, oestrogenic, anti-inflammatory, chemopreventive and antimicrobial activities [19]. The antimicrobial activity is mainly attributed to prenylated acylphloroglucinols, in particular to α-acids and β-acids (lupulone derivatives) and to prenylated chalcones, including xanthohumol (Figure 1) [20–22]. Few studies, however, describe the activity of this plant and especially of its specialized metabolites against multidrug resistant strains [14,23] and parasites [24,25]. In addition, the mechanisms of the inhibitory activities observed are not really expanded upon now.

In this context, we studied the antimicrobial potential of hop phenolic compounds against MRSA strains, *Trypanosoma brucei brucei* (Tbb) and *Leishmania mexicana mexicana* (Lmm). We opted for a fractionation using Centrifugal Partition Chromatography (CPC) and preparative High-Performance Liquid Chromatography (HPLC) to purify the major antimicrobial phenolic compounds from the most active sub-extract of hop. Purified compounds were then quantified in hop extracts. Their antibacterial potential against MRSA clinical isolates was assessed. The most promising compounds were then selected for further experiments in order to strengthen our knowledge of their action on the bacterial strains, through kill curves, post-antibiotic effects, anti-biofilm and synergy assays. The antiparasitic activity of some chalcones and acylphloroglucinols against Tbb and Lmm was also evaluated. Their cytotoxicity activity was determined on various human cell lines.

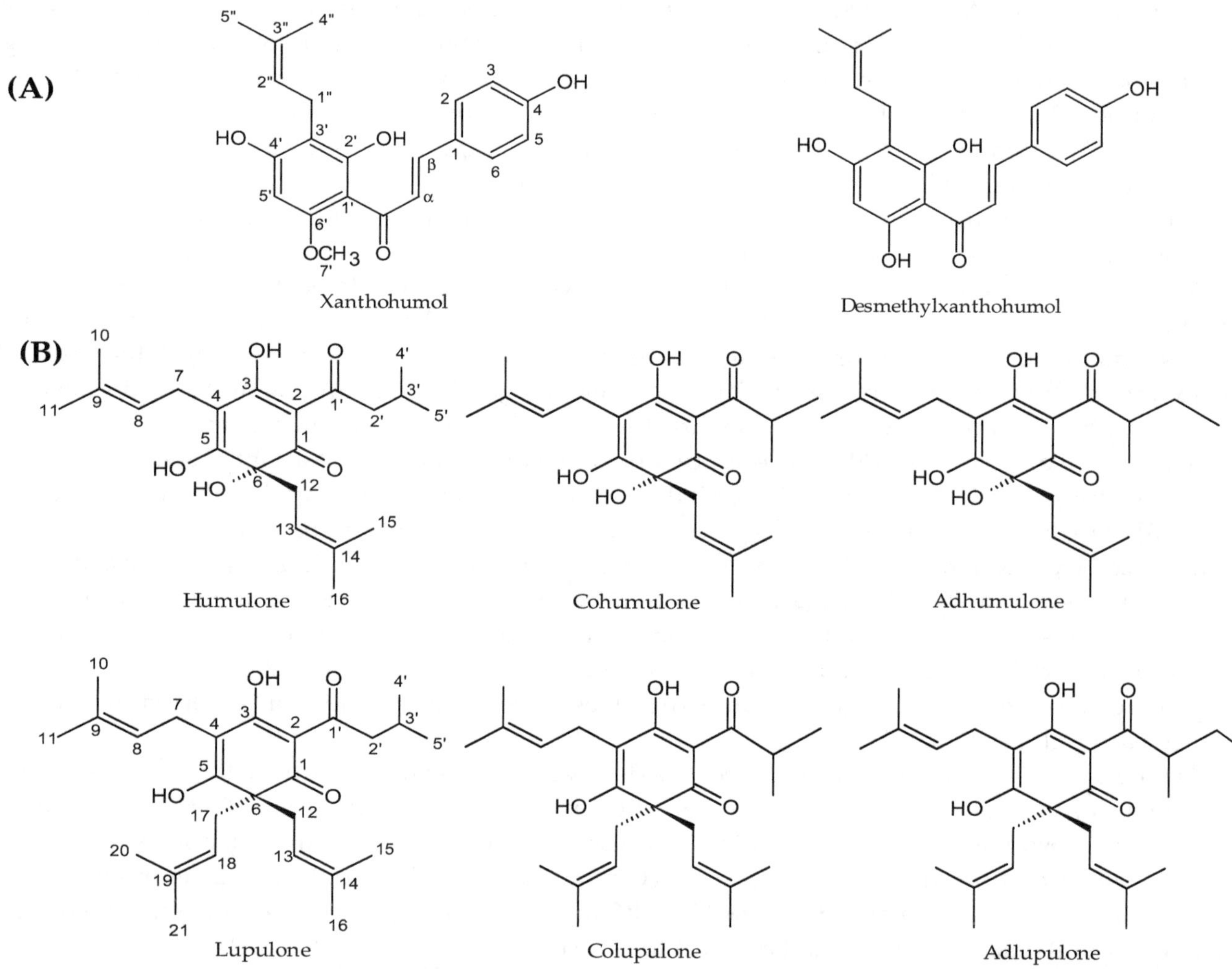

Figure 1. Structures of the main prenylated phenolic compounds from hops. (**A**) prenylated chalcones (**B**) acylphloroglucinol derivatives.

2. Results

2.1. Antimicrobial Activity of Hop Extracts and Sub-Extracts against Gram-Positive and Gram-Negative Bacteria and Parasites

We evaluated the antimicrobial activity of hop extracts and sub-extracts towards bacterial clinical isolates and parasites (Tbb and Lmm).

We first confirmed the antibacterial activity of the crude hydro-ethanolic extract of cones against Gram-positive bacteria, namely *Corynebacterium*, *Enterococcus*, *Mycobacterium*, *Staphylococcus* and *Streptococcus* strains, with MICs ranging from 39 to 156 μg/mL (Table 1). Some yeasts have also been studied. On the 36 *Candida albicans* strains tested (data not shown), only the two presented in Table 1 were susceptible to our extracts. Leaves, stems and rhizomes showed a weak antimicrobial activity. The liquid-liquid fractionation of the most active crude extract (cones) with dichloromethane

(DCM) and water led to set up a second screening only focused on Gram-positive bacteria (Table 2). This partition also led us to direct the activity towards non-polar compounds as the non-polar sub-extract was indeed more active than the crude extract. Enterococci appeared less susceptible to the DCM sub-extract than staphylococci and streptococci. *S. aureus* strains were the most susceptible with MICs ranging from 9.8 to 19.5 μg/mL (Table 2). This non-polar fraction of hops is known to contain prenylated chalcones and acylphloroglucinol derivatives (Figure 1) which were further purified to analyze their activity.

Table 1. MIC (in μg/mL) of hop hydro-ethanolic crude extracts (Co: cones, Le: leaves, St: stems, Rh: rhizomes) against some human pathogenic bacteria with their corresponding antibiotic susceptibility (S: susceptible I: intermediate, R: resistant).

Bacterial Strains and Yeasts	MIC (μg/mL)				Antibiotic and Antifungal Susceptibility		
	Co	Le	St	Rh	GEN	VAN	AMX
Gram-positive							
Corynebacterium T25-17	39	NA	NA	NA	S	S	S
Enterococcus faecalis C159-6	39	NA	NA	NA	R	S	R
Enterococcus sp. 8153	156	NA	NA	NA	R	S	S
Mycobacterium smegmatis 5003	39	NA	NA	NA	S	S	S
Staphylococcus aureus 8146	39	NA	NA	NA	S	S	I
Staphylococcus aureus 8147	39	NA	NA	NA	S	S	S
Staphylococcus epidermidis 5001	39	NA	NA	NA	S	S	S
Staphylococcus epidermidis 10282	98	NA	NA	NA	S	S	S
Staphylococcus lugdunensis T26A3	156	NA	NA	625	S	S	S
Staphylococcus warneri T12A12	39	NA	NA	625	S	R	S
Streptococcus agalactiae T25-7	39	NA	NA	NA	R	S	S
Streptococcus agalactiae T53C2	78	NA	NA	NA	S	S	S
Streptococcus dysgalactiae T46C14	39	NA	NA	NA	S	S	S
Gram-negative							
Acinetobacter baumannii 9010	NA	NA	NA	NA	S	R	R
Acinetobacter baumannii 9011	NA	NA	NA	625	R	R	R
Citrobacter freundii 11041	NA	NA	NA	NA	S	R	S
Citrobacter freundii 11042	NA	NA	NA	NA	S	R	R
Enterobacter cloacae 11050	NA	NA	NA	NA	S	R	R
Enterobacter cloacae 11051	NA	NA	NA	NA	R	R	R
Enterobacter cloacae 11053	NA	NA	NA	NA	S	R	R
Escherichia coli 8138	NA	NA	NA	NA	S	R	R
Escherichia coli 8157	NA	NA	NA	NA	S	R	R
Escherichia coli ATCC 25922	NA	NA	NA	NA	S	R	I
Klebsiella pneumoniae 11016	NA	NA	NA	NA	S	R	R
Klebsiella pneumoniae 11017	NA	NA	NA	NA	S	R	R
Proteus mirabilis 11060	NA	NA	NA	NA	S	R	R
Providencia stuartii 11038	NA	NA	NA	NA	S	R	S
Pseudomonas aeruginosa 8131	NA	NA	NA	625	S	R	R
Pseudomonas aeruginosa ATCC 27583	NA	NA	NA	625	R	R	R
Salmonella sp. 11033	NA	NA	NA	NA	S	R	R
Serratia marcescens 11056	NA	NA	NA	NA	S	R	R
Serratia marcescens 11057	NA	NA	NA	NA	R	R	R
Stenotrophomonas maltophilia	NA	NA	NA	625	S	R	R
Yeasts					AMB	FLC	VRC
Candida albicans 13203	156	625	NA	NA	S	R	R
Candida albicans ATCC 10231	<39	NA	NA	NA	S	S	S

Gentamicin (GEN) S ≤ 4, R > 8; Vancomycin (VAN) S ≤ 4, R > 16; Amoxicillin (AMX) S ≤ 4, R > 16; Amphotericin B (AMB) S ≤ 1, R > 1; Fluconazole (FLC) S ≤ 2, R > 4; Voriconazole (VRC) S ≤ 0.12, R > 0.12. NA means not active, MIC ≥ 1250 μg/mL.

Table 2. MIC (in μg/mL) of the crude extract and the dichloromethane (DCM) sub-extract of cones against Gram-positive strains with their corresponding antibiotic susceptibility (S: susceptible, I: intermediate, R: resistant).

Gram-Positive Strains	MIC (μg/mL)		Antibiotic Susceptibility		
	Crude Extract	DCM	GEN	VAN	AMX
Corynebacterium T25-17	39	19.5	S	S	S
Enterococcus faecalis C159-6	156	78	R	R	R
Enterococcus faecalis T26-B7	313	156	R	S	S
Enterococcus faecalis T34-2	313	156	S	S	S
Enterococcus faecalis T37A4	156	156	R	S	S
Enterococcus faecalis T39-C11	156	156	S	S	S
Staphylococcus aureus 8146	19.5	9.8	S	S	S
Staphylococcus aureus 8147	19.5	9.8	S	S	S
Staphylococcus aureus CIP 224	39	19.5	S	S	S
Staphylococcus aureus T1.1	39	19.5	S	S	S
Staphylococcus aureus T25.10	39	19.5	S	S	R
Staphylococcus aureus T25.3	39	19.5	S	S	R
Staphylococcus aureus T25.9	39	19.5	S	S	R
Staphylococcus aureus T26A4	39	19.5	S	S	S
Staphylococcus aureus T28.1	19.5	9.8	S	S	R
Staphylococcus aureus T36B1	39	19.5	S	S	R
Staphylococcus aureus T47A12	39	19.5	S	S	R
Staphylococcus aureus T6.7	39	9.8	S	S	R
Staphylococcus epidermidis 5001	39	19.5	S	S	S
Staphylococcus warneri T12A12	78	19.5	S	S	S
Staphylococcus lugdunensis T26A3	39	19.5	S	S	S
Staphylococcus pettenkoferi T3.3	78	39	S	S	S
Staphylococcus saprophyticus 08237	39	9.8	S	S	S
Streptococcus agalactiae 13225	39	19.5	S	S	S
Streptococcus agalactiae 13226	39	19.5	S	S	S
Streptococcus agalactiae T25.7	39	19.5	I	S	S
Streptococcus agalactiae T38.2	39	19.5	S	S	S
Streptococcus agalactiae T40A2	39	19.5	S	S	S

Gentamicin (GEN) S $\leq$ 4, R > 8; Vancomycin (VAN) S $\leq$ 4, R > 16; Amoxicillin (AMX) S $\leq$ 4, R > 16. NA means not active, MIC $\geq$ 1250 μg/mL.

Extracts and sub-extracts were also tested for their antiparasitic effect. This activity was for the first-time described here on Tbb with respective IC_{50} of 7.8 and 4.6 μg/mL for the hydro-ethanolic crude extract and the DCM sub-extract of cones. Hops is less active against Lmm with IC_{50} of 29.0 and 28.2 μg/mL, respectively.

2.2. Purification of Hops Prenylated Chalcones and Acylphloroglucinols and Quantification in Hop Samples

Major prenylated chalcones (xanthohumol and desmethylxanthohumol) and prenylated acylphloroglucinols (cohumulone, humulone, colupulone and lupulone) were purified from the active DCM sub-extract of cones by centrifugal partition chromatography (CPC) and preparative high-performance liquid chromatography (HPLC) (Figure 1). Their structure was established by comparison with their spectral data, including NMR data and mass spectra, with reported values [26–29] (Supplementary Material, Tables S2–S4). These compounds were identified in the different plant crude extracts by UHPLC-UV-MS on the basis of their retention times and their mass spectrum (Figure 2 and Supplementary Material, Figures S1–S3). They were then used for quantification in different parts of the plant and for activities testing.

Quantification was performed on crude hydro-ethanolic extracts of the cultivar 'Nugget' used for bioassays. Concerning our method, good linearity was observed for each compound over the concentration range (Supplementary Material, Table S1). Evaluation of the method on the cones extract showed acceptable intra- and inter-day precisions for xanthohumol (RSD% = 10.6, 12.0), humulone (RSD% = 12.4, 13.8) and lupulone (RSD% = 10.3, 10.7).

The contents in prenylated phenolic compounds were much higher in the crude extract of cones than in stems, roots and leaves crude extracts (Figures 2 and 3). Only xanthohumol and humulone have been quantified in the stems extract. No prenylated phenolic compounds could be quantified in the rhizome extract. Interestingly, humulone was the main compound in cones extract (147 μg/mg), with a total alpha/beta acid (humulone/lupulone derivatives) ratio of 2.4, whereas lupulone was the most abundant compound in leaves extract, with a ratio of 0.5.

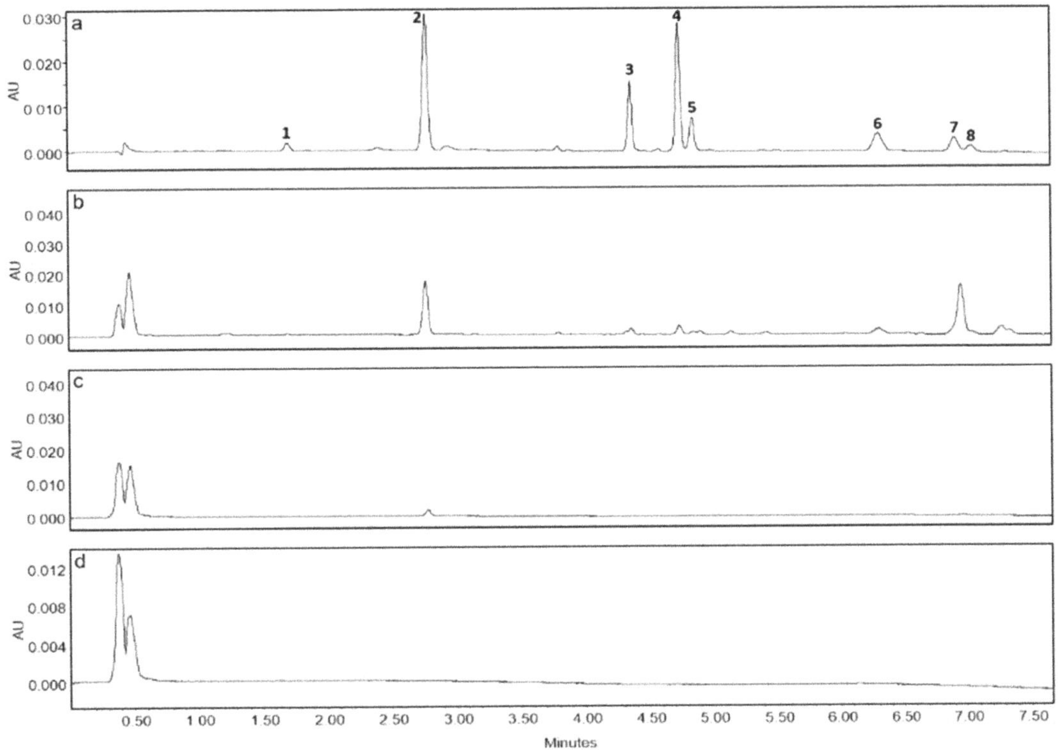

Figure 2. LC-UV chromatograms (370 nm) of crude extracts prepared at 100 μg/mL in MeOH for (**a**) cones and 1 mg/mL in MeOH for (**b**) leaves, (**c**) stems and (**d**) rhizomes. Compounds identified are as follows: desmethylxanthohumol (**1**) rt 1.70 min, xanthohumol (**2**) rt 2.78 min, cohumulone (**3**) rt 4.37 min, humulone (**4**) rt 4.75 min, adhumulone (**5**) rt 4.86 min, colupulone (**6**) rt 6.31 min, lupulone (**7**) rt 6.92 min, adlupulone (**8**) rt 7.05 min.

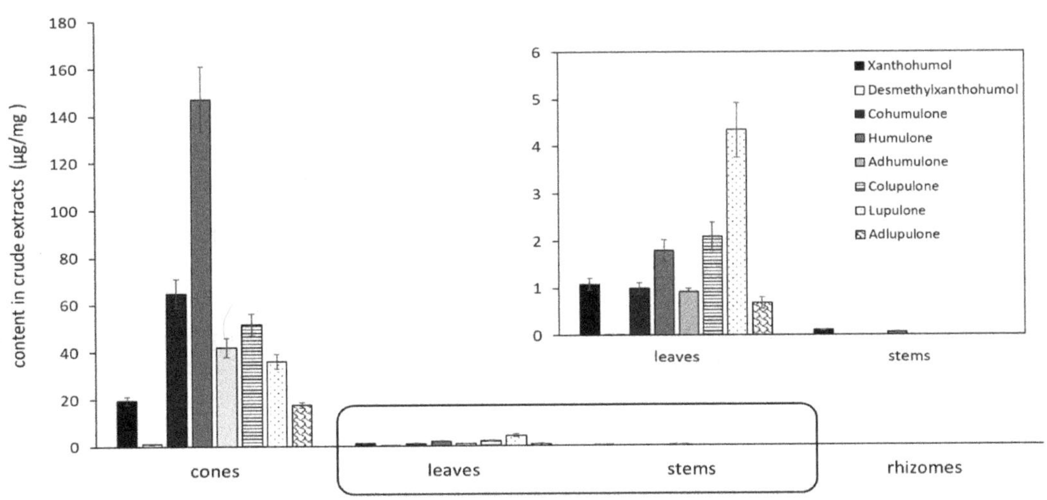

Figure 3. Content of prenylated chalcones and acylphloroglucinols in crude hydro-alcoholic extracts of different hop parts (in μg/mg) ($n = 3$, mean ± SD).

2.3. *Antibacterial Activity of Purified Prenylated Phenolic Compounds*

2.3.1. Antibacterial Activity of Purified Compounds against Selected MRSA and Methicillin-Sensitive *Staphylococcus aureus* (MSSA) Strains

All compounds tested were active against selected oxacillin susceptible and resistant *S. aureus* clinical isolates (Table 3). Indeed, methicillin resistance is routine researched by using oxacillin disks. The first strain (T28.1) was more intensively studied because it combined many pathologic features like isolation from a diabetic foot infection and harbouring genes implicated in antibiotic resistance, capsule formation and biofilm formation [30]. Lupulone was the most promising compound with MICs from 0.6 to 1.2 μg/mL towards MRSA strains. With the exception of lupulone, we demonstrated that xanthohumol and desmethylxanthohumol were more active than bitter acids, with MICs ranging from 9.8 to 19.5 and 19.5 to 39 μg/mL towards MRSA. However, desmethylxanthohumol was slightly less active than xanthohumol. MICs did not differ between MRSA and MSSA strains.

Table 3. MIC of hop chalcones and acylphloroglucinols against selected MRSA (T28.1 and T25.10) and MSSA (T26A4 and 08143) strains.

Bacteria MIC in μg/Ml (μM)	Chalcones		Acylphloroglucinols				OXA
	XN	DMX	Cohumulone	Humulone	Colupulone	Lupulone	
S. aureus T28.1	9.8 (27.7)	39 (114.7)	156 (448.3)	78 (215.5)	39 (97.5)	1.2 (2.9)	R
S. aureus T25.10	9.8 (27.7)	19.5 (57.3)	313 (899.4)	156 (430.9)	78 (195)	0.6 (1.45)	R
S. aureus T26A4	9.8 (27.7)	39 (114.7)	313 (899.4)	156 (430.9)	39 (97.5)	0.6 (1.45)	S
S. aureus 08143	19.5 (55)	39 (114.7)	313 (899.4)	156 (430.9)	78 (195)	1.2 (2.9)	S

XN: xanthohumol, DMX: desmethylxanthohumol. Positive control was oxacillin (OXA, S $\leq$ 2 μg/mL, R $\geq$ 4 μg/mL [31]).

Isoxanthohumol (Figure 4), a flavanone known to be a metabolite of xanthohumol, was also tested against the strain MRSA T28.1 and its MIC was found to be of similar activity as desmethylxanthohumol (MIC = 39 μg/mL).

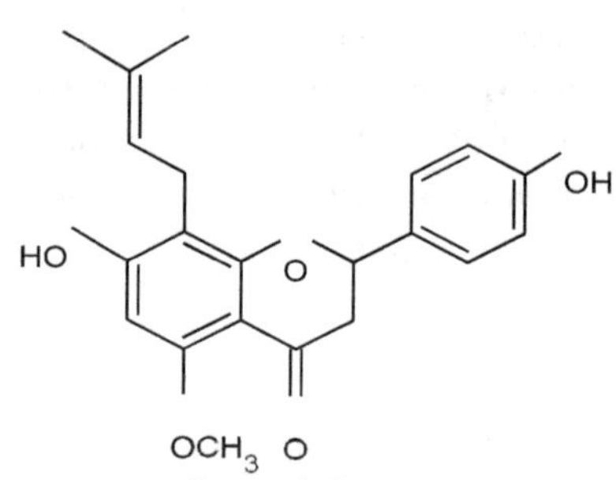

Isoxanthohumol

Figure 4. Structure of isoxanthohumol.

Xanthohumol, desmethylxanthohumol and lupulone were selected for further experiments on the *S. aureus* T28.1 clinical isolate, in order to better understand how they act on MRSA.

2.3.2. Further Experiments on MRSA T28.1 with the Most Promising Compounds Xanthohumol, Desmethylxanthohumol and Lupulone

Synergies Assessed by Checkerboard

One of the strategies employed to overcome resistant strains is the combination of current antibacterial agents with natural compounds. Hops phenolic compounds and selected antibiotics (ciprofloxacin, gentamicin, oxacillin and rifampicin) were combined using the checkerboard method, to establish the best combination of products for increasing the activity [32].

The antibacterial action of hops compounds can be enhanced by combining xanthohumol with desmethylxanthohumol or with lupulone, showing an additive effect (Table 4). In contrast, the combination of desmethylxanthohumol with lupulone was found to be antagonistic.

The combination of hops compounds with selected antibiotics highlighted interesting effects (Table 4). Xanthohumol was synergistic to additive with the four antibiotics. For example, rifampicin can be 8 times more active when combined with xanthohumol. Desmethylxanthohumol showed a synergistic activity with gentamicin, synergistic to additive with ciprofloxacin and additive with oxacillin, while sometimes antagonist effect was observed with rifampicin. The interaction of lupulone with ciprofloxacin was additive and this association was antagonist or indifferent with gentamicin and rifampicin.

Table 4. Effect of the combination of hops compounds between them and with selected antibiotics.

Association	FIC Index	Effect
XN-DMX	0.74–1	Additive
XN-Lupulone	0.75	Additive
DMX-Lupulone	5	Antagonist
CIP-XN	0.49–1	Synergistic to additive
CIP-DMX	0.38–1.5	Synergistic to indifferent
CIP-Lupulone	0.63–1	Additive
GEN-XN	0.14–1	Synergistic to additive
GEN-DMX	0.03–0.28	Synergistic
GEN-Lupulone	9	Antagonist
OXA-XN	0.28–0.75	Synergistic to additive
OXA-DMX	0.5–0.76	Additive
OXA-Lupulone	0.19–1.25	Synergistic to indifferent
RIF-XN	0.25–0.75	Synergistic to additive
RIF-DMX	1–5	Indifferent to antagonist
RIF-Lupulone	2.2–6	Indifferent to antagonist

Association can be synergistic (FIC < 0.5), additive ($0.5 \leq$ FIC ≤ 1), indifferent ($1 <$ FIC ≤ 4) or antagonist (FIC > 4). Ranges result from 3 independent experiments. XN: xanthohumol, DMX: desmethylxanthohumol, CIP: ciprofloxacin, GEN: gentamicin, OXA: oxacillin, RIF: rifampicin.

Kill Curve

Kill curves allowed the determination of time-dependent bacteriostatic and bactericidal concentrations of each product [33] (Figure 5).

Xanthohumol decreased the bacterial population by 0.5 log(CFU/mL) during the first 6 h at sub-inhibitory concentration (MIC/2) and by 2 log(CFU/mL) during 24 h at the MIC. It was bactericidal at 2xMIC, rapidly decreasing the bacterial population to around 3 log(CFU/mL) during the first 4 h which means that only 1 bacterium among 1000 initially present is still alive (Figure 5A).

Desmethylxanthohumol decreased the bacterial population during the first hours at the MIC. The bacteria grew back after 6 h of culture. However, it was bactericidal at 2 × MIC; reaching the detection threshold of 1 log(CFU/mL) after 24 h (Figure 5B).

Although lupulone was the most active compound (based on MIC of 1.2 μg/mL), it slightly decreased the bacterial population only at 4 × MIC. Lower concentrations just slowed down growth (Figure 5C) and a reduction between the control and 2 × MIC is about 3 log(CFU/mL).

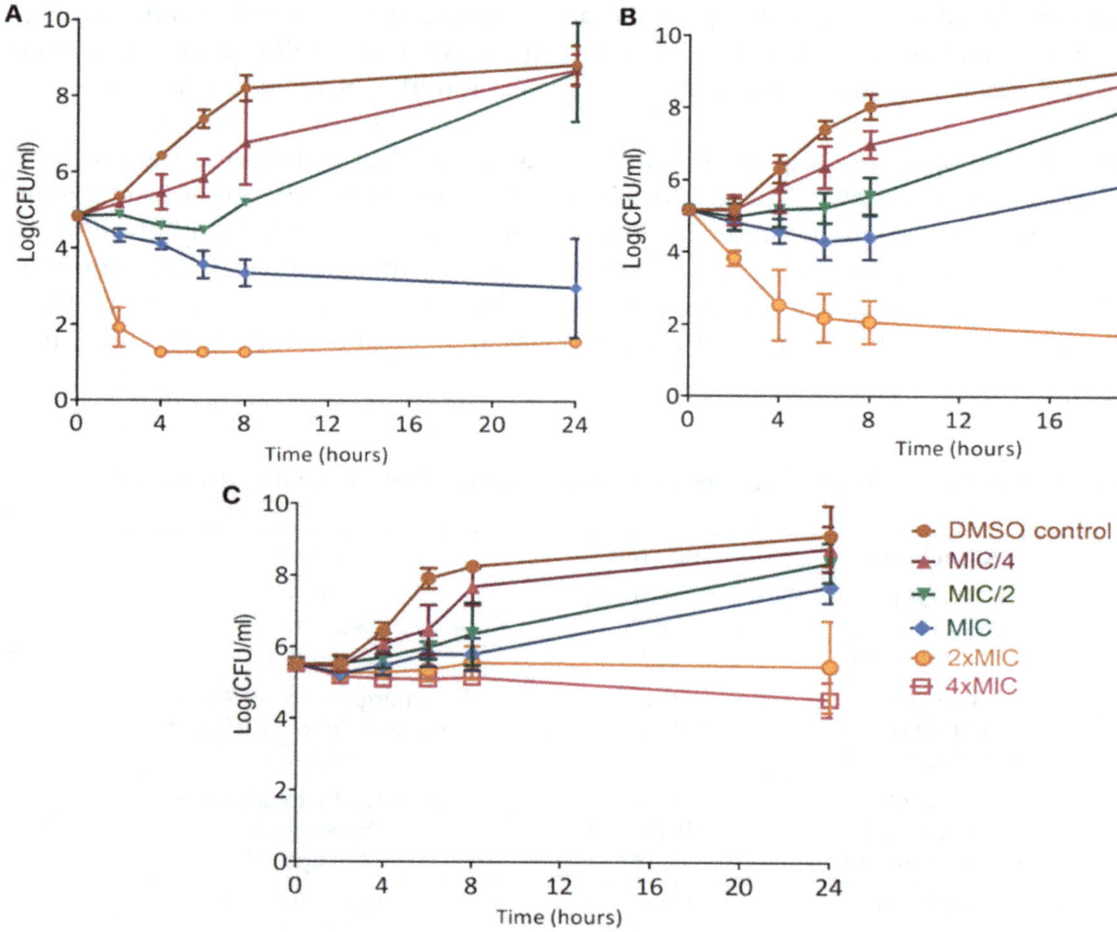

Figure 5. Kill curves showing the effect of xanthohumol (**A**), desmethylxanthohumol (**B**) and lupulone (**C**) on *S. aureus* T28.1 growing during 24 h. The detection threshold of the experiment is 1 log(CFU/mL).

Post-Antibiotic Effects

Post-antibiotic tests highlighted the fragility of the bacterial population after 2 h exposure to the active compounds followed by inactivation, which resulted in a delayed regrowth [33]. The growth retardation is quantified by the difference between the time necessary for each condition to grow from a log10 (T) and the corresponding time for the control (C). These parameters are graphically determined as shown in Figure 6.

The three compounds tested caused delayed growth at all concentrations evaluated (Table 5).

Here again, even if lupulone was the most active (based on MIC values), it caused a low effect after its inactivation with a maximum delay close to 55 min. In contrast, xanthohumol and desmethylxanthohumol caused a significant delay for regrowth. Desmethylxanthohumol inhibited bacterial regrowth for up to almost 2.5 h after pre-treatment at the MIC. Xanthohumol had the same effect at the MIC and it increased with the concentration, the delay reaching 3.29 h at 4 × MIC.

Table 5. Post-antibiotic effect on *S. aureus* T28.1 for each hops selected compound after 2 h exposure. Values are the maximum delayed growth retardation obtained after 3 independent experiments.

	Maximum Growth Retardation (h)			
	MIC/2	**MIC**	**2 × MIC**	**4 × MIC**
Xanthohumol	1.34	2.23	2.05	3.29
Desmethylxanthohumol	2.10	2.32	2.29	2.34
Lupulone	0.26	0.53	0.54	0.47

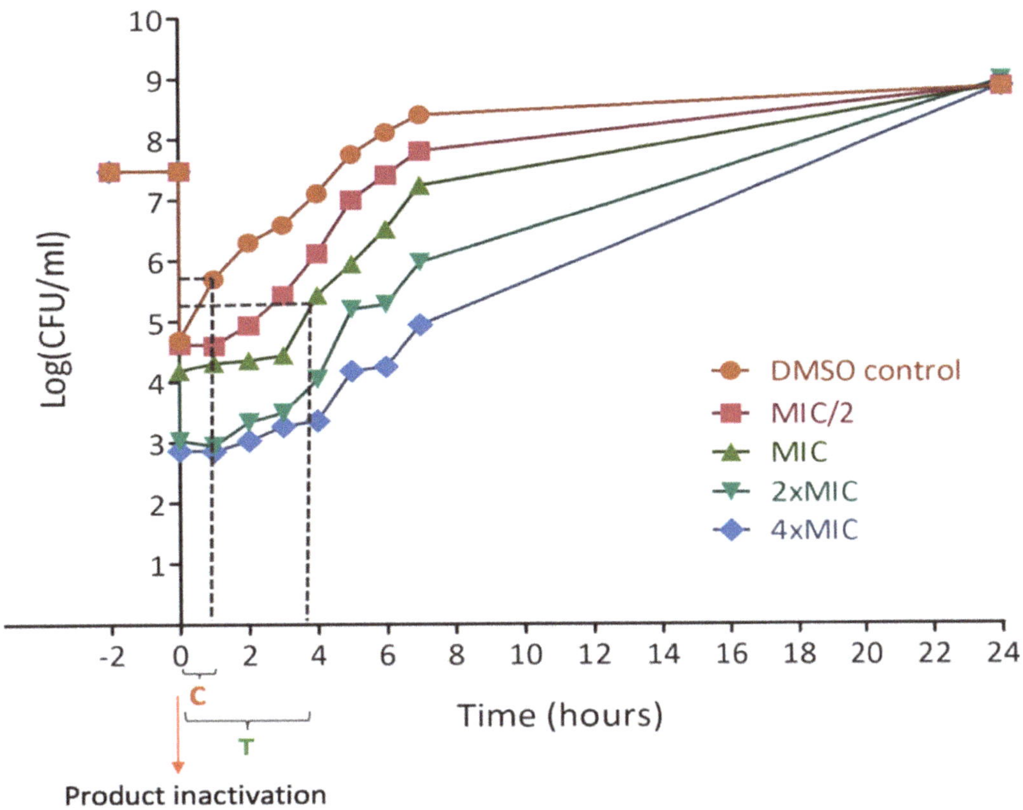

Figure 6. Post-antibiotic curve of xanthohumol indicating graphical determination of parameters for the determination of the growth delay. Time between −2 and 0 shows the pre-treatment with antibacterial product. Time 0 corresponds to the product inactivation. The growth retardation is quantified during the first hours of culture, comparing each condition with the control, using the formula: PAE = T − C. Where T is the time needed for the bacterial population to grow by 1 log10 (the present example is for the MIC) and C is the corresponding time for the control.

Anti-Biofilm Assays

Biofilms contribute to bacterial resistance, forming a complex protecting shell [34]. We initially considered the activity of hops compounds on artificial surfaces, which was confirmed on a bone substitute, the natural colonized substrate of the model strain *S. aureus* T28.1. The influence of the compounds was assessed both on the biofilm formation and on the destruction of preformed biofilms.

Xanthohumol totally inhibited the biofilm formation on artificial surface at the MIC (Figure 7A), which correlates with the bactericidal effect pointed out with kill curves (Figure 5A). Desmethylxanthohumol and lupulone showed a significant inhibition of biofilm formation at sub-inhibitory concentrations (Figure 7A). Thus, this effect seems independent of the bactericidal activity (Figure 5B,C). The same trend was observed on bone substitutes (Figure 7C). Even if the inhibition of the biofilm formation is found less intense in bone substitute, this potential remains very interesting, in particular for desmethylxanthohumol and lupulone. These last products showed a significant decrease of the biofilm formation on bone substitute discs at MIC (Figure 7C).

Hops compounds are also able to destroy the biofilm. Xanthohumol showed a non-dose-dependent activity at the MIC and above, which is similar to the inhibition dose for the biofilm formation (Figure 7B). As seen previously, desmethylxanthohumol and lupulone showed a greater anti-biofilm potential than xanthohumol. A significant biofilm destruction was also observed at sub-inhibitory concentrations, at MIC/4, with 81% and 62.8%, respectively.

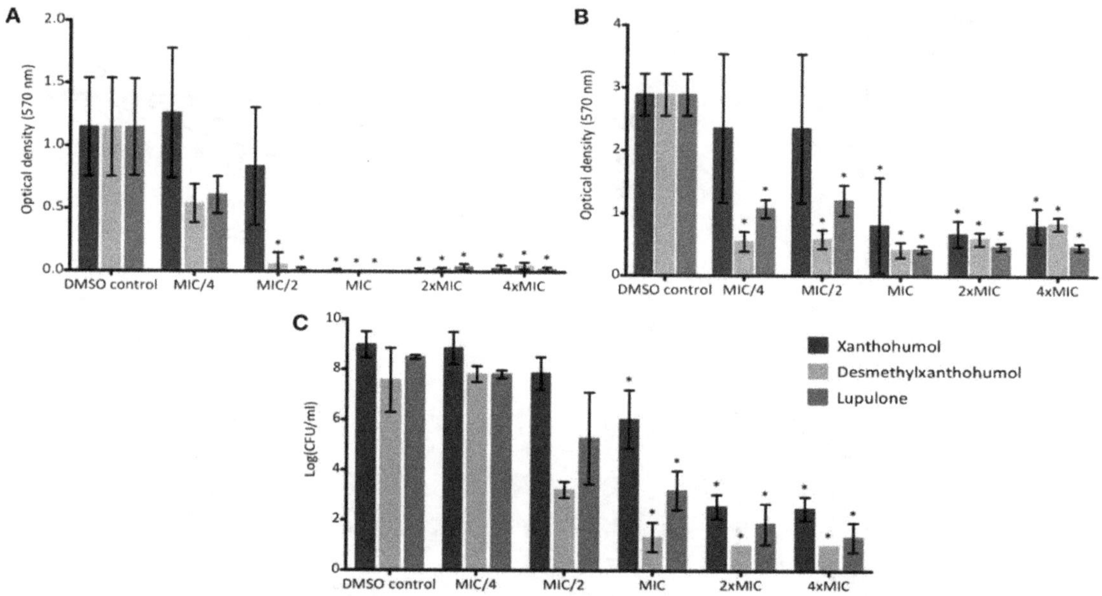

Figure 7. Effect of xanthohumol, desmethylxanthohumol and lupulone on the biofilm formation (**A**) of *S. aureus* T28.1 on artificial surface (**A**), on the biofilm destruction of *S. aureus* T28.1 on artificial surface (**B**) and on the biofilm formation of *S. aureus* T28.1 on bone substitute (**C**). According to Shapiro test, means tagged with * are significantly different from the control ($p = 0.05$) using Kruskal Wallis and Dunn's tests for (**A**) and for lupulone and desmethylxanthohumol for (**C**) or ANOVA and Tukey test for (**B**) and for xanthohumol for (**C**).

2.4. Antiparasitic Activity of Purified Prenylated Phenolic Compounds

The two chalcones, xanthohumol and desmethylxanthohumol, as well as two acylphloroglucinols, humulone and lupulone, were tested against the two parasites: *Trypanosoma brucei brucei* (Tbb) and *Leishmania mexicana mexicana* (Lmm) and were active. Lupulone is the most promising compound with IC_{50} of 0.9 and 4.7 μg/mL against Tbb and Lmm, respectively (Table 6). As for antibacterial activities, we demonstrated that xanthohumol and desmethylxanthohumol were more active than humulone on parasites, with IC_{50} from 2.4 to 6.1 and 7.7 to 26.2 μg/mL on both Tbb and Lmm.

Table 6. IC_{50} of hops chalcones and acylphloroglucinols against some *Trypanosoma brucei brucei* and *Leishmania mexicana mexicana* strains.

Parasites IC_{50} in μg/mL (μM)	XN	DMX	Humulone	Lupulone	SUR	PEN
Tbb	2.4 ± 0.2 (6.8)	7.7 ± 0.6 (22.6)	10.9 ± 0.8 (30.1)	0.9 ± 0.0 (2.2)	0.05 (0.038)	-
Lmm	6.1 ± 3.1 (17.2)	26.2 ± 1.8 (77)	28.8 ± 1.5 (77.9)	4.7 ± 0.1 (11.3)	-	0.07 (0.21)

XN: xanthohumol, DMX: desmethylxanthohumol. Positive controls were suramin (SUR) and pentamidine (PEN). ND: Not determined.

2.5. Cytotoxicity

We evaluated the antiproliferative activity of hops compounds on various cancer and non-cancer cell lines (Table 7). We showed that desmethylxanthohumol is the less toxic compound. Considering its moderate activity, active dose could be toxic. Active concentration of desmethylxanthohumol on Tbb is the only one lower than the cytotoxicity on the tested cell lines. Xanthohumol was also toxic at the antibacterial concentration on all the targeted cell lines. For both chalcones, selectivity indexes (cytotoxic IC_{50}/active IC_{50}) would be close to 1. A special attention has to be paid on lupulone, its pronounced antibacterial activity gives selectivity index > 4 compared to its cytotoxicity against MG-63 (Table 7). Antibacterial and anti-biofilm concentrations showed a cell viability close to 100%. These data make lupulone a very good candidate for a topical bone application.

Table 7. Cytotoxic activities of hops extracts and isolated compounds (chalcones and acylphloroglucinols) against WI-38, J774, Hep-G2 and MG-63 cell lines.

Cell Lines $IC_{50} \pm SD$ in μg/mL (μM)	Hydro-Alcoholic Crude Extract	MC Sub-Extract	XN	DMX	Humulone	Lupulone	CAMP
WI-38	7.6 ± 0.1	5.1 ± 1.0	6.9 ± 0.5 (19.5)	60.7 ± 2.5 (178.5)	10.5 ± 2.3 (29)	1.1 ± 0.0 (2.6)	0.06 ± 0.0 (0.17)
J774	19.7 ± 2.8	11.4 ± 2.1	3.4 ± 0.5 (9.6)	9.7 ± 1.0 (28.5)	11.5 ± 0.3 (31.7)	1.5 ± 0.1 (3.6)	0.01 ± 0.0 (0.03)
Hep-G2	6.8 ± 2.5	6.5 ± 2.1	2.5 ± 0.8 (7.1)	22.4 ± 2.9 (65.9)	ND	1.2 ± 0.5 (2.9)	0.4 ± 0.2 (1.15)
MG-63	31.4 ± 8.1	21.1 ± 0.4	10.4 ± 2.6 (29.4)	39.5 ± 3.3 (116.2)	ND	4.3 ± 0.4 (10.4)	4.4 ± 1.5 (12.6)

XN: xanthohumol, DMX: desmethylxanthohumol. Positive control was camptothecin (CAMP). ND: Not determined.

3. Discussion

Multi-drug resistance (MDR) bacteria, like methicillin-resistant *Staphylococcus aureus* (MRSA), present a major challenge for the medical community in the treatment of infections, such as diabetic foot infections [6,35]. The discovery of new antibiotics is not fast enough to offset the global spread of resistant pathogens. At the same time, we can observe a worrying emergence of resistance to some of the newer antibiotic agents [36–38]. Hence, the development of combination of current agents with other type of resistance-modifying agents, such as natural antibacterial agents, can be an alternative strategy to overcome MDR [39].

In this context, we evaluated the antibacterial potential of hop extracts and more particularly of three pure compounds isolated from hops (xanthohumol, desmethylxanthohumol and lupulone) towards MRSA, one of the most aggressive agents, with different approaches [33]. We began by a classical MIC determination, which is only an endpoint method, followed by kill-time curves assessing the time dependent effect and synergistic studies, in combination with antibiotics, giving more information on their resistance modifying potential. The checkerboard method is the preferred technique of choice to analyze these interactions, with however a certain variability in the methods of interpretation [32]. The study of a post-antibiotic effect (PAE), also applicable to substances other than antibiotics, made it possible to follow the regrowth of bacteria after inactivation of the antibacterial substance after a defined contact time at an active concentration. When damaged bacteria need some time to recover in comparison to the control, the regrowth will be lowered, which means in clinical situations that administration intervals of the antimicrobial substances can be delayed. Another innovative point is the effect on biofilms, concerning about 60% of infections. In biofilms, the bacteria are surrounded by a thick layer of extracellular polysaccharides which makes them inaccessible to antibiotics but also to defenses of the immune system. Furthermore, the lack of nutrients lowers dramatically the bacterial multiplication. As most of the antibiotics act on mechanisms implicated in multiplication, this is the second reason for their lack of action on biofilms. Influence on biofilms can be studied in two manners: destruction of established biofilms or inhibition of their formation. The first manner is more relevant for clinicians as at the time of diagnosis the biofilm is already established.

The antibacterial activity of hops has been known for many years [40,41] but has been poorly evaluated against resistant strains. We showed here their effects on *Corynebacterium*, *Enterococcus*, *Mycobacterium*, *Staphylococcus* and *Streptococcus* strains, some being resistant to antibiotics (Table 1). Their effect on *Bacillus*, *Streptomyces* and *Micrococcus* strains was previously underlined [22,41]. Hops extracts are also able to combat some human pathogenic bacteria found in food, such as *Clostridium perfringens* and *Listeria monocytogenes* [42,43]. The screening conducted on some *C. albicans* strains showed that the spectrum of activity of hops extracts against these yeasts is weak, only two strains were susceptible to our extracts. The *C. albicans* ATCC 10,231 reference strain was previously tested by Langezaal et al. [44] who also found an efficiency of cones extract. Other studies have demonstrated that hops extracts are more efficient on bacteria than yeasts, showing no effect of hops constituents on *Saccharomyces* strains [41]. Contrarily to Langezaal et al. [44] and Abram et al. [45]

who have detected a slight activity of cones extracts against *E. coli* strains, our extracts were inactive towards Gram-negative bacteria. Stems, leaves and rhizomes have been rarely studied. According to our results, their crude hydro-ethanolic extracts showed a weak antimicrobial activity in comparison with cones, as already highlighted for leaves against some bacteria [45]. Nevertheless, the rhizomes extract appeared to be more active than leaves and stems extracts (Table 1). Previous research on the quantification of the phenolic hop compounds in cones and leaves by LC-UV is reported in the literature [46]. With our method of quantification, no prenylated phenolic compounds could be quantified in the rhizome extract. Consequently, the activity of rhizomes could be related to the presence of other metabolites. The antibacterial activity of cones was mainly attributed to apolar compounds because the DCM sub-extract of cones was more active than the crude extract of the same plant part (Table 2). The content of phenolic compounds in hops is influenced in particular by the cultivar, the growth location, the field conditions, the climate, which may explain the differences in activities found in the literature [47,48].

Phenolic compounds are known to be an anti-staphylococcal class of metabolites. In our study, all purified hops prenylated chalcones and acylphloroglucinol derivatives showed an antibacterial activity towards selected *S. aureus* strains (Table 3). In the literature, the antibacterial activity of hops is mainly linked to acylphloroglucinol derivatives. This activity is enhanced by the degree of hydrophobicity of the compound [49]. The number and the length of the side chains, because of their interaction with the bacterial cell wall, is stated to influence positively the antibacterial action, so lupulone derivatives are more efficient than humulone derivatives [22,42], which is in accordance with our results. Lupulone is much more active than humulone with respective MICs ranging from 0.6 to 1.2 and 78 to 156 μg/mL towards MRSA strains (Table 3). With the exception of lupulone, we also demonstrated that xanthohumol and desmethylxanthohumol are more active than other bitter acids. Xanthohumol showed MIC ranging from 9.8 to 19.5 μg/mL against selected *S. aureus* strains. In comparison with one of the most studied promising antimicrobial chalcone, licochalcone A, which showed MIC ranging from 2 to 15 μg/mL against Gram-positive bacteria including *S. aureus* [50], the activity of xanthohumol is in the same range. Several studies have focused on the antibacterial potential of xanthohumol which showed various MICs from 2 to 125 μg/mL on *S. aureus*, depending on the strain's resistance profile and the compound's purity [14,22]. According to our results, desmethylxanthohumol was slightly less active than xanthohumol, with MICs ranging from 19.5 to 39 μg/mL against *S. aureus* strains (Table 3). The structural difference between the two molecules is the 6′-methoxyl group for xanthohumol replaced by a 6′-phenol group for desmethylxanthohumol (Figure 1). The 6′-phenol substituent is considered as a crucial group in the equilibrium chalcone-flavanone but is not expected to contribute to the activity [51]. According to Ávila et al. [51], the methylation of the 6-phenol group could lead to less active compounds, which is not the case in our study. Desmethylxanthohumol is known for its antioxidant and apoptotic activities [52] but to our knowledge, no antibacterial potential was highlighted. Olivella et al. [53] have demonstrated that chalcones have the most favorable structure for a bacteriostatic action, in comparison with flavanones. In rats, xanthohumol is partially absorbed by intestinal cells and transported in blood. The non-absorbed part of xanthohumol can be transformed into the corresponding flavanone, isoxanthohumol, by the intestinal microbiota [54]. The conversion of isoxanthohumol into 8-prenyl-naringenin occurs only in the colon and not in the stomach and small intestine [55,56]. In this context, we also tested the activity of isoxanthohumol (Figure 4) against the strain MRSA T28.1. This compound showed a MIC equal to 39 μg/mL. It is interesting to note that, even if isoxanthohumol is less active than xanthohumol, its MIC was found to be of similar than desmethylxanthohumol.

The antibacterial potential of xanthohumol, desmethylxanthohumol and lupulone against MRSA is therefore promising. Their MICs are in the same order of magnitude as those obtained for antibacterial phenolic compounds known for their important activity against MRSA strains, with MICs varying between 1.56 and 125 μg/mL [4]. Most of them are known to be antibacterial compounds but they are not used to combat strains resistant to antibiotics. Some hops metabolites also showed antibacterial activities against others strains such as: *Bacillus subtilis*, *Clostridium difficile*, *Enterococcus strains* and *Streptococcus strains* for the Gram-positive bacteria; *Bacteroides fragilis*, *Helicobacter pylori* and *Yersinia enterocolitica* for the Gram-negative bacteria [20].

To overcome bacterial resistance, one of the strategies employed is the use of a combination of drugs, such as antibiotics combined with natural products, which has already shown promising results [57]. The checkerboard is a method to establish the best combination of products increasing the activity [32,58]. The antibacterial action of hops compounds can be enhanced by combining concomitantly xanthohumol with desmethylxanthohumol or with lupulone. The effect is twice as intense because the MIC is divided by two. By contrast, the combination of desmethylxanthohumol with lupulone leads to an antagonist effect (Table 4). The combination of natural products with antibiotics may in some cases have a synergistic effect. Xanthohumol and rifampicin can be 8 times more active when they are combined. Furthermore, for both xanthohumol and lupulone, the MIC for oxacillin drops below the threshold concentration of 2 μg/mL for oxacillin resistance, which means that in the presence of these synergistic compounds the strains will no longer be classified as MRSA, so reverting their resistance. Desmethylxanthohumol has an additive effect with oxacillin but this interaction does not render the strain susceptible to this antibiotic. Desmethylxanthohumol also has a promising interaction with ciprofloxacin and gentamicin. Some authors have previously detected synergies of xanthohumol and lupulone with polymyxin, ciprofloxacin or tobramycin [59]; and of xanthohumol with oxacillin or linezolid [14].

Kill curves demonstrated a great bactericidal action of xanthohumol at the MIC, of desmethylxanthohumol from 2 × MIC, whereas lupulone is slightly bactericidal after 24 h only at 4 × MIC (Figure 5). Comparing the activity of the two chalcones, desmethylxanthohumol showed a lower bactericidal action at the MIC than xanthohumol, which is probably linked to the presence of the 6′-hydroxyl group (Figure 1). Post-antibiotic effect is a part of pharmacodynamic studies, showing that xanthohumol and desmethylxanthohumol cause a significant delay for regrowth (Table 6). It means that the bacterial growth remains inhibited even after the product has been inactivated or metabolized by the body. These data provide an indication of the delay between two applications in a clinical situation. This is the first time that PAE is analyzed for hop compounds. This effect underlines an important reduction time for recovery which means that in vivo models will have to be checked for delay in drug administration.

Xanthohumol, desmethylxanthohumol and lupulone showed an inhibition of the biofilm formation of the *S. aureus* model strain on abiotic surface, with a sub-inhibitory action for desmethylxanthohumol and lupulone (Figure 7). Rozalski et al. studied the anti-adherent potential of a hops extract enriched in xanthohumol, pure xanthohumol and a spent hops extract rich in various common flavonols and flavanols [14]. They demonstrated a potent effect of xanthohumol on the biofilm formation at the MIC with 86.5% of inhibition. In comparison, our results showed an inhibition close to 100% at the MIC for the selected MRSA clinical isolate. In addition, we have also demonstrated that a previous formation of the biofilm does not prevent hops compounds to act on bacteria. In both cases, desmethylxanthohumol and lupulone seem to be more effective than xanthohumol, with an inhibition of the biofilm formation and a biofilm destruction at sub-inhibitory concentrations (Figure 7). Bogdanova et al. [23] also showed an anti-biofilm potential of some hops compounds but lower than that of our study. This result could be related to a lower purity of their products (from 82 to 87% in Reference [23]). This potential has been confirmed on a synthetic bone substitute which is the natural colonized substrate of *S. aureus* T28.1 (Figure 7). Even if the inhibition of the biofilm formation is found somewhat less intense in bone substitute than on inert surface, this potential remains very interesting, in particular for desmethylxanthohumol and lupulone. Moreover, according to our results, the anti-biofilm effect for these two products seems to be independent of the bactericidal effect pointed out with kill curves (Figure 5). To our knowledge, the anti-biofilm effect has never been assessed for hops compounds on bone substitutes. These data confirmed the promising potential of hops compounds to tackle MRSA not only on planktonic cells (MIC, kill curves) but also on biofilms approaching clinical situations.

Diabetic foot infections (DFI) affect one ulcerated foot out of two and in many cases lead to serious complications [60]. About 50% of patients hospitalized for a DFI suffer from an osteomyelitis and the prevalence of MRSA is often associated [61]. Low diffusion in necrotic tissues emphasizes topical antibiotic therapy for the management of mildly to moderately infected diabetic foot ulcers which has shown satisfactory results in some cases, allowing high concentrations of antibiotics at the site of infection without potentially toxic systemic levels [62]. Some medical devices such as beads loaded with antibiotics can bring high concentrations of local antibiotics for a long time in the case of deep wounds [63,64]. In addition, some topical antimicrobial agents, such as impregnated wound dressings with antimicrobials, could be of interest in the prevention or possibly the treatment of mild infections [65]. DFI generates many problems in clinical practice in terms of both diagnosis and therapeutic care mainly due to formation of persistent biofilms. The anti-biofilm action of hops metabolites both on artificial surface and on a synthetic bone substitute could bring out a new perspective to treat infected diabetic foot ulcers, an emerging public health problem. Thus, hop phenolic compounds with their dual action, antibacterial and anti-biofilm, are potential agents in the treatment of infections due to MRSA. Their additive or synergistic action with antibiotics could render treatments more effective and thus could prevent potential systemic toxicity if used in topical application. In this context, we evaluated the antiproliferative activity of the three phenolic compounds on different human cell lines and in particular against the human osteoblasts MG-63 cell line. After 48 h exposure, we showed a toxicity of xanthohumol on the targeted cell line. In the literature, data on its cytotoxicity depend on the cell type used and is very variable. For example, Ho et al. and Yong et al. have determined respectively an IC_{50} of about 75 and 100 μg/mL against a human hepatocellular carcinoma [66] and a lung cell line [67]. These concentrations are higher than the active doses reported in our work. In vivo studies have also confirmed the good safety at approximately 1000 mg of xanthohumol/kg of body weight of mice [68] and up to 180 mg of compound in humans for a short intake [69]. According to our results, desmethylxanthohumol is the less toxic compound on the MG-63 osteoblastic cells. However, considering its moderate activity, bactericidal and anti-biofilm concentrations would be toxic. To our knowledge, there is no comparison data available in the literature. Special attention has to be paid on lupulone. Its very pronounced antibacterial activity makes it non-toxic at the active doses. Moreover, anti-biofilm concentrations (MIC/4 and MIC/2) lead to a cell viability close to 100%. Comparing with the literature, some authors have determined IC_{50} ranging from 3.7 to 4.4 μg/mL on prostate cancer cells, which is close to other results [70] and IC_{50} from 8.3 to 16.6 μg/mL on breast cancer cells [71]. IC_{50} values are always higher than the active doses we have identified. All these data make lupulone a very good candidate for a topical bone application. Further research could be done by combining xanthohumol or desmethylxanthohumol with antibiotics as it would reduce the dose and avoid toxicity.

In addition, we evaluated the antiparasitic activity of the main chalcones and the main acylphloroglucinols of hop against two parasites: *Trypanosoma brucei brucei* (Tbb) and *Leishmania mexicana mexicana* (Lmm). Human African trypanosomiasis and leishmaniasis are indeed two protozoan infections considered as neglected tropical diseases with a strong impact on human health because in particular fatal if untreated [16,17]. Lupulone was the most active compound and humulone the less active. The four compounds tested were more active against Tbb than against Lmm (Table 6). Data on the antiparasitic activities of hops compounds are quite limited and especially concern xanthohumol. This chalcone was active against *Plasmodium falciparum* [24] and against *Leishmania amazonensis* [72] with IC_{50} in the μM range.

4. Materials and Methods

4.1. Phytochemical Analysis

4.1.1. General Experimental Procedures

For extraction and fractionation, synthesis grade ethanol (EtOH) and dichloromethane (DCM) were furnished by VWR Prolabo® (Fontenay-sous-Bois, France). Water was bi-distilled. All organic solvents for Centrifugal Partition Chromatography (CPC) purification were High Pressure Liquid Chromatography (HPLC) grade except for the n-heptane which was synthesis grade (Carlo Erba Reagents®, Val-de-Reuil, France). Ethyl acetate (EtOAc) and methanol (MeOH) were purchased from Fisher Scientific® (Illkirch, France). Water was purified using Millipore Integral 5 (Merck®, Trosly-Breuil, France) water purification system with a resistivity of not less than 18 $M\Omega \cdot cm^{-1}$. For analyses, acetonitrile (LC-MS grade) was purchased in Carlo Erba Reagents® (Val de Reuil, France), whereas methanol (LC-MS grade) came from Fischer Scientific® (Illkirch, France). The chloroform-d6 ($CDCl_3$) and MeOD for Nuclear Magnetic Resonance (NMR) experiments was obtained from Euriso-Top® (Gif-sur-Yvette, France).

Analytical Thin Layer Chromatography (TLC) were performed on pre-coated silica gel 60 F (0.25 mm, Merck®, Darmstadt, Germany). Detection was achieved at 254 and 366 nm, then by spraying with the unspecific anisaldehyde sulphuric reagent and heating at 100 °C for 10 min.

Ultra-High Performance Liquid Chromatography (UHPLC) analyses and quantification were carried out using an Acquity UPLC® H-Class Waters® system (Waters, Guyancourt, France) equipped with a diode array detector (DAD) and an Acquity QDa ESI-Quadrupole Mass Spectrometer. The software used was Empower 3. The stationary phase was a Waters® Acquity BEH C18 column (2.1 × 50 mm, 1.7 µm) connected to a 0.2 µm in-line filter. Preparative HPLC was performed using a Shimadzu® HPLC system equipped with a LC-20AP binary high-pressure pump, a CBM-20A controller and a SPD-M20A diode array detector. The software used was LabSolution. The stationary phase was a VisionHT HL C18 (5 µm, 250 × 22 mm) column (Grace®, France).

CPC was performed using an Armen instrument 250 mL rotor (SCPC-250-L) provided by Gilson® (Saint-Avé, France). CPC analyses were monitored using Shimadzu® pump and detector.

Nuclear Magnetic Resonance (NMR) spectra were recorded on a Bruker® DPX-500 spectrometer. High Resolution Mass Spectrometry (HR-MS) analyses were carried out using a Thermo Fisher Scientific® Exactive Orbitrap Mass Spectrometer equipped with an electrospray ion source.

4.1.2. Plant Extract Preparation and Fractionation

Female hop plants (*Humulus lupulus* L., cultivar 'Nugget') were harvested at maturity stage at the Beck farm (Bailleul, Northern France), at the time of harvesting of hop by producers in September. A voucher specimen was kept at the Faculty of pharmacy in Lille (laboratory of pharmacognosy) under reference NugBeck2015. After drying for 10 days at room temperature, protected from light, rhizomes, stems, leaves and cones were powderized separately with a blender. Crude hydro-alcoholic extracts of each part were obtained after an ethanol/water (9:1; *v*/*v*; 15 mL/g) mixture-based extraction with three successive macerations of four hours and one overnight, stirring in the dark. The percentage yields (PY) on a dry weight basis of each crude extract were: 35.5% (cones), 20.3% (leaves), 21.1% (rhizomes) and 17.2% (stems). The crude extract of female cones was fractionated by a liquid-liquid separation using dichloromethane (DCM) and water to obtain two sub-extracts. The corresponding sub-extracts were obtained with percentages yields of 52% and 48% respectively

4.1.3. Purification of Phenolic Compounds

Xanthohumol, desmethylxanthohumol, humulone, cohumulone, lupulone, colupulone were purified from the DCM sub-extract of cones in several steps. A first fractionation was performed by CPC. Using the Arizona solvent system P: n-heptane/EtOAc/MeOH/water (6:5:6:5; *v*/*v*), the rotor was entirely filled at 30 mL/min with the aqueous stationary phase in the ascending mode with rotation (500 rpm). Then, the rotation speed was increased from 500 to 1600 rpm. The organic mobile phase was pumped into the column in ascending mode at a flow rate of 8 mL/min. DCM sub-extract (2 g), initially dissolved in 10 mL of the organic/aqueous phase mixture (1:1), was filtered with a Millipore (0.45 μm) syringe filter and was injected immediately after the displacement of stationary phase (approximatively 80 mL). Fractions of 8 mL were collected every min. The CPC was run in ascending mode for 60 min and then switched to extrusion mode (recovery of the stationary phase) for 10 additional minutes at 30 mL/min with the same rotor speed (1600 rpm). The content of the outgoing organic phase was monitored by online UV absorbance measurement at 254 nm and 370 nm. All the fractions were checked by TLC and developed with toluene/ethyl acetate/formic acid (73:18:9; *v*/*v*) in order to regroup 5 sub-fractions (MC1 to MC5) from ascendant mode and 3 sub-fractions (MC6 to MC8) from extrusion mode. This CPC method allowed us to purify, in one step, xanthohumol (Figure 1), with 98% purity from MC4. The other compounds were purified from other sub-fractions using preparative HPLC. The mobile phase was composed of water (solvent A) and acetonitrile (solvent B). The following proportions of solvent B were: 10–75% (0–5 min), 75% (5–30 min), 75–100% (30–35 min) and 100% (35–45 min) at 12 mL/min. Injections with 500 μL of a 60 mg/mL fraction solution in methanol were performed. This process allowed us to purify several acylphloroglucinol derivatives (α- and β-acids) from sub-fractions MC1 and MC2, as well as another chalcone, desmethylxanthohumol, from the sub-fraction MC7, with a purity greater than 95% (Figure 1). Throughout the process, we protected the samples of the light as much as possible.

4.1.4. UHPLC-UV-MS Analyses

The crude hydro-ethanolic extracts of hop parts (cones, leaves, stems and rhizomes) were analyzed by UHPLC-UV-MS. The mobile phase consisted of 0.1% formic acid in water and of 0.1% formic acid in acetonitrile. The gradient of acetonitrile was: 50% (0–1 min), 50–75% (1–3 min), 75% (3–5 min), 75–100% (5–7 min) and 100% (7–9,5 min) at 0.3 mL/min. Column temperature was set at 30 °C. Solutions of crude extracts were prepared in MeOH at 100 μg/mL for cones and 1 mg/mL for the other parts. Injection volume was 2 μL. The main chalcones and acylphloroglucinols were identified on the basis of the retention time of the purified standards and their mass spectra.

The ionization was performed in negative mode. Cone voltage was set at 10 V. Probe temperature was 600 °C. Capillary voltage was 0.8 kV. The MS-Scan mode was used from 100 to 1000 Da.

4.1.5. Quantification Using UHPLC-UV

The most abundant prenylated chalcones and acylphloroglucinol derivatives were quantified in hop crude hydro-ethanolic extracts (cones, leaves, stems and rhizomes), according to the international guidelines for analytical techniques for quality control of pharmaceuticals [73]. Quantification was performed in UV at 370 nm for chalcones and 330 nm for acylphloroglucinols. *Co*- and *ad*-acids were quantified from the respective calibration curves of the *n*-acids (humulone for alpha acids and lupulone for beta acids), using molecular weight ratio. Desmethylxanthohumol was quantified from xanthohumol calibration curve, using molecular weight ratio. Solutions of crude extracts were prepared in MeOH at 100 μg/mL for cones and 1 mg/mL for the other parts. Sample solutions were prepared in triplicate the same day. Aliquots of each solution (2 μL) were injected in triplicate.

Stock solutions of xanthohumol, humulone and lupulone, previously purified, were prepared at the concentration of 1 mg/mL in MeOH for quantification, then stored at −20 °C until use. Fifteen working solutions (100 μg/mL to 2.5 ng/mL) were daily prepared by dilutions. Three mixed solutions containing the three analytes were prepared at the concentrations of 100, 50 and 25 μg/mL from stock solutions. Then, lower concentrations were obtained from these intermediate solutions by successive dilutions in MeOH. Calibration curves were designed to cover the expected range of concentrations in samples after preliminary injection of crude extracts solutions. Nine, ten and twelve concentration levels were respectively used for calibration curves of lupulone, xanthohumol and humulone. They were built by plotting peak area (y) as a function of the nominal concentration for each calibration level (x) and then fitted by weighted ($1/x$) least square linear regression. Linearity and precision of the method, as well as the limit of detection (LOD) and the limit of quantification (LOQ) were reported in Table S1 (Supplementary Material). LOD was defined as the lowest concentration with a $S/N > 3$. LOQ was defined as the lowest concentration with a deviation <20% on back calculation. Intra and inter-day precisions were evaluated on cone sample solutions. They were prepared on three different days, in triplicate each day ($n = 3$, $k = 3$). 2 μL of each solution was injected 3 times.

4.1.6. Structural Elucidation

Structures of purified compounds were determined using NMR and HR-MS. Mono- (^{1}H and ^{13}C) and bi-dimensional (COSY, HSQC, HMBC) spectra were carried out for each compound. Prenylated chalcones were solubilized in deuterated methanol (MeOD) whereas acylphloroglucinol derivatives were solubilized in deuterated chloroform ($CDCl_3$). HR-MS analyses were carried out in positive mode with a range of m/z 100–1000 amu. Products were solubilized in methanol with a drop of DCM for the acylphloroglucinols.

4.2. Antimicrobial Bioassays

4.2.1. Antibacterial Screening of Extracts and Sub-Extracts Using Agar Dilution Method

Clinical bacterial isolates from human samples collected in Lille (France) and some collection strains were used. The first screening step on pathogenic bacteria was carried out with crude hydro-alcoholic extracts of different hop parts (Table 1). The second screening was performed using sub-extracts of cones on Gram-positive bacteria, including methicillin-sensitive *Staphylococcus aureus* (MSSA) and methicillin-resistant *Staphylococcus aureus* (MSSA) strains (Table 2). These tests were carried out on Petri dishes, Mueller-Hinton Agar (MHA) (Oxoid, UK) was mixed with the plant extract solution in MeOH at 5% (solvent control: 5% MeOH). Final extract concentrations in Petri dishes ranged from 1250 to 4.9 μg/mL. A multi-headed inoculator allowed spotting bacterial strains at 10^5 CFU/mL in cysteinated Ringer (CR) solution (Merck®, France). Minimal Inhibitory Concentrations (MICs) were visually determined after 24 h of incubation at 37 °C.

4.2.2. Antibacterial Susceptibility of Compounds Using Broth Microdilution Method

For bioassays, xanthohumol, desmethylxanthohumol, humulone, cohumulone, lupulone and colupulone were used had a minimum purity of 95% (HPLC-UV). The protocol employed was inspired by Abedini et al. [74] with some modifications. Products were solubilized in DMSO and serially diluted two-fold in MH medium. A bacterial suspension at 10^5 CFU/mL was added to obtain a final volume of 200 μL. Final phenolic product concentrations in wells ranged from 625 to 2.4 μg/mL (exception for lupulone for which dilutions were continued until 0.3 μg/mL). The susceptibility of the strain to DMSO has previously been assessed, the DMSO concentration in wells taken into account did not exceed 5% (concentration without effect on growth). Plates were incubated overnight with stirring (60 rpm) at 37 °C. The bacterial growth was indicated visually and by a developer of enzymatic activity (iodonitrotetrazolium chloride—INT, AppliChem, Germany) which reveals bacterial growth by a purple color after 15 min heating at 55 °C.

For the following experiments, the MRSA strain T28.1, isolated from a pathological sample of osteitis, was used. It was previously characterized by DNA biochips, which allowed highlighting some β-lactamases and the SCC-mec genes confirming the methicillin resistance [30]. Moreover, genes for enzymes and proteins involved in the capsule biosynthesis (capH5, capJ5 and capK5) and several intracellular adhesion proteins implicated in biofilm formation (icaA, icaC and icaD) were present.

The commercial product, isoxanthohumol, was also tested against *S. aureus* T28.1 (purity superior to 95%, Phytolab®, Germany).

4.2.3. Synergies with Selected Antibiotics (Checkerboard Method)

Checkerboard method was used to assess the potential co-action of xanthohumol, desmethylxanthohumol and lupulone between them or with some antibiotics [32,58]. Antibiotics were previously selected on the basis of a first screening using E-tests (BioMérieux®, France). They covered several classes and are currently used to treat either *S. aureus* infections or bone infections: oxacillin (purity 95%, Acros Organics, Belgium), ciprofloxacin, gentamicin and rifampicin (purity 99.9%, 65.7% and 99.2% respectively, PanReac AppliChem®, Germany). Each test was performed on a 96-well microplate using an 8-by-8 well configuration. Concentration of hops phenolic compounds and antibiotics tested ranged from MIC/4 to 4xMIC. Wells were filled with 100 µL of MH medium, 10 µL of each compound (DMSO for products and water for antibiotics) and 80 µL of a 10^5 CFU/mL bacterial suspension with appropriate solvent controls. Final concentration in DMSO was 5%, which did not affect the bacterial growth. The MIC of each product alone was checked at each test. Microplates were incubated overnight at 60 rpm and 37 °C. The bacterial growth was visually assessed and confirmed by revealing bacterial enzymatic activity by adding INT.

After visual analysis, the combination with the highest activity was determined by the calculation of the fractional inhibitory concentration (FIC) index [32], interpreted as synergistic (FIC < 0.5), additive (0.5 ≤ FIC ≤ 1), indifferent (1 < FIC ≤ 4) or antagonist (FIC > 4).

$$\text{FIC index} = \frac{\text{MIC A with B}}{\text{MIC A alone}} + \frac{\text{MIC B with A}}{\text{MIC B alone}}$$

4.2.4. Kill Curves

This experiment allowed following in time the effect of the product on a growing bacterial population, highlighting the bactericidal or bacteriostatic effect [75]. Stock solutions of xanthohumol, desmethylxanthohumol and lupulone were prepared in DMSO 20 times more concentrated than the desired final concentrations (MIC/4 to 4xMIC). An aliquot of 0.5 mL of purified product in DMSO was added to 8.5 mL of brain heart infusion (BHI) medium (Oxoid, UK). 1 mL of bacterial suspension at 10^5 CFU/mL was then introduced to the culture tube. A 5% DMSO control served as a negative control and was performed at each test. Culture tubes were incubated at 37 °C for 24 h. Counts were made every 2 h until 8 h and at 24 h by plating aliquots of serial tenfold dilutions on MHA. The determined bacterial concentrations were then converted into log(CFU/mL) and were expressed as a function of time. The detection threshold of this method was 10 CFU/mL and 1 log(CFU/mL) on graphics.

4.2.5. Post-Antibiotic Effect (PAE)

This method allows quantifying the delayed regrowth of a bacterial population following exposure to an active compound [76]. Stock solutions of xanthohumol, desmethylxanthohumol and lupulone were prepared in DMSO 20 times more concentrated than the desired final concentrations (MIC/4 to 4 × MIC). A 2 h pre-treatment with purified prenylated compounds was performed using 8.5 mL of BHI medium, 0.5 mL of purified product in DMSO and 1 mL of a bacterial suspension at 10^5 CFU/mL, incubated at 37 °C. Final concentrations in DMSO did not exceed 5%. The hop compound was then inactivated by a 1000-fold dilution. After inactivation, a growth curve was performed with counts at 30 min and every 2 h. The growth lag was quantified by comparison with the control, using the following formula:

$$\text{PAE} = \text{T} - \text{C}$$

T is the time needed for the bacterial population to grow by 1 log(CFU/mL) at the given concentration, C is the corresponding time for the control (Figure 5)

4.2.6. Anti-Biofilm Tests

These experiments were inspired and adapted from Liu et al. [77]. They were performed using a 96-well microplate with a flat bottom.

On Artificial Surface

First, the effect of xanthohumol, desmethylxanthohumol and lupulone was assessed on the biofilm formation: 180 µL of BHI medium containing glucose at 10 mg/mL was added to each well of a 96-well microplate with 10 µL of the product previously solubilized in DMSO and 10 µL of a 10^5 CFU/mL bacterial suspension. The maximum concentration in DMSO was 5%. Final concentrations of purified products were from MIC/4 to 4 × MIC. After 24 h incubation at 37 °C, wells were voided and washed 3 times with phosphate buffered saline solution (PBS, Sigma-Aldrich, Saint-Quentin Fallavier, France). Plates were then dried and 150 µL of crystal violet solution at 20 mg/mL in MeOH (Sigma-Aldrich®, Saint-Quentin Fallavier, France) were added for 15 min. After removing crystal violet, 150 µL of EtOH were added to solubilize crystal violet present in adherent bacteria. The optical density was read at 570 nm.

The effect was also evaluated after the biofilm formation in order to evaluate if the hop phenolic compounds are able to destroy it. A first culture of 24 h at 37 °C with 190 µL of BHI medium and 10 µL of a 10^5 CFU/mL bacterial suspension allowed producing the biofilm. Wells were voided and washed with PBS. The biofilm was then treated with xanthohumol, desmethylxanthohumol or lupulone diluted at 5% in the BHI medium to obtain a final volume of 200 µL. Plates were incubated for 24 h at 37 °C, then voided and colored with crystal violet as above.

On Synthetic Bone Substitute

β-Tricalcium phosphate discs (Cerasorb®, Curasan, Germany) were used as bone substitute. Non-glucose enriched BHI medium was used here, because the bacterial glucose metabolism causes an acidification of the culture medium which leads to the disintegration of the discs. Discs were introduced in a 24-well plate: 1.8 mL of BHI media were added with 0.1 mL of product in DMSO (5%) and 0.1 mL of a 10^5 CFU/mL bacterial suspension. Final concentrations of hop phenolic compounds were from MIC/4 to 4 × MIC. After 24 h at 37 °C, counts were performed in two steps. First, planktonic bacteria were counted from 100 µL of the culture supernatant by plating tenfold dilutions on MHA. Then, bacteria adhering to the discs were counted: discs were removed and washed with a CR solution, then, 10 mL of CR were added to each disk and treated 1 min by sonication (35 kHz) and 30 s by vortex. The obtained suspension was enumerated as previously. The detection threshold was also 1 log(CFU/mL).

4.2.7. Antiparasitic Activity of Hops Using Broth Microdilution Method

Tbb were cultivated in HMI9 medium containing 10% heat-inactivated foetal bovine serum (FBS) (Sigma-Aldrich), 150 mM L-cysteine and 20 mM beta-mercaptoethanol at 37 °C (CO_2 5%). Lmm (MHOM/BZ/84/BEL46) were cultivated in SDM-79 medium (Gibco) supplemented with 15% heat-inactivated FBS (Sigma-Aldrich) and 5 mg/L hemin at 28 °C (CO_2 5%). Antiparasitic bioassays were performed as described by Bero et al. [17]. Suramin (SUR) and pentamidine (PEN) were used as positive controls respectively. The hops compounds (xanthohumol, desmethylxanthohumol, humulone, lupulone) concentration that inhibits 50% of the cell viability (IC_{50}) was determined using GraphPad Prism, version 5.01 (GraphPad Software, San Diego, CA, USA).

4.3. *Antiproliferative Effect of Purified Compounds on Human Cell Lines*

Several human cell lines were used for the cytotoxic bioassays: non-cancer lung fibroblasts (WI-38), hepatocellular carcinoma (Hep-G2), osteosarcoma (MG-63) and the mouse monocyte macrophage J774. Cells were seeded into wells of a 96-well microplate in a Gibco™ Dulbecco's modified eagles medium (DMEM), except for MG-63 which were cultivated in a minimum essential medium (MEM) (ThermoFisher Scientific, Illkirch-Graffenstaden, France). Both media were enriched with 10% FBS (ThermoFisher Scientific, France) and some antibiotics (mixture penicillin/streptomycin 100 UI/mL, Sigma Aldrich). After one or two days at 37 °C (5% of CO_2), wells were emptied by suction. Cells were then treated with hops compounds (xanthohumol, desmethylxanthohumol, humulone, lupulone) in DMSO at 0.2% in the culture medium, to obtain a final volume of 100 µL in wells (negative control: 0.2% DMSO). Camptothecin was used as a positive control. After 48 to 72 h exposure, culture medium was replaced by 10% of Alamar blue or 3-(4,5-dimethylthiazol-2-yl)-2,5-diphenyltetrazolium bromide (MTT) in the medium (ThermoFisher Scientific®, Illkirch, France) and plates were incubated the time necessary to the reaction. Results were measured respectively by fluorescence (excitation 530 nm and emission 590 nm) or by optical density at 550 nm. The IC_{50} of each product was determined using GraphPad Prism (version 5.01).

4.4. Statistical Analyses

Statistical analyses were carried out using the software R, version 3.4.1 (The R Foundation for Statistical Computing, Vienna, Austria). Each experiment was performed in independent triplicates. For each distribution, the normality of the residues was assessed using Shapiro test. If the normality was accepted, an ANOVA and the Tukey HSD test were performed. If the normality was refused, Kruskal Wallis and Dunn's tests were used at a significance level of $p = 0.05$.

5. Conclusions

Xanthohumol, desmethylxanthohumol and lupulone from hops, with their dual antibacterial and anti-biofilm actions, are potential agents in the treatment of infections due to MRSA. Their additive or synergistic actions with antibiotics could render treatments more effective and thus could prevent toxicity at systemic level if used in topical application. Their chemical structures differ from current anti-staphylococcal agents and enable us to assume that they act on a different target site of action in *S. aureus*. The exact identification of this target is a future challenge. Moreover, for the first-time, activity of hops phenolic compounds was highlighted on the Tbb and Lmm parasites.

Supplementary Materials: Table S1. Linearity and sensitivity of the quantification method by UPLC-UV for xanthohumol, humulone and lupulone, Table S2. ^{1}H and ^{13}C NMR data for xanthohumol and desmethylxanthohumol in MeOD[a], Table S3. ^{1}H and ^{13}C NMR data for humulone and cohumulone in CDCl3[a], Table S4. ^{1}H and ^{13}C NMR data for lupulone and colupulone in CDCl3[a], Figure S1. Chromatograms at 370 nm of the crude hydro-ethanolic extract of cones and purified chalcones (desmethylxanthohumol and xanthohumol), Figure S2. Chromatograms at 330 nm of the crude hydro-ethanolic extract of cones and purified acylphloroglucinol derivatives (cohumulone, humulone, colupulone and lupulone), Figure S3. Total ion chromatogram of the crude hydro-ethanolic extract of cones in negative mode and selected ion recording of purified chalcones (desmethylxanthohumol and xanthohumol) and acylphloroglucinol derivatives (cohumulone, humulone, colupulone and lupulone).

Author Contributions: In this paper, L.B. (PhD student) performed the purification of hops phenolic compounds, all antibacterial bioassays and some cytotoxicity assays (Hep-G2). S.S. is one of the supervisors of L.B. and is head of the department of pharmacognosy. N.B. performed the quantification of compounds in different extracts and J.J. prepared the extracts. C.B. performed the antiparasitic bioassays and some cytotoxicity experiments (WI-38 and J774) and J.Q.-L. designed and supervised these bioassays. S.M. helped L.B. in the realization of antibacterial experiments and C.N. conceived and supervised these bioassays. V.R. supervised cytotoxicity assays against Hep-G2. S.B. and T.H. contributed in the realization of a few experiments. F.C. conceived and performed cytotoxicity experiments against MG-63. J.S. helped L.B. in the purification of compounds and the realization of some antibacterial bioassays. C.R. is the supervisor of L.B. and is at the origin of the project. She obtained the funding of the PhD fellowship of L.B. She designed the entire project and she mainly supervised the phytochemistry part. C.R., L.B., C.N., J.Q.-L. and N.B. contributed to the writing of the paper and all of the authors approved the manuscript.

Acknowledgments: The authors wish to thank Beck family (Bailleul, France) to supply hop samples each year. They are grateful to PSM (University of Lille, France, J.F. Goossens) and LARMN (University of Lille, France, N. Azaroual), as well as the laboratory of bacteriology (LIRIC, France) and the laboratory of toxicology (S. Anthérieu) for access to equipment. They also acknowledge Charlotte Maillet and Isabelle Houcke (LIRIC, France) and Maude Bourlet (UCL) for their skillful technical assistance. The authors wish to thank Eric Senneville (Centre Hospitalier Gustave Dron, Department of Infectious Diseases) for his helpful comments on the manuscript.

References

1. OMS. Global Action Plan on Antimicrobial Resistance. 2015. Available online: www.wpro.who.int/entity/drug_resistance/resources/global_action_plan_eng.pdf (accessed on 4 March 2019).
2. ANSES; ANSM; Santé Publique France. Consommation D'antibiotiques et Résistance aux Antibiotiques en France: Nécessité D'une Mobilisation Déterminée et Durable. 2016. Available online: http://invs.santepubliquefrance.fr/Publications-et-outils/Rapports-et-syntheses/Maladies-infectieuses/2016/Consommation-d-antibiotiques-et-resistance-aux-antibiotiques-en-France-necessite-d-une-mobilisation-determinee-et-durable (accessed on 4 March 2019).
3. Kavanagh, K.T.; Abusalaim, S.; Calderon, L.E. The incidence of MRSA infections in the United States: Is a more comprehensive tracking system needed? *Antimicrob. Resist. Infect. Control* **2017**, *6*, 34. [CrossRef] [PubMed]
4. Gibbons, S. Anti-staphylococcal plant natural products. *Nat. Prod. Rep.* **2004**, *21*, 263–277. [CrossRef] [PubMed]
5. Abreu, A.C.; McBain, A.J.; Simões, M. Plants as sources of new antimicrobials and resistance-modifying agents. *Nat. Prod. Rep.* **2012**, *29*, 1007–1021. [CrossRef] [PubMed]
6. European Centre for Disease Prevention and Control. *Surveillance of Antimicrobial Resistance in Europe 2016*; Annual Report of the European Antimicrobial Resistance Surveillance Network (EARS-Net); ECDC: Stockholm, Sweden, 2017.
7. Cosgrove, S.E.; Sakoulas, G.; Perencevich, E.N.; Schwaber, M.J.; Karchmer, A.W.; Carmeli, Y. Comparison of mortality associated with methicillin-resistant and methicillin-susceptible *Staphylococcus aureus* bacteremia: A meta-analysis. *Clin. Infect. Dis.* **2003**, *36*, 53–59. [CrossRef] [PubMed]
8. Hanberger, H.; Walther, S.; Leone, M.; Barie, P.S.; Rello, J.; Lipman, J.; Marshall, J.C.; Anzueto, A.; Sakr, Y.; Pickkers, P.; et al. Increased mortality associated with meticillin-resistant *Staphylococcus aureus* (MRSA) infection in the Intensive Care Unit: Results from the EPIC II study. *Int. J. Antimicrob. Agents* **2011**, *38*, 331–335. [CrossRef] [PubMed]
9. Dunyach-Remy, C.; Ngba Essebe, C.; Sotto, A.; Lavigne, J.P. *Staphylococcus aureus* Toxins and Diabetic Foot Ulcers: Role in Pathogenesis and Interest in Diagnosis. *Toxins* **2016**, *8*, 209. [CrossRef] [PubMed]
10. Stavri, M.; Piddock, L.J.; Gibbons, S. Bacterial efflux pump inhibitors from natural sources. *J. Antimicrob. Chemother.* **2007**, *59*, 1247–1260. [CrossRef] [PubMed]
11. Handzlik, J.; Matys, A.; Kieć-Kononowicz, K. Recent Advances in Multi-Drug Resistance (MDR) Efflux Pump Inhibitors of Gram-Positive Bacteria *S. aureus*. *Antibiotics* **2013**, *2*, 28–45. [CrossRef]
12. Brincat, J.P.; Broccatelli, F.; Sabatini, S.; Frosini, M.; Neri, A.; Kaatz, G.W.; Cruciani, G.; Carosati, E. Ligand Promiscuity between the Efflux Pumps Human P-Glycoprotein and *S. aureus* NorA. *ACS Med. Chem. Lett.* **2012**, *3*, 248–251. [CrossRef]
13. Gould, I.M.; David, M.Z.; Esposito, S.; Garau, J.; Lina, G.; Mazzei, T.; Peters, G. New insights into meticillin-resistant *Staphylococcus aureus* (MRSA) pathogenesis, treatment and resistance. *Int. J. Antimicrob. Agents* **2012**, *39*, 96–104. [CrossRef]
14. Rozalski, M.; Micota, B.; Sadowska, B.; Stochmal, A.; Jedrejek, D.; Wieckowska-Szakiel, M.; Rozalska, B. Antiadherent and Antibiofilm Activity of *Humulus lupulus* L. Derived Products: New Pharmacological Properties. *BioMed Res. Int.* **2013**, *2013*, 7. [CrossRef]
15. Keita, M.; Bouteille, B.; Enanga, B.; Vallat, J.M.; Dumas, M. *Trypanosoma brucei brucei*: A Long-Term Model of Human African Trypanosomiases in Mice, Meningo-Encaphalitis, Astrocytosis, and Neurological Disorders. *Exp. Parasitol.* **1997**, *85*, 183–192. [CrossRef]

16. Ponte-Sucre, A. An Overview of *Trypanosoma brucei* Infections: An Intense Host-Parasite Interaction. *Front. Microbiol.* **2016**, *7*, 2126. [CrossRef]
17. Bero, J.; Hannaert, V.; Chataigne, G.; Hérent, M.F.; Quetin-Leclercq, J. In vitro antitrypanosomal and antileishmanial activity of plants used in Benin in traditional medicine and bio-guided fractionation of the most active extract. *J. Ethnopharmacol.* **2011**, *137*, 998–1002. [CrossRef]
18. Steenackers, B.; De Cooman, L.; De Vos, D. Chemical transformations of characteristic hop secondary metabolites in relation to beer properties and the brewing process: A review. *Food Chem.* **2015**, *172*, 742–756. [CrossRef]
19. Bocquet, L.; Sahpaz, S.; Hilbert, J.L.; Rambaud, C.; Rivière, C. *Humulus lupulus* L., a very popular beer ingredient and medicinal plant: Overview of its phytochemistry, its bioactivity, and its biotechnology. *Phytochem. Rev.* **2018**, *17*, 1047–1090. [CrossRef]
20. Bocquet, L.; Sahpaz, S.; Rivière, C. An Overview of the Antimicrobial Properties of Hop. In *Natural Antimicrobial Agents*; Mérillon, J.M., Rivière, C., Eds.; Series Sustainable Development and Biodiversity; Springer International Publishing AG: Cham, Switzerland, 2018; Volume 19, pp. 31–54.
21. Teuber, M.; Schmalreck, A.F. Membrane leakage in *Bacillus subtilis* 168 induced by the hop constituents lupulone, humulone, isohumulone and humulinic acid. *Arch. Für Mikrobiol.* **1973**, *94*, 159–171. [CrossRef]
22. Gerhäuser, C. Broad spectrum anti-infective potential of xanthohumol from hop (*Humulus lupulus* L.) in comparison with activities of other hop constituents and xanthohumol metabolites. *Mol. Nutr. Food Res.* **2005**, *49*, 827–831. [CrossRef]
23. Bogdanova, K.; Röderova, M.; Kolar, M.; Langova, K.; Dusek, M.; Jost, P.; Kubelkova, K.; Bostik, P.; Olsovska, J. Antibiofilm activity of bioactive hop compounds humulone, lupulone and xanthohumol toward susceptible and resistant staphylococci. *Res. Microbiol.* **2018**, *169*, 127–134. [CrossRef]
24. Frölich, S.; Schubert, C.; Bienzle, U.; Jenett-Siems, K. In Vitro Antiplasmodial activity of prenylated chalcone derivatives of hops (*Humulus lupulus*) and their interaction with Haemin. *J. Antimicrob. Chemother.* **2005**, *55*, 883–887. [CrossRef]
25. Srinivasan, V.; Goldberg, D.; Haas, G.J. Contribution to the Antimicrobial Spectrum of Hop Constituents. *Econ. Bot.* **2004**, *58*, 230–238. [CrossRef]
26. Höltzel, A.; Schlotterbeck, G.; Albert, K.; Bayer, E. Separation and characterisation of hop bitter acids by HPLC-^{1}H NMR coupling. *Chromatographia* **1996**, *42*, 499–505. [CrossRef]
27. Zhang, X.; Liang, X.; Xiao, H.; Xu, Q. Direct characterization of bitter acids in a crude hop extract by liquid chromatography-atmospheric pressure chemical ionization mass spectrometry. *J. Am. Soc. Mass Spectrom.* **2004**, *15*, 180–187. [CrossRef] [PubMed]
28. Vogel, S.; Ohmayer, S.; Brunner, G.; Heilmann, J. Natural and non-natural prenylated chalcones: Synthesis, cytotoxicity and anti-oxidative activity. *Bioorg. Med. Chem.* **2008**, *16*, 4286–4293. [CrossRef]
29. Intelmann, D.; Haseleu, G.; Hofmann, T. LC-MS/MS quantitation of hop-derived bitter compounds in beer using the ECHO technique. *J. Agric. Food Chem.* **2009**, *57*, 1172–1182. [CrossRef] [PubMed]
30. Senneville, E.; Brière, M.; Neut, C.; Messad, N.; Lina, G.; Richard, J.L.; Sotto, A.; Lavigne, J.P.; The French Study Group on the Diabetic Foot. First report of the predominance of clonal complex 398 *Staphylococcus aureus* strains in osteomyelitis complicating diabetic foot ulcers: A national French study. *Clin. Microbiol. Infect.* **2014**, *20*, O274–O277. [CrossRef]
31. EUCAST, European Committee on Antimicrobial Susceptibility Testing. Comité de l'Antibiogramme de la Société Française de Microbiologie. Recommandations. 2019. Available online: File:///C:/Users/celine/Desktop/CASFM2019_V1.0.pdf (accessed on 4 March 2019).
32. Bonapace, C.R.; Bosso, J.A.; Friedrich, L.V.; White, R.L. Comparison of methods of interpretation of checkerboard synergy testing. *Diagn. Microbiol. Infect. Dis.* **2002**, *44*, 363–366. [CrossRef]
33. Mahieux, S.; Nieto-Bobadilla, M.S.; Houcke, I.; Neut, C. How to Study Antimicrobial Activities of Plant Extracts: A Critical Point of View. In *Natural Antimicrobial Agents*; Mérillon, J.M., Rivière, C., Eds.; Series Sustainable Development and Biodiversity; Springer International Publishing AG: Cham, Switzerland, 2018; Volume 19, pp. 55–71.
34. Stoodley, P.; Sauer, K.; Davies, D.G.; Costerton, J.W. Biofilms as Complex Differentiated Communities. *Annu. Rev. Microbiol.* **2002**, *56*, 187–209. [CrossRef] [PubMed]

35. Centers for Disease Control and Prevention. *Antibiotic Resistance Threats in the United States, 2013*; Centers for Disease Control and Prevention: Atlanta, GA, USA, 2013. Available online: http://www.cdc.gov/drugresistance/threat-report-2013/pdf/ar-threats-2013-508.pdf (accessed on 4 March 2019).
36. Tacconelli, E.; Carrara, E.; Savoldi, A.; Harbarth, S.; Mendelson, M.; Monnet, D.L.; Pulcini, C.; Kahlmeter, G.; Kluytmans, J.; Carmeli, Y.; et al. Discovery, research, and development of new antibiotics: The WHO priority list of antibiotic-resistant bacteria and tuberculosis. *Lancet. Infect. Dis.* **2018**, *18*, 318–327. [CrossRef]
37. Arias, C.A.; Murray, B.E. A New Antibiotic and the Evolution of Resistance. *N. Engl. J. Med.* **2015**, *372*, 1168–1170. [CrossRef]
38. Ventola, C.L. The Antibiotic Resistance Crisis. Part 1: Causes and Threats. *PT* **2015**, *40*, 277–283.
39. Bollenbach, T. Antimicrobial interactions: Mechanisms and implications for drug discovery and resistance evolution. *Curr. Opin. Microbiol.* **2015**, *27*, 1–9. [CrossRef]
40. Mizobuchi, S.; Sato, Y. Antifungal Activities of Hop Bitter Resins and Related Compounds. *Agric. Biol. Chem.* **1985**, *49*, 399–403.
41. Schmalreck, A.F.; Teuber, M. Structural features determining the antibiotic potencies of natural and synthetic hop bitter resins, their precursors and derivatives. *Can. J. Microbiol.* **1975**, *21*, 205–212. [CrossRef]
42. Larson, A.E.; Yu, R.R.Y.; Lee, O.A.; Price, S.; Haas, G.J.; Johnson, E.A. Antimicrobial activity of hop extracts against *Listeria monocytogenes* in media and in food. *Int. J. Food Microbiol.* **1996**, *33*, 195–207. [CrossRef]
43. Cermak, P.; Olsovska, J.; Mikyska, A.; Dusek, M.; Kadleckova, Z.; Vanicek, J.; Nyc, O.; Sigler, K.; Bostikova, V.; Bostik, P. Strong antimicrobial activity of xanthohumol and other derivatives from hops (*Humulus lupulus* L.) on gut anaerobic bacteria. *APMIS* **2017**, *125*, 1033–1038. [CrossRef]
44. Langezaal, C.R.; Chandra, A.; Scheffer, J.J.C. Antimicrobial screening of essential oils and extracts of some *Humulus lupulus* L. cultivars. *Pharmaceutisch Weekblad. Sci. Ed.* **1992**, *14*, 353–356. [CrossRef]
45. Abram, V.; Čeh, B.; Vidmar, M.; Hercezi, M.; Lazić, N.; Bucik, V.; Mozina, S.S.; Kosir, I.J.; Kac, M.; Demsar, L.; et al. A comparison of antioxidant and antimicrobial activity between hop leaves and hop cones. *Ind. Crops Prod.* **2015**, *64*, 124–134. [CrossRef]
46. Prencipe, F.P.; Brighenti, V.; Rodolfi, M.; Mongelli, A.; d'all'Asta, C.; Ganino, T.; Bruni, R.; Pellati, F. Development of a new high-performance liquid chromatography method with diode array and electrospray ionization-mass spectrometry detection for the metabolite fingerprinting of bioactive compounds in *Humulus lupulus* L. *J. Chromatogr. A* **2014**, *1349*, 50–59. [CrossRef]
47. Čeh, B.; Kač, M.; Košir, I.J.; Abram, V. Relationships between Xanthohumol and Polyphenol Content in Hop Leaves and Hop Cones with Regard to Water Supply and Cultivar. *Int. J. Mol. Sci.* **2007**, *8*, 989–1000. [CrossRef]
48. Farag, M.A.; Porzel, A.; Schmidt, J.; Wessjohann, L.A. Metabolite profiling and fingerprinting of commercial cultivars of *Humulus lupulus* L. (hop): A comparison of MS and NMR methods in metabolomics. *Metabolomics* **2012**, *8*, 492–507. [CrossRef]
49. Simpson, W.J.; Smith, A.R. Factors affecting antibacterial activity of hop compounds and their derivatives. *J. Appl. Bacteriol.* **1992**, *72*, 327–334. [CrossRef]
50. Tsukiyama, R.I.; Katsura, H.; Tokuriki, N.; Kobayashi, M. Antibacterial activity of licochalcone A against spore-forming bacteria. *Antimicrob. Agents Chemother.* **2002**, *46*, 1226–1230. [CrossRef]
51. Ávila, H.P.; Smânia, E.F.; Monache, F.D.; Smânia, A., Jr. Structure-activity relationship of antibacterial chalcones. *Bioorg. Med. Chem.* **2008**, *16*, 9790–9794. [CrossRef]
52. Teng, Y.; Li, X.; Yang, K.; Li, X.; Zhang, Z.; Wang, L.; Deng, Z.; Song, B.; Yan, Z.; Zhang, Y.; et al. Synthesis and antioxidant evaluation of desmethylxanthohumol analogs and their dimers. *Eur. J. Med. Chem.* **2017**, *125*, 335–345. [CrossRef]
53. Olivella, M.S.; Zarelli, V.E.P.; Pappano, N.B.; Debattista, N.B. A comparative study of bacteriostatic activity of synthetic hydroxylated flavonoids. *Braz. J. Microbiol.* **2001**, *32*, 229–232. [CrossRef]
54. Legette, L.; Ma, L.; Reed, R.L.; Miranda, C.L.; Christensen, J.M.; Rodriguez-Proteau, R.; Stevens, J.F. Pharmacokinetics of xanthohumol and metabolites in rats after oral and intravenous administration. *Mol. Nutr. Food Res.* **2012**, *56*, 466–474. [CrossRef]
55. Żołnierczyk, A.K.; Mączka, W.K.; Grabarczyk, M.; Wińska, K.; Woźniak, E.; Anioł, M. Isoxanthohumol—Biologically active hop flavonoid. *Fitoterapia* **2015**, *103*, 71–82. [CrossRef]

56. Possemiers, S.; Bolca, S.; Grootaert, C.; Heyerick, A.; Decroos, K.; Dhooge, W.; De Keukeleire, D.; Rabot, S.; Verstraete, W.; Van de Wiele, T. The prenylflavonoid isoxanthohumol from hops (*Humulus lupulus* L.) is activated into the potent phytoestrogen 8-prenylnaringenin in vitro and in the human intestine. *J. Nutr.* **2006**, *136*, 1862–1867. [CrossRef]
57. Hemaiswarya, S.; Kruthiventi, A.K.; Doble, M. Synergism between natural products and antibiotics against infectious diseases. *Phytomedicine* **2008**, *15*, 639–652. [CrossRef]
58. Hsieh, M.H.; Yu, C.M.; Yu, V.L.; Chow, J.W. Synergy assessed by checkerboard a critical analysis. *Diagn. Microbiol. Infect. Dis.* **1993**, *16*, 343–349. [CrossRef]
59. Natarajan, P.; Katta, S.; Andrei, I.; Babu Rao Ambati, V.; Leonida, M.; Haas, G.J. Positive antibacterial co-action between hop (*Humulus lupulus*) constituents and selected antibiotics. *Phytomedicine* **2008**, *15*, 194–201. [CrossRef]
60. Lipsky, B.A.; Peters, E.J.; Senneville, E.; Berendt, A.R.; Embil, J.M.; Lavery, L.A.; Urbančič-Rovan, V.; Jeffcoate, W.J. Expert opinion on the management of infections in the diabetic foot. *Diabetes Metab. Res. Rev.* **2012**, *1*, 163–178. [CrossRef] [PubMed]
61. Nicodème, J.D.; Nicodème Paulin, E.; Zingg, M.; Uçkay, I.; Malacarne, S.; Suva, D. Pied diabétique infecté: Du diagnostic à la prise en charge. *Rev. Méd. Suisse* **2015**, *11*, 1238–1241.
62. Lipsky, B.A.; Hoey, C. Topical Antimicrobial Therapy for Treating Chronic Wounds. *Clin. Infect. Dis.* **2009**, *49*, 1541–1549. [CrossRef] [PubMed]
63. Barth, R.E.; Vogely, H.C.; Hoepelman, A.I.; Peters, E.J.; Peters, E.J. To bead or not to bead? Treatment of osteomyelitis and prosthetic joint associated infections with gentamicin bead chains. *Int. J. Antimicrob. Agents* **2011**, *38*, 371–375. [CrossRef]
64. Roeder, B.; Van Gils, C.C.; Maling, S. Antibiotic beads in the treatment of diabetic pedal osteomyelitis. *J. Foot Ankle Surg.* **2000**, *39*, 124–130. [CrossRef]
65. O' Meara, S.M.; Cullum, N.A.; Majid, M.; Sheldon, T.A. Systematic review of antimicrobial agents used for chronic wounds. *Br. J. Surg.* **2001**, *88*, 4–21. [CrossRef]
66. Ho, Y.C.; Liu, C.H.; Chen, C.N.; Duan, K.J.; Lin, M.T. Inhibitory effects of xanthohumol from hops (*Humulus lupulus* L.) on human hepatocellular carcinoma cell lines. *Phytother. Res.* **2008**, *22*, 1465–1468. [CrossRef]
67. Yong, W.K.; Ho, Y.F.; Malek, S.N. Xanthohumol induces apoptosis and S phase cell cycle arrest in A549 non-small cell lung cancer cells. *Pharmacogn. Mag.* **2015**, *11*, 275–283.
68. Dorn, C.; Bataille, F.; Gaebele, E.; Heilmann, J.; Hellerbrand, C. Xanthohumol feeding deas not impair organ function and homeostasis in mice. *Food Chem. Toxicol.* **2010**, *48*, 1890–1897. [CrossRef] [PubMed]
69. Legette, L.C.; Karnpracha, C.; Reed, R.L.; Choi, J.; Bobe, G.; Christensen, J.M.; Rodriguez-Proteau, R.; Purnell, J.; Stevens, J.F. Human pharmacokinetics of xanthohumol, an anti-hyperglycemic flavonoid from hops. *Mol. Nutr. Food Res.* **2014**, *58*, 248–255. [CrossRef]
70. Mouratidis, P.X.E.; Colston, K.W.; Tucknott, M.L.; Tyrrell, E.; Pirianov, G. An Investigation into the Anticancer Effects and Mechanism of Action of Hop β-Acid Lupulone and Its Natural and Synthetic Derivatives in Prostate Cancer Cells. *Nutr. Cancer* **2013**, *65*, 1086–1092. [CrossRef] [PubMed]
71. Tyrrell, E.; Archer, R.; Tucknott, M.; Colston, K.; Pirianov, G.; Ramanthan, D.; Dhillon, R.; Sinclair, A.; Skinner, G.A. The synthesis and anticancer effects of a range of natural and unnatural hop β-acids on breast cancer cells. *Phytochem. Lett.* **2012**, *5*, 144–149. [CrossRef]
72. Monzote, L.; Lackova, A.; Staniek, K.; Steinbauer, S.; Pichler, G.; Jäger, W.; Gille, L. The antileishmanial activity of xanthohumol is mediated by mitochondrial inhibition. *Parasitology* **2017**, *144*, 747–759. [CrossRef]
73. *International Conference on Harmonization of Technical Requirements for the Registration of Pharmaceuticals for Human Use (ICH), Guideline Q2(R1)-Validation of Analytical Procedures: Text and Methodology*; ICH Secretariat, c/o; IFPMA: Geneva, Switzerland, 2005.
74. Abedini, A.; Roumy, V.; Mahieux, S.; Biabiany, M.; Standaert-Vitse, A.; Rivière, C.; Sahpaz, S.; Bailleul, F.; Neut, C.; Hennebelle, T. Rosmarinic Acid and Its Methyl Ester as Antimicrobial Components of the Hydromethanolic Extract of *Hyptis atrorubens* Poit. (Lamiaceae). *Evid. Based Complement. Altern. Med.* **2013**, *2013*, 1–11. [CrossRef]
75. Zwietering, M.H.; Jongenburger, I.; Rombouts, F.M.; van't Riet, K. Modeling of the Bacterial Growth Curve. *Appl. Environ. Microbiol.* **1990**, *56*, 1875–1881.

Analysis of Flavonoids Bioactivity for Cholestatic Liver Disease: Systematic Literature Search and Experimental Approaches

Juan Carlos Sánchez-Salgado [1,2,*], Samuel Estrada-Soto [2,*], Sara García-Jiménez [2], Sergio Montes [3], Jaime Gómez-Zamudio [4] and Rafael Villalobos-Molina [5,6]

1 Instituto de Medicina Molecular y Ciencias Avanzadas, Mexico City 01900, Mexico
2 Facultad de Farmacia, Universidad Autónoma del Estado de Morelos, Cuernavaca, MOR 62209, Mexico; saragarcia@uaem.mx
3 Instituto Nacional de Neurología y Neurocirugía, Mexico City 14269, Mexico; montesergio@yahoo.com
4 Unidad de Investigación Médica en Bioquímica, Hospital de Especialidades, Centro Médico Nacional Siglo XXI, IMSS, México City 06720, Mexico; jaime_gomez_zamudio@hotmail.com
5 Unidad de Biomedicina, Facultad de Estudios Superiores-Iztacala, Universidad Nacional Autónoma de México, Tlalnepantla 54090, Mexico; villalobos@campus.iztacala.unam.mx
6 Departamento de Bioquímica, Facultad de Medicina, Universidad Nacional Autónoma de México, Ciudad de México 04510, México
* Correspondence: juanc.sanchez@immca.com.mx (J.C.S.-S.); enoch@uaem.mx (S.E.-S.);

Abstract: Flavonoids are naturally occurring compounds that show health benefits on the liver. However, there is little investigation about identification and evaluation of new flavonoid-containing drugs for cholestatic liver disease, one of the most common liver illnesses. We aimed to a systematic search regarding efficacy of flavonoids for treatment of cholestatic liver disease, and then evaluate naringenin (NG) as representative flavonoid in an obstructive cholestasis model. We searched for information of experimental and clinical studies in four major databases without time and language limits. Intervention was defined as any flavonoid derivate compared with other flavonoid, placebo, or without comparator. In addition, we evaluated NG on a bile duct-ligated model in order to contribute evidence of its actions. Eleven experimental reports that support the efficacy of flavonoids in cholestatic liver disease were identified. However, there was no homogeneity in efficacy endpoints evaluated and methodology. On the other hand, NG showed beneficial effects by improving specific metabolic (cholesterol and lipoproteins) and liver damage (bilirubin and alkaline phosphatase) biomarkers. The review lacks homogeneous evidence about efficacy of flavonoids in experimental settings, and is susceptible to risk for bias. NG only showed improvements in specific disease biomarkers. More investigation is still needed to determine its potential for drug development.

Keywords: flavonoids; systematic review; cholestasis

1. Introduction

Liver disease is a prominent health problem with an important epidemiological and economic burden worldwide, accounting for 25% of prevalence [1,2]. However, this estimation is inconsistent since there is no reliable and applicable diagnostic test yet [2].

Cholestasis is an impaired bile flow from liver to duodenum that triggers unspecific cellular damage, which initiates inflammatory and fibro-genic processes in the liver, as well as cirrhosis and hepatocellular cancer in advanced stages [3]. This alteration might be provoked by an impaired export of bile acids to bile canaliculi (intrahepatic cholestasis), or by physical obstruction of bile flow due to gall stones, parasites, or biliary tumor growth (extrahepatic cholestasis) [4].

The most accepted and well established experimental model that reproduces pathobiochemical alterations is the bile duct-ligated (BDL) rodent model [3,5]. The surgical bile duct ligation induces an obstructive cholestatic damage, which results in typical phenotype as in human cholestasis [3,5,6]. In this context, there are exhaustive efforts to found new therapeutic agents able to decrease pathological severity and progression of cholestatic liver diseases. Despite this, there are limited approved drug interventions for the treatment of this disease, i.e., ursodeoxycholic acid (UDCA) is the only approved oral drug for cholestatic liver diseases, such as primary biliary cirrhosis and obstructive cholestasis [7,8]. Additionally, silymarin, a mixture of flavolignans from Silybum marianum (milk thistle), has been proposed as an alternative for primary biliary cirrhosis due to its antioxidant and hepatoprotective properties [9–11].

Systematic reviews and meta-analysis have become increasingly important in decision making for drug discovery. In fact, this technique is a powerful evidence-based strategy to ensure there is justification for further research on bioactive molecules or re-planning research objectives [12]. A little investigation has been carried out on flavonoid efficacy in disease. Only a systematic review summarizes biological activities of prenylated flavonoids and suggests the structural implications for their bioactivities [13]. However, there is no information about efficacy of these compounds on cholestatic liver disease despite previous evidence for silymarin.

Previously we reported the beneficial effects of flavonoid-rich extract of *Cochlospermum vitifolium* bark for improvement of liver enzymes activity in BDL rat [14]. Then, HPLC analysis showed that one of its main bioactive compounds was naringenin (NG), a widely spread flavonoid in nature [15]. Recently, a chemical analysis revealed the presence of other flavonoids in the bark extract of this species [16].

This work summarizes and compares the efficacy endpoints reported for flavonoids in cholestatic liver disease, taking into account clinical and experimental settings, by systematic literature search in four major databases. Moreover, we evaluated the efficacy of NG in a BDL Wistar rat model in order to compare retrieved information from literature. To the best of our knowledge, this is the first systematic search of flavonoids as candidates for cholestasis therapy, as well as to show the biological effects of NG on the BDL rat.

2. Materials and Methods

2.1. *Systematic Review*

2.1.1. Sources

We conducted a systematic search for peer-reviewed articles in four major databases: Pubmed (Medline), Cochrane Library, Trip Database, and Lilacs. PRISMA statement was followed in order to establish the evidence-based minimum set of items for reporting on systematic reviews.

2.1.2. Eligibility Criteria

A PICO strategy was developed as described in Table S1. Briefly, the databases were searched using combinations of the following terms: flavonoid, cholestasis, and bile duct ligated. A species filter for human or animal was applied to identify clinical trials or experimental assays, respectively. Simple literature reviews, case reports, editorial letters, comments, as well as duplicated or no abstract articles were excluded. The searching did not consider time and language limits.

2.1.3. Studies Selection

The inclusion criteria for the selection of manuscripts were: all articles containing keywords in title, abstract or full-text, as well as those reporting clinical trials or experimental studies of isolated flavonoids for the treatment of cholestatic liver diseases (primary biliary cirrhosis, primary sclerosing cholangitis, biliary atresia, or Alagille syndrome). Only with BDL were selected in order to compare our experimental data. The selection was conducted by two independent reviewers, who analyzed the articles for discrepancies.

2.1.4. Meta-Analysis

A meta-analysis of the retrieved data could not be carried out due to methodological heterogeneity such as dosing, mode of administration, animal species, and time of exposure.

2.1.5. Risk of Bias Assessment

In order to assess the risk of biases of the animal studies reported in this systematic review, we applied a modified version of Cochrane's RoB tool denominated Systematic Review Centre for Laboratory animal Experimentation (SYRCLE). This tool considers six types of biases: Selection, performance, detection, attrition, reporting, and other biases, comprised of 10 items [17].

2.2. Experimental Studies

2.2.1. Reagents and Materials

Naringenin ~95% were purchased from Sigma-Aldrich Co. (St. Louis, MO, USA). Other reagents and surgical supplies were purchased from local sources.

2.2.2. Sample Preparation

Briefly, test samples were dissolved using a 10% aqueous solution of dimethylsulfoxide (DMSO). Dose of NG used was 50 mg/kg/day; the control group received 2 mL of vehicle.

2.2.3. Animal Model

Male Wistar rats (250–300 g, b.w.) were used under laboratory conditions with standard rodent diet and water ad libitum. All of the protocols were conducted as established by Federal Regulations for Animal Experimentation and Care (NOM-062-ZOO-1999, SAGARPA) and approved by Scientific and Bioethics Committee of Facultad de Farmacia (UAEM).

All animals were anesthetized by intraperitoneal injection of sodium pentobarbital (35 mg/kg), shaved and sanitized using a surgical disinfecting solution. A 1 cm incision below xiphoid process was made to extract gastrohepatic epiplon and locate duodenum segment. Once bile duct was cleaned for connective tissue, a triple ligation was made on bile duct using non-absorbable monofilament nylon suture (Farmacéutica Internacional S.A. de C.V., Mexico City, Mexico), and cut in two segments. Unconscious animals were gently sutured and allocated in warmed room until recovery. Sham animals (surgery control group) were subjected to the same protocol, but without ligation.

After 24 h post-surgery, animals were randomly allocated in three experimental groups ($n = 10$ animals per group) and began to receive the treatment. The experimental groups were: Sham + vehicle, BDL + vehicle, and BDL + NG. Aseptic cleaning was made along experiments using povidone-iodine 10% solution as palliative care. After 10 days of treatment all animals were sacrificed by dislocation and blood samples extracted by cardiac puncture. ARRIVE guidelines were followed for reporting this assay.

2.2.4. Biomarkers Quantification

Fresh collected blood samples were centrifuged at 3000 g for 10 min. Serum was separated from cell fraction and stored at −20 °C until analysis. Non-specific cholestasis biomarkers alanine transaminase (ALT), aspartate transaminase (AST), alkaline phosphatase (AP), and γ-glutamyltranspeptidase (GGT) activities) were determined as described by Rivera-Macías et al. [18].

Additionally, metabolic biomarkers were determined such as glucose, total cholesterol, triglycerides, very low-density lipoprotein (VLDL), high-density lipoprotein (HDL), and low-density lipoprotein (LDL). Quantitative enzymatic spectrophotometry was carried out using commercial kits (Wiener Labs, Mexico City, Mexico).

2.2.5. Data Analysis and Statistics

Data shown are expressed as mean ± standard error of the mean (SEM) obtained from three independent experiments. Plots were constructed with Microcal™ Origin 6.0 software (Microcal Software Inc., Northampton, MA, USA). Statistical analysis was done with IBM® SPSS® software (IBM Corporation, Somer, NY, USA) by Student's t-test and One-way ANOVA. Statistical significance was established when $p < 0.05$. Bonferroni post-hoc analysis was used for ANOVA.

3. Results

3.1. Systematic Review

Of all ninety articles identified in the primary search (Pubmed = 76, Trip Database = 5, Lilacs = 9, Cochrane Library = 0), we selected 12 of the experimental studies and one clinical trial (a pilot study on primary biliary cirrhosis). After full-text revision, we selected 11 articles for data discussion (Figure 1). All of them were on experimental studies on BDL rodents, as described in Table 1. Despite use of synonyms terms to retrieve a larger number of articles, we did not have more available information. Meta-analysis was not possible because of different animal species, route of administration, time of exposure, or methodology.

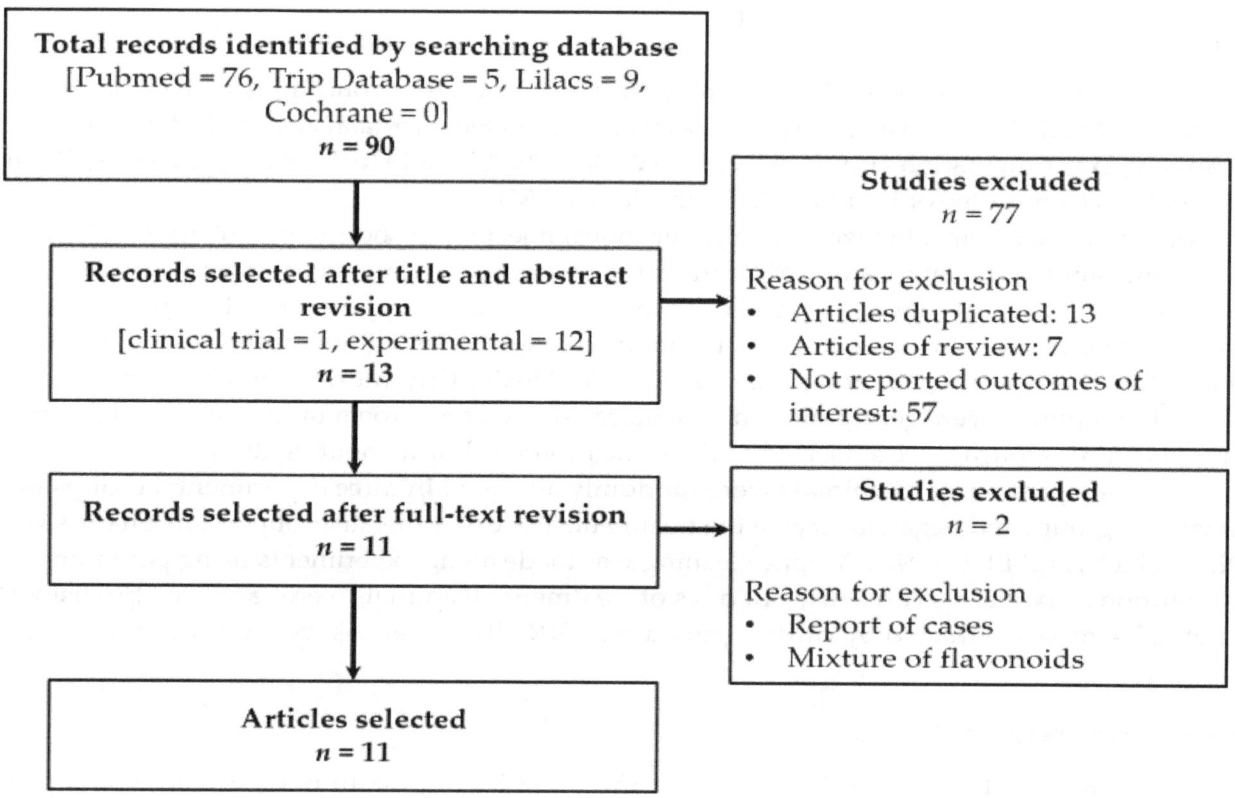

Figure 1. Flowchart showing the selection process for included studies on this systematic review.

Table 1. Efficacy endpoints studied on selected articles of systematic review.

No	Chemical Structure	Compound Name	Dose Applied	Species	Efficacy Endpoints: Liver Function	Efficacy Endpoints: Fibrosis	Efficacy Endpoints: Oxidative Stress	Efficacy Endpoints: Inflammation	Reference
1	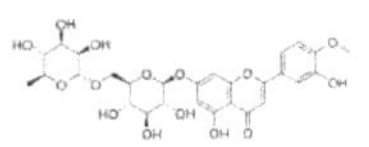	Diosmin	100 mg/kg/day, p.o. for 28 days	Wistar rat	X	X	X	X	Ali et al 2018
2			30 mg/kg/day p.o. for 28 days	Wistar rat	X	X	X		Kabirifar et al 2017
3	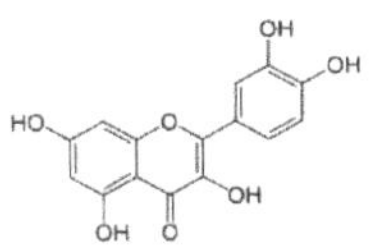	Quercetin	25 mg/kg/day p.o. for 28 days *	Sprague Dawley rat	X	X	X	X	Lin et al 2014
4			75, 150, 300 μmol/kg/day i.p. for 28 days	Wistar rat	X	X	X		Peres et al 2000
5	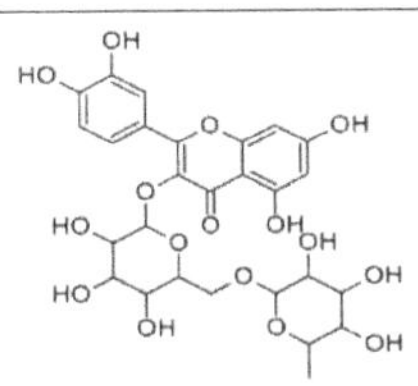	Rutin	25mg/kg/day p.o. for 28 days *	Sprague Dawley rat	X	X	X	X	Pan et al 2014
6	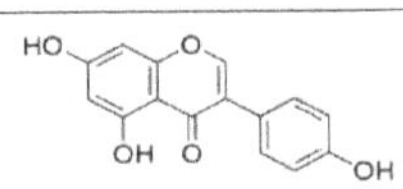	Genistein	5 μg/rat/day p.o. for 56 days	Wistar rat	X	X			Salas et al 2007
7	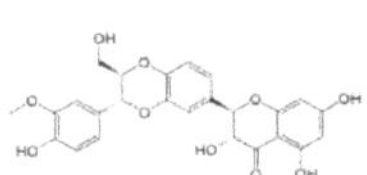	Silybin/ Silibinin	0.4g/kg ad libitum p.o. for 28 days	Wistar rat			X		Serviddio et al 2014
8			Dose not determined for 28 days	Wistar rat				X	Stanca et al 2013
9	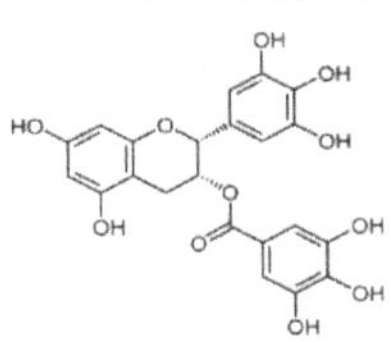	Epigallo-catechin 3-gallate	30mg/kg/day i.p. for 14 days **	C57BL/6 mice		X	X	X	Shen et al 2015
10			25 mg/kg/day p.o. for 14 days	Sprague Dawley rat	X	X		X	Yu et al 2015
11	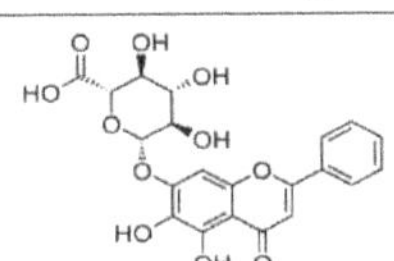	Baicalin	50 mg/kg/day i.p. for 14 days **	C57BL/6 mice		X	X	X	Shen et al 2017

* Compound administration began 1 week before surgery and 3 weeks postoperative. ** Compound administration began 2 h before surgery and 14 days postoperative.

The major flavonoids identified from this search were diosmin, bacailin, quercetin, epigallocatechin 3-gallate, silybin or silibinin (major active component of silymarin), rutin (quercetin-3-O-rutinoside), and genistein (Table 1). Interestingly, no evidence was found about NG, one of the most naturally occurring flavonoid studied due of its health benefits on metabolic and cardiovascular diseases (Figure 2). This no evidence scenario encouraged us to evaluate NG as candidate for drug discovery, and contribute to experimental pharmacological data of flavonoids.

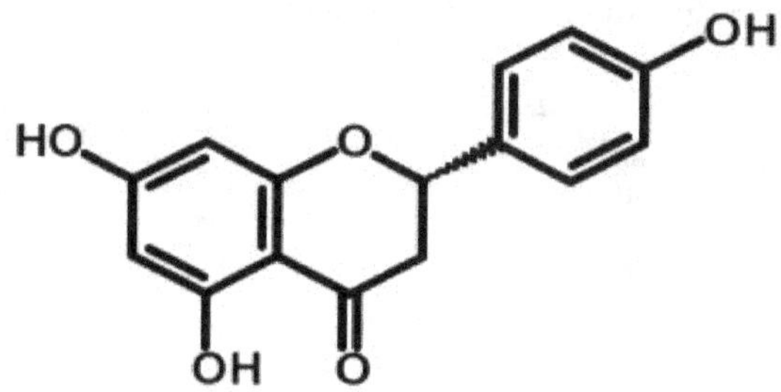

Figure 2. Chemical structure of naringenin (NG).

The biological processes altered on obstructive cholestasis are liver function, extracellular matrix components processing, redox status, and inflammation balance [3]. In this context, only diosmin, quercetin and rutin were evaluated for all these components (Table 1). Lin et al. showed that quercetin supplementation produced alleviation of liver histological integrity, serum biomarkers stabilization, reduction of fibrotic and inflammatory processes, and resolution of oxidative stress probably by modulation of bile duct proliferation and ductal reaction, blockade of mitogenic and fibrogenic signaling, and antioxidant effect [19]. Additionally, they evaluated rutin (quercetin-3-O-rutinoside), the O-glycoside compound that combine quercetin and disaccharide rutinose, on the same model and evaluated the same endpoints. The evidence showed that rutin had similar effects taking into account that it is converted to quercetin during metabolism [20].

On the other hand, Ali et al. reported data on efficacy of diosmin alone or in combination with sildenafil (erectile dysfunction approved drug with antioxidant and anti-inflammatory properties [21,22]) on the same model. Interestingly, diosmin alone was able to restore redox homeostasis by regulation of antioxidant enzymes GSR and SOD, a putative mechanism proposed for this molecule [23].

In order to compare parameters of the liver function and metabolic status on BDL-treated animals, we show tables of percentage change of each parameter vs. untreated cholestatic rats (Tables 2 and 3). It should be noticed that only one study reported mortality as valid endpoint for evaluation of experimental efficacy [23]. Additionally, ductal enzymes AP and GGT were missing on several studies despite these biomarkers are pivotal for cholestasis diagnostic [24].

Table 2. Percentage changes of liver function parameters induced by flavonoids on BDL model.

No	Reference	Compound	Change %					
			ALT	**AST**	**AP**	**GGT**	**Total Bilirubin**	**Mortality**
1	Ali et al 2018	Diosmin	48.77	48.32	50.53	46.37	56.77	20%
2	Kabirifar et al 2017	Quercetin	32.89	34.32	44.44	ND	ND	ND
3	Lin et al 2014	Quercetin	30.05	35.98	ND	55.87	36.26	ND
4	Peres et al 2000 *	Quercetin	55.81	78.57	49.86	ND	ND	ND
5	Pan et al 2014	Rutin	37.16	44.55	ND	63.49	40.66	ND
6	Salas et al 2007	Genistein	51.53	ND	59.88	73.68	68.97	ND
7	Serviddio et al 2014	Silybin/Silibinin	ND	ND	ND	ND	ND	ND
8	Stanca et al 2013	Silybin/Silibinin	30.76	23.68	27.78	ND	39.76	ND
9	Shen et al 2015	Epigallocatechin 3-Gallate	ND	ND	ND	ND	ND	ND
10	Yu et al 2015	Epigallocatechin 3-Gallate	−29.77	3.66	ND	ND	-4.64	ND
11	Shen et al 2017	Baicalin	ND	ND	ND	ND	ND	ND
12	Current article	NG	−6.79	−40.02	19.78	−7.82	38.91	30%

ND, not determined; NG, Naringenin; ALT, alanine transaminase; AST, aspartate transaminase; AP, alkaline phosphatase; GGT, gamma glutamyltranspeptidase. * Only was considered dose 150 μg/mL for this analysis since this dose was administered for 28 days. Negative values means an augmentation of the parameter in comparison with untreated cholestatic animals.

Table 3. Percentage changes of metabolic parameters induced by flavonoids on BDL model.

No	Reference	Compound	Change %						
			Glucose	Cholesterol	Triglycerides	Insulin	VLDL	LDL	HDL
3	Lin et al 2014	Quercetin	ND	14.78	26.47	ND	ND	ND	ND
5	Pan et al 2014	Rutin	ND	19.13	25.00	ND	ND	ND	ND
10	Yu et al 2015	Epigallocatechin 3-Gallate	ND	0.69	ND	ND	ND	0.74	−18.52
12	Current article	NG	−2.51	36.33	29.43	44.44	29.43	58.44	−48.50

ND, not determined; NG, naringenin; VLDL, very low density lipoprotein; LDL, low density lipoprotein; HDL, high density lipoprotein. Negative values means an augmentation of the parameter in comparison with untreated cholestatic animals.

Flavonoids showed a good performance in hepatoprotection since almost all compounds showed a marked serum decrease of the liver and ductal enzymes (about 50% on average). In accordance with these data, it seems that genistein (5 μg/rat/day, p.o.) and quercetin (150 μmol/kg/day, i.p.) had a better performance than other flavonoids; however, intraperitoneal high dose (about 45 mg daily), and a confusing mode of administration (it began four weeks before biliary obstruction and was continued for a further four weeks) were inconclusive [25,26].

It is important to mention that quantification of metabolic biomarkers such as cholesterol, depicts indirect improvements on bile acid synthesis; however, metabolites such as glucose, triglycerides, and lipoproteins might determine a correct function of the liver, since this organ plays a central role in lipid and carbohydrate metabolism [24]. As seen above, few investigations consider metabolic parameters as pivotal endpoints for the evaluation of efficacy. Only three studies measured serum cholesterol, two measured triglycerides, and one measured lipoprotein content (LDL and HDL) (Table 3).

Further, it was remarkable to consider that risk of bias assessment show that the majority of studies assessed had a high risk for selection, performance, and detection biases (Figure S1). This evidence exposes an unmet need to improve the quality of the experimental protocols for most confident information in drug discovery. This was another reason for not including a meta-analysis in this investigation.

3.2. *Experimental Study*

3.2.1. Signature of Obstructive Cholestasis in the Rat

As reported, bile duct obstruction produced significant alterations in serum biomarkers concentration compared with sham-operated rats. Major alterations were decrease of glucose (Figure 3a) and HDL (Figure 3d), as well as increase of total cholesterol (Figure 3b), LDL (Figure 3d), and bilirrubin (Figure 4d) in comparison with the sham group. Triglycerides and VLDL concentrations were unaltered similar to the report by Stedman et al. [27]. Increase of liver enzymes ALT and AST, and bile ductal enzymes GGT and AP were determinant for cholestatic liver disease signature in BDL (Figure 4), due to hepatocellular damage produced by high concentrations of toxic bile acids [28].

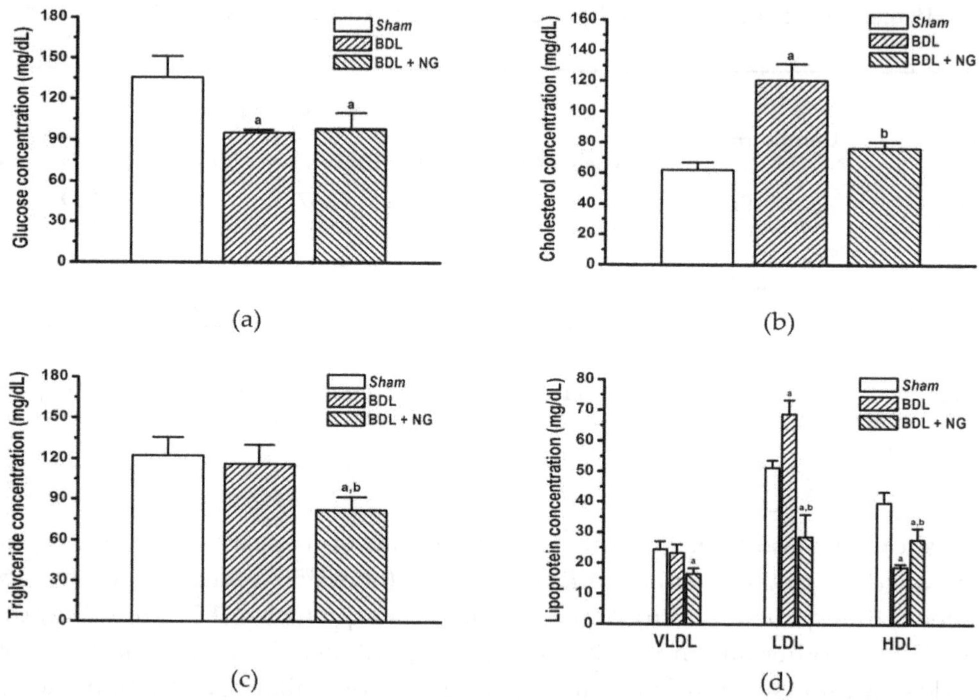

Figure 3. Metabolic biomarkers quantified on bile duct-ligated (BDL) model after administration of naringenin (NG, 50 mg/kg/day) for 10 days. (**a**) Glucose, (**b**) total cholesterol, (**c**) triglycerides, (**d**) lipoprotein (very low-density lipoprotein (VLDL), low-density lipoprotein (LDL), and high-density lipoprotein (HDL)). Data are expressed as means ± SEM (n = 8–10). a: Significantly different from sham control group at $p < 0.05$, and b: Significantly different from BDL group at $p < 0.05$.

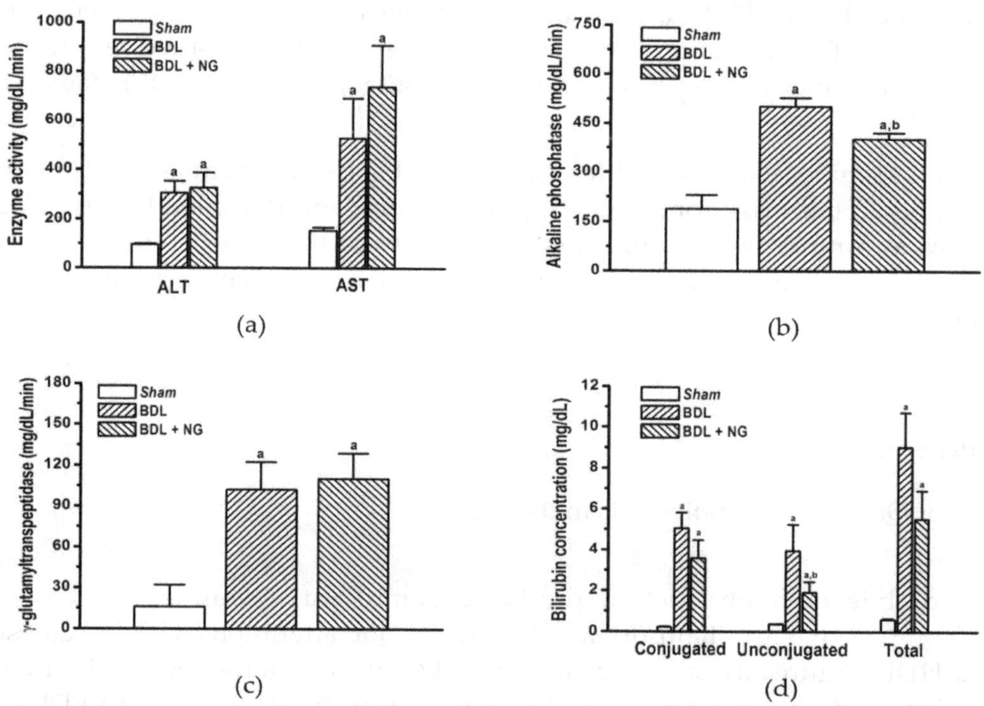

Figure 4. Liver function and cholestasis biomarkers quantified on bile duct-ligated (BDL) model after administration of naringenin (NG, 50 mg/kg/day) for 10 days. (**a**) Transaminases (ALT and AST), (**b**) alkaline phosphatase, (**c**) γ-glutamyltranspeptidase (**d**), and bilirubin were expressed from each group. Data are expressed as means ± SEM (n = 8–10). a: Significantly different from sham control group at p < 0.05, and b: Significantly different from BDL group at $p < 0.05$.

3.2.2. Efficacy of NG in Obstructive Cholestasis

Naringenin significantly improved serum cholesterol (Figure 4b) and low and high-density lipoproteins (Figure 4d) in the BDL model. Interestingly, despite triglycerides and VLDL were not modified on cholestatic damage, this flavonoid decreased both parameters. Additionally, significant decrease in bilirubin (Figure 4d) and AP activity (Figure 4b) suggests an improvement of liver and bile duct damage.

Finally, biochemical improvements attributed to NG allowed reduced mortality. By contrast, body weight changes along time had no modification. In fact, treated BDL rats suffered more weight loss than the BDL group (Figure 5).

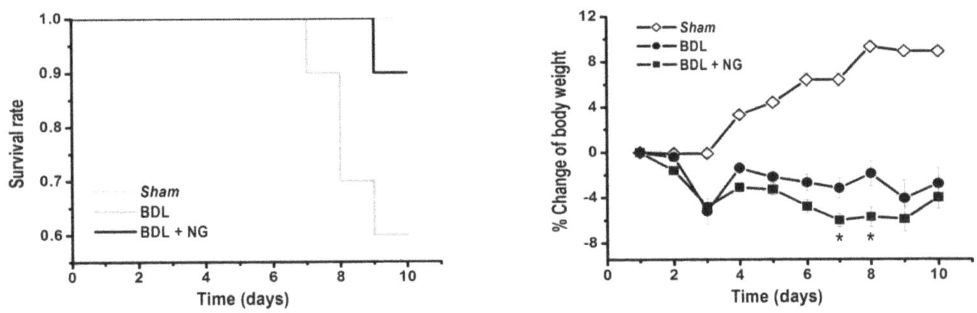

(a) (b)

Figure 5. Survival rate (**a**), and percentage change of body weight (**b**) measured after administration of naringenin (NG, 50 mg/kg/day) for 10 days. *Significantly different from bile duct-ligated (BDL) group at $p < 0.05$ ($n = 10$ animals/group).

4. Discussion

Flavonoids are naturally occurring compounds with beneficial health effects in chronic diseases, being cardiovascular and metabolic diseases that are better characterized. Further, higher intake of these compounds has been associated with lower mortality rates from specific vascular diseases and cancer [29]. The importance of flavonoid-rich foods consumption in preventing cholestasis mortality remains uncertain. For this reason, we aimed to show the state-of-the-art of flavonoids for the drug design of new anti-cholestatic agents through a systematic review.

Currently, some articles have applied systematic searching in order to analyze proficiency of natural products on specific illnesses (e.g. triterpenes on wound healing) [30]. Recently, Chen et al. reviewed phenylated flavonoids and their biological effects; this investigation focused on structural properties of the phenylated flavonoids and the implication in biological activity. However, no evidence was found on cholestatic liver disease or liver disease related abnormalities [13]. For this reason, the anti-cholestatic effect of flavonoids remains an outstanding issue in drug discovery.

Silymarin has been the most studied flavonoid for liver disease. This extract has been characterized as a potent antioxidant, immunomodulatory, and anti-fibrotic agent indicated as adjuvant treatment for all-causes liver disorders [11]. Our analysis shows that one major component of this extract, silibinin or silybin, improved serum transaminase, AP, and bilirubin in BDL model; which is possible by a decrease of pro-inflammatory lipids (platelet-activating factor, PAF), and improved activity and expression of both lysophosphatidylcholine acyltransferase LPCAT1 and LPCAT2, key enzymes in PAF remodeling [31]. Despite evidence, there is no more investigation about flavonoid-based therapeutic interventions for the treatment of cholestasis. This situation suggests an opportunity for medicinal chemists, computer-aided designers, or organic chemists to evaluate flavonoid as a potential scaffold for new lead compounds.

Our database search shows no evidence for evaluation of flavonoids efficacy and safety in a clinical setting. Only a pilot study ($n = 27$) was found where oral silymarin was assessed in UDCA non-responsive primary biliary cirrhosis (PBC) patients. Despite UDCA therapy for 52.6 $\pm$ 10.4

months, elevation of AP activity (2 times above normal) was persistent, neither adjuvant therapy with silymarin improved clinical endpoints [11]. In this context, diosmin, quercetin, or genistein should be good options since these flavonoids decreased AP activity 40–50% (Table 2). However, more clinical investigation is still needed to assess this potential.

On the other hand, eleven reports were retrieved from systematic search. The analysis showed a variety of administration and time framework, i.e., some reported pre-operative (one week) and post-operative (three weeks) administration [19,20]. This approach might bias in the therapeutic effect assessment, since it began one week before a cholestatic pattern is established. Additionally, animal species were different and possibly crucial for biological behavior. The most used is the Wistar rat (six studies) followed by Sprague Dawley (three studies). Despite Sprague Dawley was developed from Wistar strain, data show that Wistar strain is prone for metabolic impairments [32]. This should be relevant in taking into account the metabolic component of cholestasis [33,34].

As mentioned, metabolic impairment is a pivotal alteration on obstructive cholestasis. Alterations in glucose, cholesterol, LDL, and HDL were observed in the BDL group (Figure 4). Modification of cholesterol and lipoprotein on cholestasis by bile duct ligation surgery is known [35]; also, high concentration of plasma insulin [36,37] and low concentration of glucose [38] have been reported for this model. In contrast, other studies reported contradictory values suggesting a wide metabolic disparity between species, rodent strain, and time of damage exposure [38,39]. In addition, it has been established that intrahepatic cholestasis of pregnancy (ICP) and PBC are associated with impaired metabolic profile, including glucose intolerance and dyslipidemia [33,34]. Our analysis showed few data on metabolic parameters for BDL (Table 3).

This is the first time that NG is evaluated in a BDL model, despite that a simple review about beneficial effects of this flavonoid in ethanol- and carbon tetrachloride-induced liver diseases and its putative mechanisms was published with no evidence about obstructive cholestasis [40]. Mulvihill and colleagues reported similar effects in their studies using LDL receptor-null ($LDL^{-/-}$) mice fed with a Western high caloric diet, which expressed metabolic impairments as dyslipidemia (increased VLDL and LDL), hyperinsulinemia, and weight gain vs. wild-type littermates. Treatment with NG 1% or 3% (wt/wt) improved triglyceride, total cholesterol, and lipoprotein concentrations after four weeks. In contrast, HDL was unaltered in animals with the Western diet, and NG did not modify this condition [41]. Our findings contribute for the beneficial metabolic effects induced by this flavonoid, taking into account that cholestasis have a distinct etiology and target organ than the diet-induced dyslipidemia.

Finally, the precise mechanism by which flavonoids exert their hepatoprotective effects is unclear yet. However, there is evidence suggesting that flavonoids might improve imbalance in oxidant/antioxidant status. For example, Kabirifar et al. reported that quercetin might improve the antioxidant capacity of the liver tissue by decreasing the activity of NADPH oxidase 1 (NOX1), a major intracellular producer of reactive oxygen species [42], and the expression of its activator Rac1. Further, an increase of the antioxidant enzymes catalase and glutathione superoxide dismutase (SOD) was reported [43]. Lin et al. showed similar evidences where an elevated mRNA expression of Mn-SOD, Cu/Zn-SOD, and catalase was observed. [19] On the other hand, it has been reported that flavonoids exert a regulation of inflammatory response and deposition of extracellular matrix by the decrease of mitogenic IL-1β and fibrogenic TGF-β1 expression and down-regulated BDL-induced hepatic Smad2/3 phosphorylation. [19] More investigation must be encouraged to promote comprehensive studies that describe the beneficial effects of flavonoids and its mechanism.

5. Conclusions

Flavonoids comprise a group of natural products with promising efficacy for the management of cholestatic liver disease. More clinical and experimental investigation should be driven to promote the drug design of flavonoid-based pharmaceuticals for the treatment of these pathologies with the lowest risk of bias. Naringenin is a flavonoid with specific beneficial effects on liver function and metabolic flow altered in cholestasis. Further investigation needs is required to characterize its pharmacological mechanism and applicability in a clinical setting.

Author Contributions: J.C.S.-S.; methodology, data curacy, writing first draft, S.E.-S; validation, supervision, administration of the project, S.G.-J; methodology, S.M.; methodology, J.G.-Z; methodology, and R.V.-M.; supervision, verification.

Acknowledgments: Juan Carlos Sánchez-Salgado and Samuel Estrada-Soto belong to Red Nacional de Investigación Preclínica de Productos Naturales.

References

1. Williams, R. Global challenges in liver disease. *Hepatology* **2006**, *44*, 521–526. [CrossRef]
2. Araújo, A.R.; Rosso, N.; Bedogni, G.; Tiribelli, C.; Bellentani, S. Global epidemiology of non-alcoholic fatty liver disease/non-alcoholic steatohepatitis: What we need in the future. *Liver Int.* **2018**, *38*, 47–51. [CrossRef]
3. Abshagen, K.; König, M.; Hoppe, A.; Müller, I.; Ebert, M.; Weng, H.; Holzhütter, H.-G.; Zanger, U.M.; Bode, J.; Vollmar, B.; et al. Pathobiochemical signatures of cholestatic liver disease in bile duct ligated mice. *BMC Syst. Biol.* **2015**, *9*, 83. [CrossRef] [PubMed]
4. Heathcote, E.J. Diagnosis and management of cholestatic liver disease. *Clin. Gastroenterol. Hepatol.* **2007**, *5*, 776–782. [CrossRef] [PubMed]
5. Bosoi, C.R.; Oliveira, M.M.; Ochoa-Sanchez, R.; Tremblay, M.; Ten Have, G.A.; Deutz, N.E.; Rose, C.F.; Bemeur, C. The bile duct ligated rat: A relevant model to study muscle mass loss in cirrhosis. *Metab. Brain Dis.* **2017**, *32*, 513–518. [CrossRef] [PubMed]
6. Wang, H.; Vohra, B.P.S.; Zhang, Y.; Heuckeroth, R.O. Transcriptional profiling after bile duct ligation identifies PAI-1 as a contributor to cholestatic injury in mice. *Hepatology* **2005**, *42*, 1099–1108. [CrossRef] [PubMed]
7. Rudic, J.S.; Poropat, G.; Krstic, M.N.; Bjelakovic, G.; Gluud, C. Ursodeoxycholic acid for primary biliary cirrhosis. *Cochrane Database Syst. Rev.* **2012**, *12*, CD000551. [CrossRef] [PubMed]
8. Thompson, J.N.; Cohen, J.; Blenkharn, J.I.; McConnell, J.S.; Barr, J.; Blumgart, L.H. A randomized clinical trial of oral ursodeoxycholic acid in obstructive jaundice. *Br. J. Surg.* **1986**, *73*, 634–636. [CrossRef]
9. Federico, A.; Dallio, M.; Loguercio, C. Silymarin/Silybin and Chronic Liver Disease: A Marriage of Many Years. *Molecules* **2017**, *22*, 191. [CrossRef] [PubMed]
10. Crocenzi, F.A.; Roma, M.G. Silymarin as a new hepatoprotective agent in experimental cholestasis: New possibilities for an ancient medication. *Curr. Med. Chem.* **2006**, *13*, 1055–1074. [CrossRef]
11. Angulo, P.; Patel, T.; Jorgensen, R.A.; Therneau, T.M.; Lindor, K.D. Silymarin in the treatment of patients with primary biliary cirrhosis with a suboptimal response to ursodeoxycholic acid. *Hepatology* **2000**, *32*, 897–900. [CrossRef] [PubMed]
12. Schuler, J.; Hudson, M.L.; Schwartz, D.; Samudrala, R. A Systematic Review of Computational Drug Discovery, Development, and Repurposing for Ebola Virus Disease Treatment. *Molecules* **2017**, *22*, 177. [CrossRef] [PubMed]
13. Chen, X.; Mukwaya, E.; Wong, M.-S.; Zhang, Y. A systematic review on biological activities of prenylated flavonoids. *Pharm. Biol.* **2014**, *52*, 655–660. [CrossRef]
14. Sánchez-Salgado, J.C.; Ortiz-Andrade, R.R.; Aguirre-Crespo, F.; Vergara-Galicia, J.; León-Rivera, I.; Montes, S.; Villalobos-Molina, R.; Estrada-Soto, S. Hypoglycemic, vasorelaxant and hepatoprotective effects of Cochlospermum vitifolium (Willd) Sprengel: A potential agent for the treatment of metabolic syndrome. *J. Ethnopharmacol.* **2007**, *109*, 400–405.
15. Sánchez-Salgado, J.C.; Castillo-España, P.; Ibarra-Barajas, M.; Villalobos-Molina, R.; Estrada-Soto, S. Cochlospermum vitifolium induces vasorelaxant and antihypertensive effects mainly by activation of NO/cGMP signaling pathway. *J. Ethnopharmacol.* **2010**, *130*, 477–484. [CrossRef] [PubMed]

16. Aguilar-Guadarrama, A.B.; Rios, M.Y. Flavonoids, Sterols and Lignans from Cochlospermum vitifolium and Their Relationship with Its Liver Activity. *Molecules* **2018**, *23*, 1952. [CrossRef] [PubMed]
17. Hooijmans, C.R.; Rovers, M.M.; de Vries, R.B.M.; Leenaars, M.; Ritskes-Hoitinga, M.; Langendam, M.W. SYRCLE's risk of bias tool for animal studies. *BMC Med. Res. Methodol.* **2014**, *14*, 43. [CrossRef]
18. Rivera-Mancía, S.; Montes, S.; Méndez-Armenta, M.; Muriel, P.; Ríos, C. Morphological changes of rat astrocytes induced by liver damage but not by manganese chloride exposure. *Metab. Brain. Dis.* **2009**, *24*, 243–255. [CrossRef]
19. Lin, S.-Y.; Wang, Y.-Y.; Chen, W.-Y.; Chuang, Y.-H.; Pan, P.-H.; Chen, C.-J. Beneficial effect of quercetin on cholestatic liver injury. *J. Nutr. Biochem.* **2014**, *25*, 1183–1195. [CrossRef]
20. Pan, P.-H.; Lin, S.-Y.; Wang, Y.-Y.; Chen, W.-Y.; Chuang, Y.-H.; Wu, C.-C.; Chen, C.-J. Protective effects of rutin on liver injury induced by biliary obstruction in rats. *Free Radic. Biol. Med.* **2014**, *73*, 106–116. [CrossRef]
21. Zahran, M.H.; Hussein, A.M.; Barakat, N.; Awadalla, A.; Khater, S.; Harraz, A.; Shokeir, A.A. Sildenafil activates antioxidant and antiapoptotic genes and inhibits proinflammatory cytokine genes in a rat model of renal ischemia/reperfusion injury. *Int. Urol. Nephrol.* **2015**, *47*, 1907–1915. [CrossRef] [PubMed]
22. Kaur, M.; Singh, A.; Kumar, B.; Singh, S.K.; Bhatia, A.; Gulati, M.; Prakash, T.; Bawa, P.; Malik, A.H. Protective effect of co-administration of curcumin and sildenafil in alcohol induced neuropathy in rats. *Eur. J. Pharmacol.* **2017**, *805*, 58–66. [CrossRef]
23. Ali, F.E.M.; Azouz, A.A.; Bakr, A.G.; Abo-Youssef, A.M.; Hemeida, R.A.M. Hepatoprotective effects of diosmin and/or sildenafil against cholestatic liver cirrhosis: The role of Keap-1/Nrf-2 and P38-MAPK/NF-κB/iNOS signaling pathway. *Food Chem. Toxicol.* **2018**, *120*, 294–304. [CrossRef] [PubMed]
24. Lawrence, Y.A.; Steiner, J.M. Laboratory Evaluation of the Liver. *Vet. Clin. North Am. Small Anim. Pract.* **2017**, *47*, 539–553. [CrossRef] [PubMed]
25. Salas, A.L.; Ocampo, G.; Fariña, G.G.; Reyes-Esparza, J.; Rodríguez-Fragoso, L. Genistein decreases liver fibrosis and cholestasis induced by prolonged biliary obstruction in the rat. *Ann. Hepatol.* **2007**, *6*, 41–47.
26. Peres, W.; Tuñón, M.J.; Collado, P.S.; Herrmann, S.; Marroni, N.; González-Gallego, J. The flavonoid quercetin ameliorates liver damage in rats with biliary obstruction. *J. Hepatol.* **2000**, *33*, 742–750. [CrossRef]
27. Stedman, C.; Liddle, C.; Coulter, S.; Sonoda, J.; Alvarez, J.G.; Evans, R.M.; Downes, M. Benefit of farnesoid X receptor inhibition in obstructive cholestasis. *Proc. Natl. Acad. Sci. USA* **2006**, *103*, 11323–11328. [CrossRef]
28. Higuchi, H.; Gores, G.J. Bile acid regulation of hepatic physiology: IV. Bile acids and death receptors. Am. J. Physiol. Gastrointest. *Liver Physiol.* **2003**, *284*, G734–G738.
29. Ivey, K.L.; Jensen, M.K.; Hodgson, J.M.; Eliassen, A.H.; Cassidy, A.; Rimm, E.B. Association of flavonoid-rich foods and flavonoids with risk of all-cause mortality. *Br. J. Nutr.* **2017**, *117*, 1470–1477. [CrossRef]
30. Agra, L.C.; Ferro, J.N.S.; Barbosa, F.T.; Barreto, E. Triterpenes with healing activity: A systematic review. *J. Dermatolog. Treat.* **2015**, *26*, 465–470. [CrossRef]
31. Stanca, E.; Serviddio, G.; Bellanti, F.; Vendemiale, G.; Siculella, L.; Giudetti, A.M. Down-regulation of LPCAT expression increases platelet-activating factor level in cirrhotic rat liver: potential antiinflammatory effect of silybin. *Biochim. Biophys. Acta.* **2013**, *1832*, 2019–2026. [CrossRef] [PubMed]
32. Marques, C.; Meireles, M.; Norberto, S.; Leite, J.; Freitas, J.; Pestana, D.; Faria, A.; Calhau, C. High-fat diet-induced obesity Rat model: A comparison between Wistar and Sprague-Dawley Rat. *Adipocyte* **2015**, *5*, 11–21. [CrossRef] [PubMed]
33. Menżyk, T.; Bator, M.; Derra, A.; Kierach, R.; Kukla, M. The role of metabolic disorders in the pathogenesis of intrahepatic cholestasis of pregnancy. *Clin. Exp. Hepatol.* **2018**, *4*, 217–223. [CrossRef] [PubMed]
34. Vignoli, A.; Orlandini, B.; Tenori, L.; Biagini, M.R.; Milani, S.; Renzi, D.; Luchinat, C.; Calabrò, A.S. The metabolic signature of Primary Biliary Cholangitis and its comparison with Coeliac Disease. *J. Proteome Res.* **2018**, *18*, 1228–1236. [CrossRef] [PubMed]
35. Bauer, J.E.; Meyer, D.J.; Campbell, M.; McMurphy, R. Serum lipid and lipoprotein changes in ponies with experimentally induced liver disease. *Am. J. Vet. Res.* **1990**, *51*, 1380–1384.
36. Jessen, N.; Buhl, E.S.; Schmitz, O.; Lund, S. Impaired insulin action despite upregulation of proximal insulin signaling: novel insights into skeletal muscle insulin resistance in liver cirrhosis. *J. Hepatol.* **2006**, *45*, 797–804. [CrossRef] [PubMed]
37. Lin, S.-Y.; Sheu, W.H.-H.; Chen, W.-Y.; Lee, F.-Y.; Huang, C.-J. Stimulated resistin expression in white adipose of rats with bile duct ligation-induced liver cirrhosis: relationship to cirrhotic hyperinsulinemia and increased tumor necrosis factor-alpha. *Mol. Cell. Endocrinol.* **2005**, *232*, 1–8. [CrossRef]

38. Enochsson, L.; Isaksson, B.; Strömmer, L.; Erlanson-Albertsson, C.; Permert, J. Bile duct obstruction is associated with early postoperative upregulation of liver uncoupling protein-2 and reduced circulating glucose concentration in the rat. *Nutrition* **2010**, *26*, 405–410. [CrossRef]
39. Catala, J.; Daumas, M.; Chanh, A.P.; Lasserre, B.; Hollande, E. Insulin and glucagon impairments in relation with islet cells morphological modifications following long term pancreatic duct ligation in the rabbit–a model of non-insulin-dependent diabetes. *Int. J. Exp. Diabetes Res.* **2001**, *2*, 101–112. [CrossRef]
40. Hernández-Aquino, E.; Muriel, P. Beneficial effects of naringenin in liver diseases: Molecular mechanisms. *World J. Gastroenterol.* **2018**, *24*, 1679–1707. [CrossRef]
41. Mulvihill, E.E.; Allister, E.M.; Sutherland, B.G.; Telford, D.E.; Sawyez, C.G.; Edwards, J.Y.; Markle, J.M.; Hegele, R.A.; Huff, M.W. Naringenin prevents dyslipidemia, apolipoprotein B overproduction, and hyperinsulinemia in LDL receptor-null mice with diet-induced insulin resistance. *Diabetes* **2009**, *58*, 2198–2210. [CrossRef] [PubMed]
42. Choi, S.S.; Sicklick, J.K.; Ma, Q.; Yang, L.; Huang, J.; Qi, Y.; Chen, W.; Li, Y.-X.; Goldschmidt-Clermont, P.J.; Diehl, A.M. Sustained activation of Rac1 in hepatic stellate cells promotes liver injury and fibrosis in mice. *Hepatology* **2006**, *44*, 1267–1277. [CrossRef] [PubMed]
43. Kabirifar, R.; Ghoreshi, Z.-A.-S.; Safari, F.; Karimollah, A.; Moradi, A.; Eskandari-Nasab, E. Quercetin protects liver injury induced by bile duct ligation via attenuation of Rac1 and NADPH oxidase1 expression in rats. *HBPD INT* **2017**, *16*, 88–95. [CrossRef]

9

Insights into the Phytochemistry of the Cuban Endemic Medicinal Plant *Phyllanthus orbicularis*: Fideloside, a Novel Bioactive 8-*C*-glycosyl 2,3-Dihydroflavonol

Antonio Francioso [1,2,3,*], Katrin Franke [1], Claudio Villani [4], Luciana Mosca [2], Maria D'Erme [2], Stefan Frischbutter [5,6], Wolfgang Brandt [1], Angel Sanchez-Lamar [3] and Ludger Wessjohann [1,*]

1 Department of Bioorganic Chemistry, Leibniz Institute of Plant Biochemistry, 06120 Halle (Saale), Germany
2 Department of Biochemical Sciences "A. Rossi Fanelli", Sapienza University of Rome, 00185 Roma, Italy
3 Department of Plant Biology, Faculty of Biology, University of Havana, 10 200 La Habana, Cuba
4 Department of Chemistry and Technology of Drugs, Sapienza University of Rome, 00185 Roma, Italy
5 Department of Dermatology and Allergy, Charité, Universitätsmedizin Berlin, 10117 Berlin, Germany
6 German Rheumatism Research Centre, a Leibniz Institute, 10117 Berlin, Germany
* Correspondence: Antonio.francioso@uniroma1.it (A.F.); Ludger.Wessjohann@ipb-halle.de (L.W.)

Academic Editor: Pinarosa Avato

Abstract: *Phyllanthus orbicularis* (Phyllanthaceae) is an endemic evergreen tropical plant of Cuba that grows in the western part of the island and is used in traditional medicine as an infusion. The aqueous extract of this plant presents a wide range of pharmacological activitiessuch as antimutagenic, antioxidant and antiviral effects. Given the many beneficial effects and the great interest in the development of new pharmacological products from natural sources, the aim of this work was to investigate the phytochemistry of this species and to elucidate the structure of the main bioactive principles. Besides the presence of several known polyphenols, the major constituent was hitherto not described. The chemical structure of this compound, here named Fideloside, was elucidated by means of HR-ESIMS/MS^n, 1D/2D NMR, FT-IR, and ECD as (2*R*,3*R*)-(−)-3′,4′,5,7-tetrahydroxydihydroflavonol-8-*C*-β-D-glucopyranoside. The compound, as well as the plant aqueous preparations, showed promising bioactive properties, i.e., anti-inflammatory capacity in human explanted monocytes, corroborating future pharmacological use for this new natural C-glycosyl flavanonol.

Keywords: *Phyllanthus orbicularis*; *C*-glycoside; flavonoid; natural products; traditional medicine; Cuba; *Phyllanthus chamacristoides*; chromatography; mass spectrometry; NMR; circular dichroism; stereochemistry; Fideloside; cytokines; anti-inflammatory activity

---

1. Introduction

Natural products represent a very important traditionalsource of novel drugs. They are also a relevant inspiration for the synthesis of novel molecules of pharmaceutical interest. Among the plethora of potential pharmaceutical and nutritional plant-derived molecules, phenolics represent a dominant group of compounds with crucialnatural antioxidantsand flavors [1–4].

With 7500 species of flowering plants, of which 50% are endemic, Cuba hosts more than half of all Caribbean flora [5], that is also the reason why the use of "green" medicine to prevent or treat different illnesses is deeply rooted in Cuban popular traditions. About 1250 species in180 families from Cuba are used as medicinal plants, in which the Euphorbiaceae family is one of the most broadly represented [6,7]. Euphorbiaceae and the segregated Phyllanthraceae are commonly very rich in bioactive metabolites. The genus *Phyllanthus* of this family includes Cuban endemic species which are widely used by traditional medical practitioners for the treatment of different types of diseases [8]. Indeed, other *Phyllanthus* species have worldwide applications including reports from China, the Philippines, Nigeria, East and West Africa, and Latin America comprising further Caribbean countries [9]. Several therapeutic properties have been attributed to this genus, such as antipyretic, antibacterial, antiparasitic, anticontraceptive, and antiviral activities [10,11]. Crude extracts of species such as *Phyllanthus amarus* and *Phyllanthus emblica* have been reported to provide antioxidant and anti-genotoxic activities [12].

Phyllanthus orbicularis Kunth is an endemic evergreen plant of Cuba that grows in the western side of the island in Pinar del Rio district. This plant, commonly known as "Alegrìa", is used in traditional medicine as an infusion for its anti-pyretic and antiviral properties [13–15]. In vitro tests showed that the aqueous extract from this species has a marked antiviral activity [16]. In sight of this, several preclinical studies have been carried out with the aim to use this extract as a pharmacological alternative in hepatitis B and human herpes virus type-2 therapy [15,17]. In addition, *P. orbicularis* aqueous extract has anti-mutagenic properties against hydrogen peroxide-induced clastogenicity and mutagenicity exhibiting protective effects against pro-mutagenic aromatics [18–20]. Moreover, the extract exhibits a photo-protective activity against γ-radiation, both in pre- and post-irradiation treatments [21,22]. Recent data demonstrated the protective effect of aqueous extracts from Cuban endemic *P. orbicularis* against UV-light induced DNA damage and genotoxicity [23–25].

To gain insight into the chemical principles responsible for the biological effects, a complete characterization of the phytochemical profile of Cuban endemic *Phyllanthus* species is required. To date only limited data are available, obtained by GC/MS and HPLC analyses of organic or aqueous extracts, which demonstrate the presence of known bioactive terpenoids and flavonoids [15,26]. *P. orbicularis* aqueous extract is the most interesting preparation from a pharmacological point of view, being the most effective and most studied in biological models, and the most relevant in application. However, despite its beneficial biological activities, the phytochemical composition of this plant is still not completely known. Of all previous works describing *P. orbicularis* aqueous extract chemistry, none offer a complete profile and a detailed chemical characterization. Given its common use in Cuba and the many beneficial effects of the plant, and the still increasing interest in the development of new pharmacological products from natural sources, the aim of this work is to investigate the phytochemistry of the Cuban endemic *P. orbicularis* compared to the endemic *P.chamacristoides*, which is not used in traditional medicine. The focus will be laid on the elucidation of the structures of the still unknown main bioactive principles.

2. Results

2.1. Phytochemical Characterization of Cuban Phyllanthus Species

UPLC-DAD profiles (280 nm) of aqueous extracts from two endemic Cuban *Phyllanthus* species (*P. orbicularis* and *P. chamacristoides*) analyzed at the same concentration and in the same chromatographic conditionsare shown in Figure 1. We compared the metabolite profile of the medicinal plant *Phyllanthus orbicularis* with that from *Phyllanthus chamacristoides* not used in traditional medicine. The chromatograms can be divided virtually in three regions, representing three different classes of molecules. From the beginning of the chromatographic run to 3.5 min there is the elution of hydrophilic phenolic acids, the central part of the chromatogram (from 3.5 to 4.8 min) is characterized by the presence of catechins and procyanidins (monomers and polymers), and from 4.8 min to the end of the gradient the last eluting molecules of these extracts are represented by more complex flavonoids. Analyzed compounds were numbered from **1** to **9** (Suppl., Figure S1) in order of their retention times and correspond to the major compounds detected (Table 1). In accordance with previously reported data, our results reveal the presence of catechin (peak **4**, Rt 3.85 min), procyanidin B2 (peak **5**, Rt 4.07 min), epicatechin (peak **6**, Rt 4.23 min) and rutoside (peak **8**, Rt 4.51 min) in *P. orbicularis*. The identity of these compounds was confirmed by the analysis of authentic analytical standards. As Figure 1 shows, peak **3** is the major compound in *P. orbicularis* and is present only in this species. Negative mode HRESIMS analyses of the other eluting peaks evidenced deprotonated ions $[M-H]^-$ ($UV\lambda_{max}$) at *m/z* 315.0717 (255,sh290 nm), *m/z* 355.0668 (326 nm), *m/z* 465.1039(290 nm), *m/z* 865.1984 (280 nm), and *m/z* 593.1514 (255 and 354 nm) corresponding, respectively, to compounds **1**, **2**, **3**, **7** and **9**. Collected samples were first submitted to direct infusion ESI-MS/MS fragmentation and then the whole extracts were analyzed by LC-HRESI-MS^n for further structural elucidations. Molecular fragments obtained by both methods were in accordance with standards and literature data for all compounds investigated. The UV-Vis absorption features of compound **1** ($C_{13}H_{16}O_9$, Rt 3.49 min) fit with the presence of a protocatechuic moiety (255 nm; sh 290 nm). The MS^2 fragmentation pattern of the parent ion (*m/z* 315.0717) is consistent with protocatechuic acid glucoside, showing the presence of the major fragment at *m/z* 153.0196 derived from the loss of the sugar moiety. MS^3 of this fragment gives rise to an ion at *m/z* 109 in accordance with the structure of this molecule [27,28]. Compound **2** ($C_{15}H_{16}O_{10}$, Rt 3.52 min) shows an UV-Vis spectrum with λ_{max} at 326 nm typical of hydroxycinnamate conjugated systems. ESI-MS^2 fragmentation of the pseudomolecular ion at *m/z* 355.0668 generates fragments at *m/z* 147.0301 and *m/z* 163.0405, resulting from two different cleavages of the ester bond, and two complementary fragments at *m/z* 209.0304 ($C_6H_9O_8^-$) and *m/z* 191.0198, referring to glucaric acid and its dehydration product, respectively [29–31]. MS^3 of the fragment at *m/z* 191 gives rise to subsequent glucaric acid decarboxylation products at *m/z* 147.1865 and *m/z* 85.0297. Peak **2** was consequently identified as *p*-cumaroyl-glucaric acid. Compounds **7** (Rt 4.35 min) and **9** (Rt 4.6 min) were already detected in *Phyllanthus orbicularis* extracts and were re-identified by means of their chromatographic behavior, spectroscopic features and ESI-HRMS/MS^n fragmentation patterns [15]. Compound **7** shows a molecular ion at *m/z* 865.1986 and a UV-vis λ_{max} at 281 nm. This molecule was previously identified in this extract as the epicatechin trimer procyanidin C1. The MS/MS fragmentation of the precursor ion generates the dimer at *m/z* 577.1353 with the same subsequent MS/MS fragmentation pattern as procyanidin B1/B2 type molecules, confirming the nature of this compound [32]. Peak **9** was identified as the flavonol glycoside nicotiflorin in accordance to the literature data for this plant constituent. MS/MS fragmentation of the pseudomolecular ion (*m/z* 593.1514 $[M-H]^-$) gives rise to the aglycone part at *m/z* 285.0403, corresponding to a kaempferol moiety. Further MS/MS of the fragment at *m/z* 285 generates fragments at *m/z* 255, 227 and 151 [33].

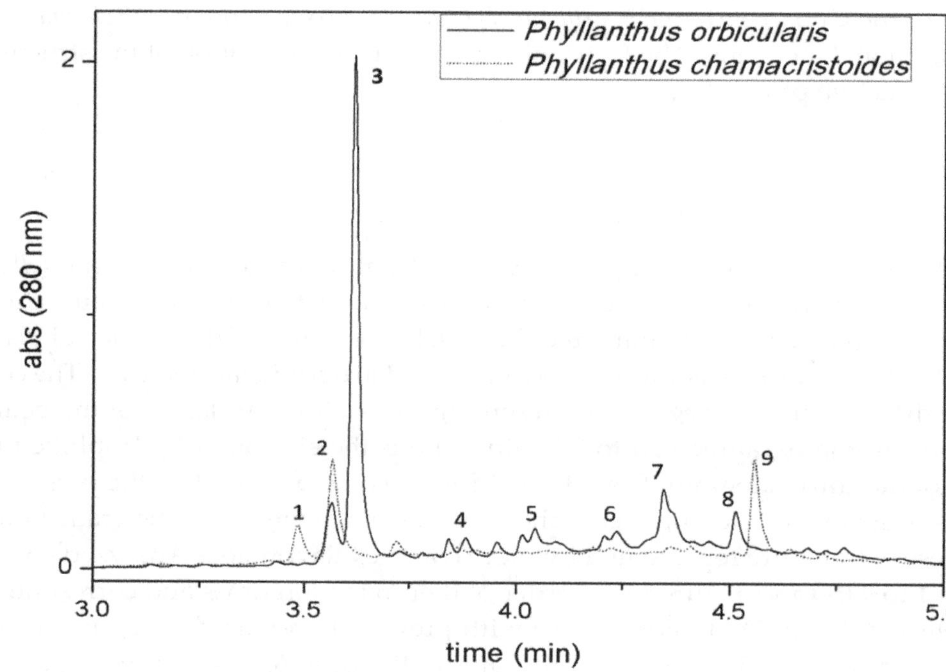

Figure 1. UPLC-DAD (280 nm) chromatograms of *Phyllanthus orbicularis* and *Phyllanthus chamacristoides* aqueous extracts and assignments of eluting peaks.

Table 1. Spectroscopic and spectrometric data of identified compounds.

Peak	Retention Time (min)	Compound	Molecular Formula	λ_{max}abs(nm)	MS[1] [M − H]⁻(*m/z*)	MS[2] [M − H]⁻(*m/z*)	MS[3][M − H]⁻(*m/z*)
1	3.49	Protocatechuic acid glucoside	$C_{13}H_{16}O_9$	290	315.0717	153.0196	109
2	3.52	*p*-Cumaroyl-glucaric acid	$C_{15}H_{16}O_{10}$	326	355.0668	191.0198	147; 85
3	**3.65**	**Fideloside**	$C_{21}H_{22}O_{12}$	**290**	**465.1039**	**345.0620**	**277; 179; 167**
4 *	3.85	Catechin	$C_{15}H_{14}O_6$	278	289.0720	271.0620; 245.0825	
5 *	4.07	Procyanidin B2	$C_{30}H_{26}O_{12}$	280	577.1352	451.1036; 425.088; 289.0720	
6 *	4.23	Epicatechin	$C_{15}H_{14}O_6$	278	289.0720	271.0620; 245.0825	
7	4.35	Procyanidin C1	$C_{45}H_{38}O_{18}$	281	865.1986	847.1882; 739.1667; 695.1407; 577.1353	[865 → 577] 289
8 *	4.51	Rutoside	$C_{27}H_{30}O_{16}$	355	609.1460		
9	4.60	Nicotiflorin	$C_{27}H_{30}O_{15}$	343	593.1514	285.0403	255; 227; 151

* confirmed by analytical standard injection.

2.2. Structure Elucidation of Compound 3 (Fideloside)

Although compound **3** is the major metabolite of *P. orbicularis* (*m/z* 465.1039 [M-H]⁻, Rt 3.65 min), no previous chemical identification was reported [17]. The UV-Vis absorption features of this molecule (λ_{max} at 290 nm) suggested a not completely conjugated flavonoid system and the HRESI-MS derived molecular formula of $C_{21}H_{22}O_{12}$ indicates the presence of one hexose moiety. MS/MS fragmentation of the precursor ion at *m/z* 465.1039 [M-H]⁻ gives rise to a *m/z* 345.0620 [(M − H) − 120]⁻ fragment, generated by the cleavage in the glycoside portion on position 2″. These data are consistent with a C-type glycosidic structure [34,35]. Further MS/MSof *m/z* 345 generates ions at *m/z* 179and 167 resulting from the retro-Diels–Alder fragmentation of flavonoid ring C, indicating the position of the glycoside moiety to be on ring A. Another ion generated by MS[3] fragmentation of *m/z* 345 is the *m/z* 277 ion generated by a cleavage in the B ring (Figure 2).

For completechemical characterization, compound **3** was isolated and the structure was elucidated by means of $^{1}H/^{13}C$ 1D and 2D NMR and IR spectroscopy. Table 2 reports NMR data for compound **3**. ^{1}H/NMR and ^{13}C/NMR spectra in DMSO-d6 display an array of signals in agreement with the hypothesized structure and consistent with literature data of similar flavonoid *C*-glycosides (Suppl., Figures S2–S7) [35–37]. HMBC correlations from the anomeric sugar proton (H-1″) to C-8, C-7 and C-9 established the presence of the glycosidic moiety at C-8. The diaxial coupling of H-2 and H-3 in the ^{1}H NMR spectrum indicates a *trans*-type dihydro-saturation at positions C-2 and C-3. Furthermore, NOESY experiments suggest the positions of phenolic OH groups at C-3′ and C-4′ (Figure 3). The infrared spectrum of compound **3** (Suppl., Figure S8) is in agreement with the structure, showing representative IR vibrational bands at 3233 cm^{-1} (O–H stretching), 1633 cm^{-1} (C=O stretching), 1362 cm^{-1} (phenolic C–O and O–H vibrational modes), 1277 cm^{-1} (C–O–C stretching in =C–O–C– groups) [38].

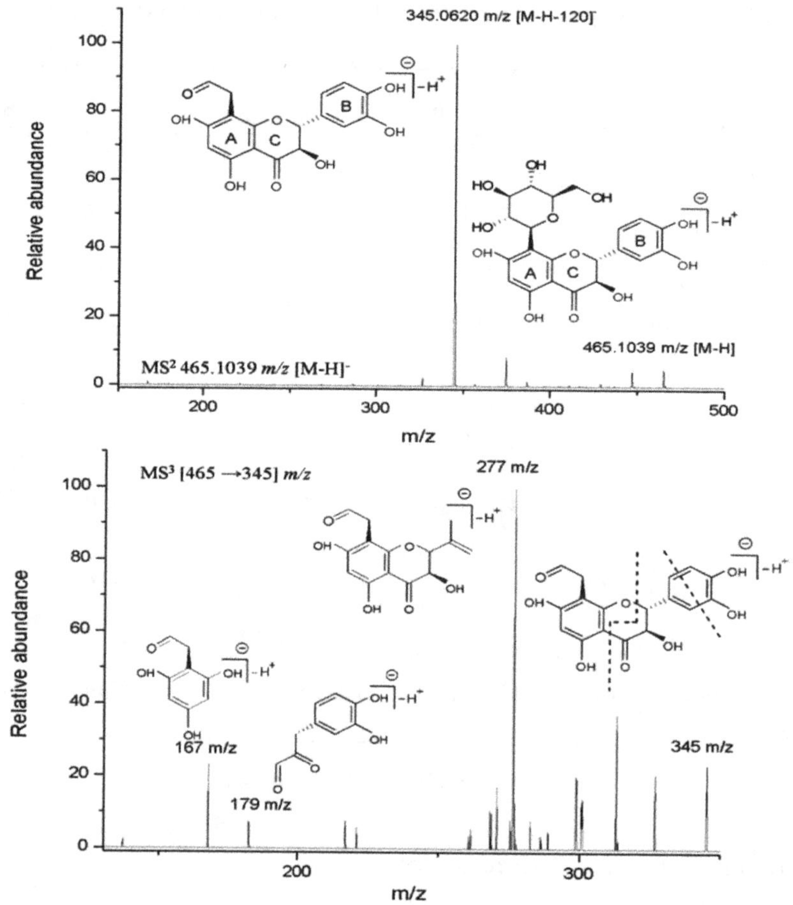

Figure 2. Fideloside (**3**) MS/MS^n fragmentation.

Table 2. 1D and 2D $^1H/^{13}C$ NMR data of Fideloside (**3**) in DMSO-d6 as solvent.

Nr.	δ c	DEPT	δ H (J in Hz)	^1H-^1H COSY	NOESY	HMBC
2	82.1	CH	5.02 (d, 11.02)	H-3	H-3-; H-6′; H-2′	H-2′;H-6′; OH-3
3	72.1	CH	4.25 (m)	H-2; OH-3	H-2′, H-6′; OH-3	OH-3; H-2
4	197.9	C				H-2; H-6;OH-3
5	162.1	C				H-6; OH-5
6	95.6	CH	6.04 (s)			OH-5
7	165.7	C				H-6; H-1″
8	105.5	C				H-6; H-1″-H; H-2″
9	161.4	C				H-2; H-1″
10	100.5	C				H-6; OH-5
1′	128.4	C				H-2; H-5′; H-2′
2′	115.0	CH	6.94 (brs)	H-6′	H-3; H-2	H-2; H-5′
3′	144.6	C				H-5′
4′	145.1	C				H-2′; H-6′
5′	115.0	CH	6.73 (d, 8.09)	H-6′	H-6′	H-2′; H-6′
6′	118.3	CH	6.84 (brd, 8.09)	H-2′; H-5′	H-2; H-5′; H-3	H-2′; H-2
1″	73.0	CH	4.45 (d, 9.63)	H-2″	H-3″	H-2″; H-6
2″	70.2	CH	3.82 (brt, 9.53)	H-1″; H-3″, OH-2″	H-4″; H-3″; H-1″	H-1″
3″	78.6	CH	3.11 (m)	H-2″; H-4″; OH-3″	H-1″; H-2″	H-1″; H-2″
4″	70.4	CH	2.95 (br)	H-3″; H-5″; OH-4″	H-2″; OH-4; H_2-6″	H-5″; H-3″; H-1″
5″	81.3	CH	3.09 (m)	H-6″	H-2″; Hb-6″	H-1″
6″	61.7	CH_2	Ha: 3.70 (m) Hb: 3.43 (m)	H-5″; H-6″; OH-6″	H-6″; H-4″	
3-OH			5.82(d, 6.13)	H-3	H-3	
5-OH			12.01(s)		H-6	
7-OH			-			
3′-OH			8.87 (brs)		H-2′	
4″-OH			9.00 (brs)		H-5′	
2″-OH			4.62 (brs)	H-2″		
3″-OH			4.83 (brs)	H-3″	H-2″, H-4″	
4″-OH			4.84 (brs)	H-4″		
6″-OH			4.57 (brs)	H_2-6″		

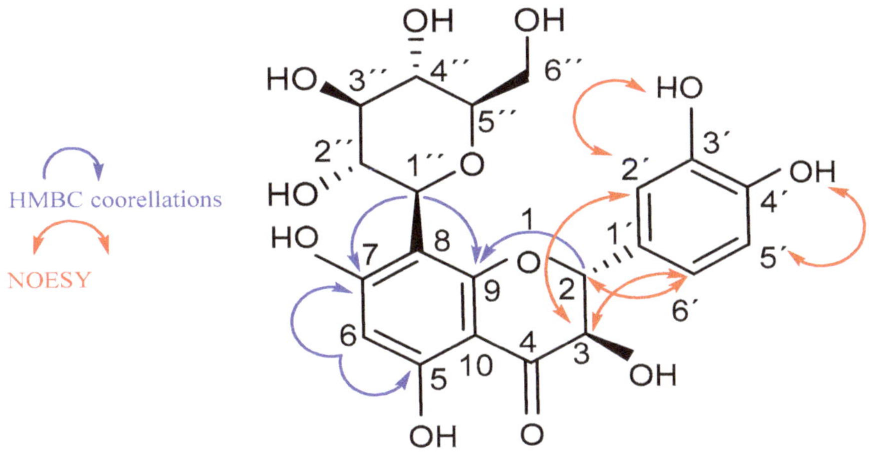

Figure 3. Fideloside (**3**) chemical structure with selected key NMR correlations.

The absolute configuration was elucidated by comparison of experimental and calculated circular dichroism spectra. The measured spectrum shows the presence of a negative Cotton effect at 295 nm and positive Cotton effect at 331 nm, which correspond to the (2*R*,3*R*) isomer (Figure 4), as previously reported for flavanonols [37,39,40].

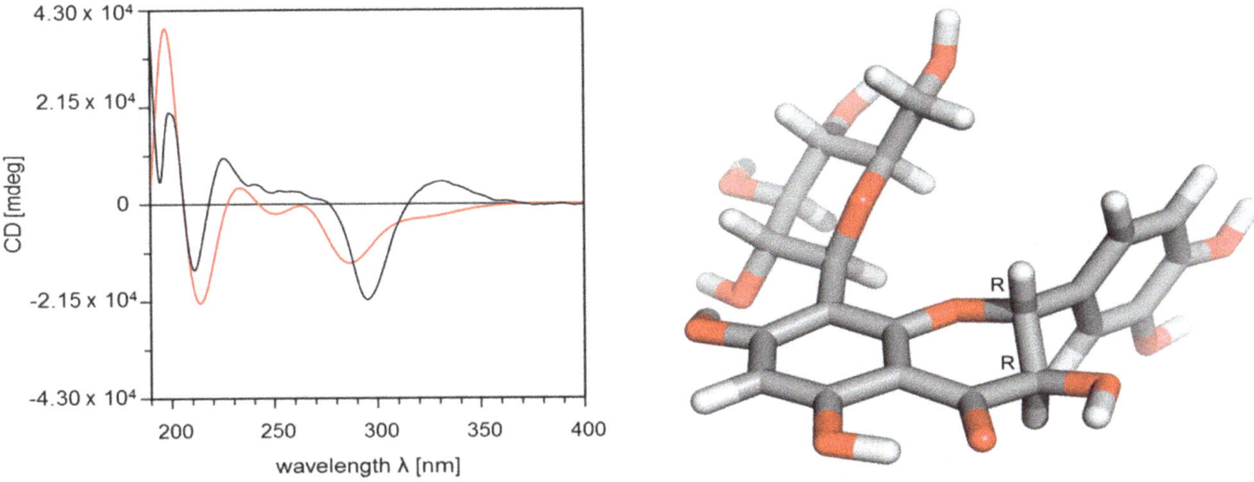

Figure 4. Left: comparison of experimental CD spectrum (black line) with Boltzmann weighted calculated CD spectrum for the (2*R*,3*R*)-enantiomer of compound **3** with a similarity factor S = 0.7099 for sigma = 0.3 eV and 18 nm shift. Right: calculated most stable conformation of the (2*R*,3*R*)-enantiomer.

The calculated relative conformational energies of the DFT optimized structures are listed in Table 3. The comparison of the Boltzmann weighted calculated CD spectra with the experimental ones clearly indicate that compound **3** adopts a (2*R*,3*R*)-configuration, since the fit with the experimental spectrum for this configuration is much better (Figure 4) than for the (2*S*,3*S*)-configuration (Suppl., Figure S9, Table S1).

Table 3. Results of DFT calculations for the (2*R*,3*R*) enantiomer of compound **3**.

Conformation	O-C2-C1′-C2′ (in°)	C2′-C3′-O-H (in°)	Energy (kcal/mol)	Boltzmann Weight	CD-Fit
1	−61.8	−179.5	0	59.4	0.6757
2	122.8	2.4	0.66	19.5	0.5712
3	−54.7	1.0	0.97	11.5	0.7065
4	121.9	−179.0	1.08	9.6	0.5974
Boltzmann					**0.7099**

On the basis of all experimental and calculated data, the chemical structure of this molecule is elucidated as (2*R*,3*R*)-(−)-3′,4′,5,7-tetrahydroxydihydroflavonol-8-*C*-*β*-D-glucopyranoside, a structure never reported previously for the genus *Phyllanthus* or in any other plant. We suggest to name this new natural compound *'Fideloside'* as the start of our work on this Cuban natural product coincided with the death of the long term Cuban leader Fidel Castro Ruz (Birán, 1927–La Habana, 2016).

2.3. Modulation of Cytokine Production

Since flavonoids can act in multiple way on inflammatory processes and Fideloside comprises the bioactive aglycon taxifolin, we investigated whether it is able to modulate interleukin production in human monocytes. Figure 5 shows a first biological assessment of pro-inflammatory (IL-1beta, IL-6) and anti-inflammatory (IL-10) cytokine production in human monocytes treated with poly-IC as a pro-inflammatory stimulus.

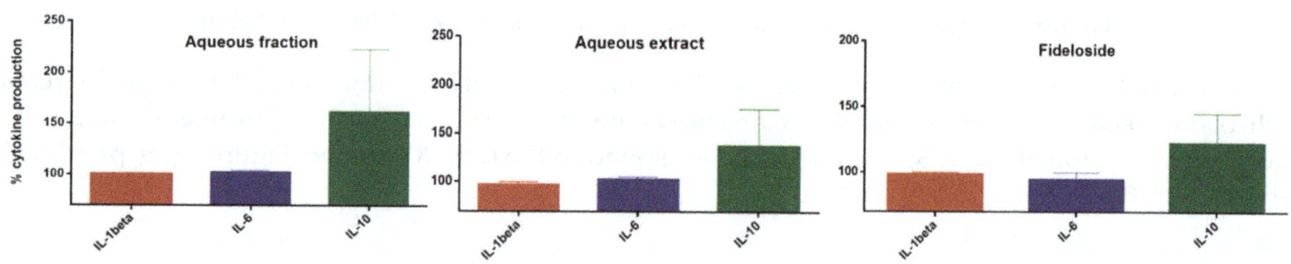

Figure 5. Anti-inflammatory capacity of extracts (3 μg/mL) and isolated Fideloside (1 μM) from *Phyllanthus orbicularis*. Levels of pro- and anti-inflammatory cytokines after poly-IC stimuli (CTRL+, 100%) of human monocytes.

These initial results show that the profile of interleukins secretion, in particular IL-10, seems to be modulated by Fideloside similarly to the aqueous extract and aqueous fraction suggesting a crucial role for this compound in the aqueous preparation used in Cuban traditional medicine.

3. Discussion

As expected, different polyphenols are the main secondary metabolites in both Cuban *Phyllanthus* species, i.e., *P. orbicularis* and *P. chamacristoides*. *P. orbicularis* presents a more diverse profile of polyphenolic compounds compared to *P. chamacristoides*, and especially a before unidentified dominating compound. Alvarez and co-workers investigated *P. orbicularis* extracts by bioactivity-guided fractionation and determined some phenolic compounds, like catechins and procyanidins, as anti HSV-2 compounds [15]. However, these authors did not characterize the main compound, which together with the identification of several minor constituents, was still lacking [15,17]. Our results demonstrate the presence of phenolic compounds unidentified in previous investigations in the two plant species and, most importantly, of a new C-glycoside flavonoid from *P. orbicularis* which represents the main component (circa 70%) of the aqueous infusion. This compound, and C-glycoside flavonoids in general, were not described for the genus *Phyllanthus* until now. C-glycoside flavonoids are a rare and very interesting class of organic natural compounds, considering that many of them have demonstrated their effectiveness as therapeutic agents such as anti-inflammatory, antioxidant, anticancer and antidiabetic drugs [41]. Compared to common glycosides (*O*- and *N*-), *C*-glycosides present minimal conformational differences with the advantage of being resistant to enzymatic or acidic hydrolysis, since the anomeric center of the acetal group is converted to an ether moiety.

Our finding is highly relevant from both a pharmacological and an analytical point of view, because of its potential as a chemotaxonomic and drug quality analysis tool for the recognition and distinction of effective *P. orbicularis* extracts versus, e.g., closely related species. The other consideration rises up from the evidence that *P. orbicularis* is used in traditional medicine as an aqueous extract whereas *P. chamacristoides* is not. Other than *O*-glycosides, *C*-glycosides are much more stable to hydrolysis during extraction and especially stomach passage (acidic cleavage), as well as in the further absorption and metabolism in humans, i.e., in terms of an increased bioavailability and half-life time in vivo [41]. *C*-linked glycosides, as well as the enzymes involved in their metabolism (*C*-glycosyltranferases and *C*-glycosidases), are extremely rare in nature and absent in human metabolism. These features can confer to the molecule a very unique pharmacokinetic profile and distribution.

Fideloside (**3**) as major flavonoid was tested for its anti-inflammatory capacity on human monocytes and demonstrated an increasing effect on the production of IL-10 anti-inflammatory cytokine with respect to pro-inflammatory mediators. The aqueous extract and the aqueous fraction of *P. orbicularis* show a closely related activity profile, suggesting that the newly discovered natural product could act as the major compound responsible for the pharmacological properties of this medicinal plant. In addition to the biochemical features, its physico-chemical properties are very interesting and promising from a pharmacological point of view. The C-glycosidic moiety strongly increases the water solubility and the bioavailability of the molecule, and, as pointed out above, suggests that its amphiphilic behavior could be longer retained if applied orally. For the same reason, its "green"water extraction is possible not only for direct consumption as in traditional applications, but also should allow for easier processing into standardized formulations. Fideloside is the *C*-8-glycosylated form of taxifolin, a well-known flavanonol found in a wide range of vegetables with strong antioxidant capacity and recently published interesting bioactive properties, including anti-inflammatory activity [42–45]. To date, the only known natural *C*-glycosylated taxifolin is the *C*-6 glycoside with (2*S*,3*S*) stereochemistry (Ulmoside), which biological activity is still under investigation [37,46].

As mentioned before, *C*-linked glycosidic phenols are a very unique class of compounds with future potential in different fields. These modifications of plant secondary metabolites are biochemically and evolutionally not well studied and characterized. Enzymes involved in C-glycosyl bond formation are very little known, or minor amounts of C-glycosides are formed as minor byproduct of O-glycosylation [47]. The latter case is highly unlikely here, thus the elucidation of this new peculiar product from the Cuban endemic *Phyllanthus orbicularis* can represent a starting point for the study and characterization of novel enzymes involved in *C*-glycosyl phenolics biosynthesis.

4. Materials and Methods

4.1. Chemicals, Reagents and General Procedures

TLC was carried out on silica gel 60 F_{254} plates (Merck, Germany). Spots were visualized under UV light (254 and 365 nm) or by heating after spraying with 2% vanillin solution (in 96%H_2SO_4). Low resolution ESI-MS analyses were performed on a SCIEX API-3200 instrument (Applied Biosystems, Concord, Ontario, Canada) combined with a HTC-XT autosampler (CTC Analytics, Zwingen, Switzerland). The samples were introduced via autosampler and 2 μL loop injection. ^{1}H, ^{13}C NMR and 2D (COSY, HSQC, HMBC and NOESY) spectra were recorded on an Agilent DD2 400 NMR spectrometer and the chemical shifts were referenced to TMS or the solvent residual peak. UV spectra were measured with a Jasco V-560 UV/Vis spectrophotometer. CD spectra were acquired on a Jasco J-815 CD spectrophotometer and the specific rotation was measured with a Jasco P-2000 polarimeter. Infrared spectra (ATR) were recorded using a Thermo Nicolet 5700 FT-IR spectrometer. Rutoside, (+)-catechin and (−)-epicatechin analytical standards were obtained from Sigma Aldrich (Germany). Procyanidin B2 was used from the IPB-NWC in-house reference compound library (isolated from *Bumelia sartorum* Mart.) [48]. All the reagents and solvents used were of analytical and LC-MS grade.

4.2. Plant Material

Phyllanthus orbicularis Kunth was collected in February 2007 from Cajálbana, Pinar del Río, Cuba. The specimens were authenticated and stored at the Cuban Botanical Garden (No.7/220 HAJB). *Phyllanthus chamaecristoides* was collected in spring 2011 from Guantánamo region, Cuba (20° 28″ 32.7″″

N, 74° 43″ 45.4″″ W). The specimens were authenticated by specialists of Cuban Botanical Garden, and stored in this scientific institution as: *Phyllanthus chamaecristoides* Urbano subsp. *baracoensis* (TB4452).

4.3. Extraction and Compound Isolation

The plant material aerial parts were extracted with two different methods according to literature data affording an aqueous extract (AE) and a crude methanolic extract (CE).

The aqueous extracts (AEs) were obtained from dried aerial parts (ground leaves and stems) following previously described methods [16,25]. Briefly, dry plant material was extracted in bi-distilled water under continuous shaking (1 g: 7.5 mL) for 4 h at 37 °C, or 2 h at 70 °C. After filtration and lyophilization, the material was stored in a dry, cool place until subsequent analyses.

Crude extracts (CEs) were obtained by extracting grounddry plant aerial parts with 10 volumes (*w*/*v*) of aqueous methanol (80% MeOH). After an initial 15 min of ultrasonication (bath), the plant material was extracted other two times for 2h with 10 volumes each of 80%MeOH at room temperature without sonication and one last time overnight at room temperature with the same procedure. The combined extracts were filtered and the solvents were evaporated to dryness under reduced pressure using a rotary evaporator. The isolation and purification of compound **3** was performed as follows: 25 g of *Phyllanthus orbilucularis* dry material were extracted with 80% MeOH as described above to obtain CE. The dry extract was resuspended in H_2O and partitioned by liquid–liquid extraction, first with *n*-hexane and then with ethyl acetate, to give the respective H_2O fraction (AF, 2.2 gr), *n*-hexane fraction (HF, 129 mg) and EtOAc fraction (EF 159 mg). Before purification, every fraction was dissolved to the same concentration and checked by TLC and UHPLC-DAD-MS. Then, 550 mg of AF were chromatographed on a Sephadex LH-20 (Pharmacia) column using pure MeOH as eluent to obtain 20 mg of **3** (Rf 0.43; silica gel;EtOAc:MeOH:H_2O/6:1:1) (2*R*,3*R*)-(−)-3′,4′,5,7-tetrahydroxydihydroflavonol-8-C-β-D-glucopyranoside (Fideloside):

Yellow amorphous. $[\alpha]^{25}{}_{D}$−10.46 (c 0.5; MeOH). CD (c 0.005; MeOH) $[\theta]_{295}$−21,139, $[\theta]_{331}$ +5001. UV λ_{max};MeOH: 290 nm. IR data: 3233 cm^{-1}, 1633 cm^{-1}, 1362 cm^{-1}, 1277 cm^{-1}.^{1}H NMR: (DMSO-d6, 400 MHz) and δ: ^{13}C NMR: (DMSO-d6, 101 MHz) see Table 2 HRESIMS $[M-H]^-$ calculated for $C_{21}H_{21}O_{12}{}^-$: 465.1038, found 465.1039.

4.4. UPLC-DAD-MS and ESI-MS/MS

UPLC-DAD-MS was performed on a Waters Acquity H-Class UPLC system (Waters, Milford, MA, USA), including a quaternary solvent manager (QSM),a sample manager with a flow through needle system (FTN), a photodiode array detector (PDA) anda single-quadruple mass detector with electrospray ionization source (ACQUITY QDa). Chromatography was performed on a Waters C18 HSST3 column (100 mm × 2.1 mm i.d., 1.7 μm particle size). Solvent A was 0.1% aqueous HCOOH and solvent B was 0.1% HCOOH in CH_3CN. Flow rate was 0.5 mL/min and column temperature was set at 25 °C. Elution was performed isocratically for the first minute with 2% B; from minute 1 to minute 6 solvent B was linearly increased to 55%; from 6 to 10 min 20%A and 80%B; then, in 0.5 min solvent B was set at 100% and maintained for 2 min. The column was re-equilibrated with 98% A and 2%B before the next injection. Samples were dissolved in the mobile phase and 10 μL injected through the needle. The PDA detector was set up in the range 200 to 600nm. Mass spectrometric detection was performed in the negative electrospray ionization mode using nitrogen as nebulizer gas. Analyses were performed in the Total Ion Current (TIC) mode in a mass range 50–1000 *m*/*z*. Capillary voltage was 0.8 kV, cone voltage 30 V, ion source temperature 120°C and probe temperature 600 °C. Direct infusion ESI-MS/MS analyses were performed on UHPLC-DAD collected pure peaks.

4.5. LC-High Resolution-MS^n

Separations were performed with the same chromatographic method described above ona Waters C18 HSST3 column (100 mm × 1 mm i.d., 1.7 μm particle size) using a Dionex Ultimate 3000 UHPLC System, equipped with a quaternary pump, autosampler (100 μL sample loop, partial injection mode,

2 μL injection volume, sample temperature 8 °C), and DAD Detector (Thermo Fisher Scientific, Bremen, Germany). The effluent from the PDA detector was connected on-line to an LTQ-Orbitrap Elite mass spectrometer equipped with a high-temperature electrospray ionization (HESI) ion source, controlled by the Excalibur 2.7 software (Thermo Fisher Scientific, Bremen, Germany) and operated in the negative ion mode. The ion spray voltage was set to 4.0 kV, sheath and auxiliary gases on 20 and 5 psi, respectively. The Orbitrap-MS spectra were acquired within the *m*/*z* range of 50–2000 and resolution of 30,000. The tandem mass spectra were acquired by collision induced dissociation (CID) in linear ion trap (LIT) at 35% normalized collision energy and isolation width of 2.0 *m*/*z*. The fragments were detected at anFT-resolution of 30,000.

4.6. Molecular Modeling and DFT Calculations

NMR-measurements of compound **3** clearly indicate a *trans* conformation for C2-C3 hydrogen atoms, which are possible only for a (2*S*,3*S*) or (2*R*,3*R*) configuration even when an axial orientation of the dihydroxybenzyl moiety is taken into consideration. Therefore, CD-spectra where calculated for the two enantiomers and compared with the experimental one. The models were constructed using the Molecular Operating Environment (MOE) software and energy optimized using the MMFF94 molecular mechanics force field [49,50]. Conformational analysis was performed with the low mode conformational search module implemented in MOE. As first result, four conformations for each enantiomer with almost identical energies appeared for the dihydroxybenzyl moiety. The resulting most stable conformation for the sugar moiety was incorporated in an identical fashion for all further calculations. For validation of the obtained results for the entire compounds, corresponding calculations were performed with removed sugar moiety. All four low energy conformations of each enantiomer were optimized by using density functional theory (DFT) with BP86 functional and the def2-TZVPP basis set implemented in the ab initio ORCA 3.0.3 program package [51–56]. The influence of the solvent MeOH was included in the DFT calculations using the COSMO model [56]. For the simulation of the CD spectra, the first 50 excited states of each enantiomer were calculated by applying the long-range corrected hybrid functional TD CAM-B3LYP with the def2-TZVP(-f) and def2-TZVP/J basis sets. The CD curves were visualized and compared with the experimental ones with the help of the software SpecDis 1.64 [57].

4.7. Human Monocyte Isolation andAssessment of Cytokine Release

PBMCs (peripheral blood mononuclear cells) were isolated from the fresh blood of healthy donors (DRK Berlin, in accordance with the recommendations of the local ethics committee on human studies, Charité, Berlin, Germany) by density gradient centrifugation. Briefly, blood was added to Leucosep tubes (Greiner Bio-one GmbH, Frickenhausen, Germany) containing 15 mL of Leukocyte separation medium (Ficoll-Paque Plus, GE Healthcare Biosciences AB, Uppsala, Sweden) and centrifuged at 840× *g* for 20 min without breaks at room temperature. The interphase (PBMCs) was harvested and washed two times with PBS/BSA/EDTA (PBS + 0.2% BSA + 2 mM EDTA) and centrifuged (20 °C, 15 min, 200× *g*) to remove platelets. Monocytes were isolated using the monocyte isolation Kit II (Miltenyi Biotech GmbH Bergisch Gladbach, Germany) following the manufacturer's instructions. The purity of monocytes as assessed by flow cytometry was between 90% and 95% (±2%). Cells were seeded at 1 × 105 cells/well in serum free medium (X-Vivo 15, Lonza, Verviers, Belgium) in a round-bottom 96 well plate (Sarstedt AG & Co. KG, Nümbrecht, Germany) in the presence of the extracts or compounds or 0.1% DMSO (as control) and activated with 3 μg/mL poly-IC (Sigma Aldrich, Taufkirchen, Germany). Extracts or compound concentrations used for anti-inflammatory activity assay were previously assessed non-toxic for the cells by flow cytometry analyses. After 24 h of incubation at 37 °C supernatants were harvested and cytokine release was measured using a bead-based multiplex cytokine assay (Cytokine 25-Plex human Procarta Plex Panel 1B, Thermo Fisher Scientific, Darmstadt, Germany) and the Bioplex 200 system (Bio-Rad Laboratories GmbH, München, Germany).

5. Conclusions

Our results demonstrate the presence of a new bioactive natural product, (2*R*,3*R*)-(−)-3′,4′,5,7-tetrahydroxydihydroflavonol-8-*C*-*β*-D-glucopyranoside (Fideloside, **3**), here reported for the first time, belonging to the rare but highly-valued class of *C*-glycosylated phenols. The compound was isolated and purified from the endemic Cuban medicinal plant *Phyllanthus orbicularis*, and the chemical structure was unequivocally assessed as C8-glucoside of (2*R*,3*R*)-taxifolin by means of spectrometric, experimental and molecular modeling techniques. While is already taxifolin endowed with antioxidant and anti-inflammatory activities, the *C*-glycosylation could give to this derivative even better pharmacological and pharmaceutical properties. Preliminary experimental results on human monocytes demonstrated a promising bioactivity profile, with a positive modulation of anti-inflammatory mediators with respect to pro-inflammatory ones after cellular pro-inflammatory stimulus. In view of the above, Fideloside and *P. orbicularis* represent an important starting point for further bioactivity studies and of both the development of a standardized phytopharmaceutical product and the biochemistry of *C*-glycosylation.

Author Contributions: Conceptualization, A.F., L.W., A.S.-L. and L.M.; methodology, A.F., A.S.-L., K.F., S.F., C.V. and W.B.; software, A.F., L.W. and W.B.; validation, L.M., K.F. and M.D.; formal analysis, K.F. and A.F.; investigation, A.F.; resources, L.W. and A.S.-L.; data curation, A.F., W.B. and S.F.; writing—original draft preparation, A.F.; writing—review and editing, K.F., L.M., A.F., M.D., L.W. and A.S.-L.; visualization, A.F.; supervision, A.F., L.M., K.F., A.S.-L. and L.W.; project administration, A.F. and L.W.; funding acquisition, A.F. and L.W.", please turn to the CRediT taxonomy for the term explanation. Authorship is limited to those who have contributed substantially to the work reported.

Acknowledgments: The authorsthankAndrea Porzel for NMR spectral analyses, and Aldrin Vasco-Vidal, Manuel Garcia-Ricardo, Alfredo Rodriguez-Puentesand TuvshinjargalBudragchaafortheir technical support.

References

1. Shahidi, F.; Ambigaipalan, P. Phenolics and polyphenolics in foods, beverages and spices: Antioxidant activity and health effects—A review. *J. Funct. Foods* **2015**, *18*, 820–897. [CrossRef]
2. Mastromarino, P.; Capobianco, D.; Cannata, F.; Nardis, C.; Mattia, E.; De Leo, A.; Restignoli, R.; Francioso, A.; Mosca, L. Resveratrol inhibits rhinovirus replication and expression of inflammatory mediators in nasal epithelia. *Antiviral Res.* **2015**, *123*, 15–21. [CrossRef] [PubMed]
3. Lim, C.-G.; Koffas, M.A.G. Bioavailability and Recent Advances in the Bioactivity of Flavonoid and Stilbene Compounds. *Curr. Org. Chem.* **2010**, *14*, 1727–1751. [CrossRef]
4. Mattioli, R.; Francioso, A.; d'Erme, M.; Trovato, M.; Mancini, P.; Piacentini, L.; Casale, A.; Wessjohann, L.; Gazzino, R.; Costantino, P.; et al. Anti-Inflammatory Activity of A Polyphenolic Extract from Arabidopsis thaliana in In Vitro and In Vivo Models of Alzheimer's Disease. *Int. J. Mol. Sci.* **2019**, *20*, 708. [CrossRef] [PubMed]
5. Menes, M.D.O. Dos nuevasvariedades de *Portulaca brevifolia* Urb. (Portulacaceae) para la Flora de Cuba. *FeddesRepert* **2007**. [CrossRef]
6. Hammer, K.; Esquivel, M.; Fuentes, V.; Lima, H.; Knüpffer, H. Additional notes to the cheklist of cuban cultivated plants (1). *Die Kult.* **1990**, *38*, 325–343. [CrossRef]
7. Riverón-Giró, F.B.; Sánchez, C. Two new species of Tectaria (Tectariaceae) from Cuba. *Willdenowia* **2015**, *45*, 189–196. [CrossRef]
8. Ihantola-Vormisto, A.; Summanen, J.; Kankaanranta, H.; Vuorela, H.; Asmawi, Z.M.; Moilanen, E. Anti-inflammatory activity of extracts from leaves of *Phyllanthus emblica*. *Planta Med.* **1997**, *63*, 518–524. [CrossRef]

9. Thyagarajan, S.P.; Thirunalasundari, T.; Subramanian, S.; Venkateswaran, P.S.; Blumberg, B.S. Effect of phyllanthusamarus on chronic carriers of hepatitis b virus. *Lancet* **1988**, *332*, 764–766. [CrossRef]
10. Kuttan, R.; Harikumar, K.B. *Phyllanthus Species: Scientific Evaluation and Medicinal Applications*; CRC Press: Boca Raton, FL, USA, 2011; ISBN 1439821445.
11. Joy, K.L.; Kuttan, R. Inhibition by *Phyllanthus amarus* of Hepatocarcinogenesis Induced by N-Nitrosodiethylamine. *J. Clin. Biochem. Nutr.* **2011**, *24*, 133–139. [CrossRef]
12. Gowrishanker, B.; Vivekanandan, O.S. In vivo studies of a crude extract of *Phyllanthus amarus* L. in modifying the genotoxicity induced in *Viciafaba* L. by tannery effluents. *Mutat. Res. Toxicol.* **1994**, *322*, 185–192. [CrossRef]
13. Gaitén, Y.I.G.; Martínez, M.M.; Alarcón, A.B.; Vãzquez, M.M.; Hernãndez, J.L.F.; Roche, L.D.; Rastrelli, L. Anti-inflammatory and antioxidant activity of a methanolic extract of phyllanthus orbicularis and its derived flavonols). *J. Essent. Oil Res.* **2011**, *23*, 50–53. [CrossRef]
14. Quintero, A.R.; Gutiérrez, I.S.; Díaz, L.M.; del Barrio Alonso, G. Effect of Phyllanthus orbicularis on the cell viability and the hepatitis B surface antigen in PLC/PRF/5 cells. *Rev. Cuba. Farm.* **2011**, *45*, 536–544.
15. Álvarez, Á.L.; Dalton, K.P.; Nicieza, I.; Diñeiro, Y.; Picinelli, A.; Melón, S.; Roque, A.; Suárez, B.; Parra, F. Bioactivity-guided fractionation of phyllanthus orbicularis and identification of the principal anti HSV-2 compounds. *Phyther. Res.* **2012**, *26*, 1513–1520. [CrossRef] [PubMed]
16. Del Barrio, G.; Parra, F. Evaluation of the antiviral activity of an aqueous extract from Phyllanthus orbicularis. *J. Ethnopharmacol.* **2000**, *72*, 317–322. [CrossRef]
17. Álvarez, Á.L.; del Barrio, G.; Kourí, V.; Martínez, P.A.; Suárez, B.; Parra, F. In vitro anti-herpetic activity of an aqueous extract from the plant *Phyllanthus orbicularis*. *Phytomedicine* **2009**, *16*, 960–966. [CrossRef] [PubMed]
18. Sànchez-Lamar, A.; Fiore, M.; Cundari, E.; Ricordy, R.; Cozzi, R.; De Salvia, R. Phyllanthus orbicularis aqueous extract: Cytotoxic, genotoxic, and antimutagenic effects in the CHO cell line. *Toxicol. Appl. Pharmacol.* **1999**, *161*, 231–239. [CrossRef] [PubMed]
19. Ferrer, M.; Sánchez-Lamar, A.; Fuentes, J.L.; Barbé, J.; Llagostera, M. Studies on the antimutagenesis of *Phyllanthus orbicularis*: Mechanisms involved against aromatic amines. *Mutat. Res. Genet. Toxicol. Environ. Mutagen.* **2001**, *498*, 99–105. [CrossRef]
20. Ferrer, M.; Cristófol, C.; Sánchez-Lamar, A.; Fuentes, J.L.; Barbé, J.; Llagostera, M. Modulation of rat and human cytochromes P450 involved in PhIP and 4-ABP activation by an aqueous extract of *Phyllanthus orbicularis*. *J. Ethnopharmacol.* **2004**, *90*, 273–277. [CrossRef]
21. Vernhes, M.; González-Pumariega, M.; Alonso, A.; Baly, L.; Menck, C.F.M.; Sánchez-Lamar, A. Photoprotective effect phyllanthus orbicularis HBK in *E. coli* cells. *Vaccimonitor* **2010**, *19*, 233.
22. Alonso, A.; Fuentes, J.L.; Sánchez-Lamar, A.; Llagostera, M. Antimutagenic Effect of Phyllanthus orbicularis against γ-radiation. *Lat. Am. J. Pharm.* **2010**, *29*, 148–152.
23. Vernhes, M.; González-Pumariega, M.; Passaglia, A.; Martins, F.C.; Sánchez-Lamar, A. Aqueous extract of *Phyllanthus orbicularis* K protects the plasmid DNA from the damage induced by ultraviolet radiation. *Ars Pharm.* **2013**, *54*, 1.
24. Tamayo, M.V.; Schuch, A.P.; Yagura, T.; Gil, L.B.; Menck, C.F.M.; Sánchez-Lamar, A. Genoprotective Effect of *Phyllanthus orbicularis* Extract Against UVA, UVB, and Solar Radiation. *Photochem. Photobiol.* **2018**, *94*, 1026–1031. [CrossRef] [PubMed]
25. Menéndez-Perdomo, I.M.; Wong-Guerra, M.; Fuentes-León, F.; Carrazana, E.; Casadelvalle, I.; Vidal, A.; Sánchez-Lamar, A. Antioxidant, photoprotective and antimutagenic properties of *Phyllanthus* spp. from Cuban flora. *J. Pharm. Pharmacogn. Res.* **2017**, *5*, 251–261.
26. Gutiérrez, Y.; Miranda, M.; Henriques, A.; del Barrio, G. Flavonoids analysis of a butanol fraction obtained from *Phyllanthus orbicularis* HBK. *Univ. Revista Cubana de Farmacia* **2010**, *44*, 367–373.
27. Catarino, M.D.; Silva, A.M.S.; Saraiva, S.C.; Sobral, A.J.F.N.; Cardoso, S.M. Characterization of phenolic constituents and evaluation of antioxidant properties of leaves and stems of *Eriocephalus africanus*. *Arab. J. Chem.* **2018**, *11*, 62–69. [CrossRef]
28. Jaiswal, R.; Halabi, E.A.; Karar, M.G.E.; Kuhnert, N. Identification and characterisation of the phenolics of *Ilex glabra* L. Gray (Aquifoliaceae) leaves by liquid chromatography tandem mass spectrometry. *Phytochemistry* **2014**, *106*, 141–155. [CrossRef] [PubMed]

29. Elliger, C.A.; Lundin, R.E.; Haddon, W.F. Caffeyl esters of glucaric acid in *Lycopersiconesculentum* leaves. *Phytochemistry* **1981**, *20*, 1133–1134. [CrossRef]
30. Coutinho, I.D.; Baker, J.M.; Ward, J.L.; Beale, M.H.; Creste, S.; Cavalheiro, A.J. Metabolite profiling of sugarcane genotypes and identification of flavonoid glycosides and phenolic acids. *J. Agric. Food Chem.* **2016**, *64*, 4198–4206. [CrossRef]
31. Risch, B.; Herrmann, K.; Wray, V. (E)-O-p-Coumaroyl-, (E)-O-Feruloyl-derivatives of glucaric acid in citrus. *Phytochemistry* **1988**, *27*, 3327–3329. [CrossRef]
32. Lin, L.Z.; Sun, J.; Chen, P.; Monagas, M.J.; Harnly, J.M. UHPLC-PDA-ESI/HRMSnprofiling method to identify and quantify oligomeric proanthocyanidins in plant products. *J. Agric. Food Chem.* **2014**, *62*, 9387–9400. [CrossRef] [PubMed]
33. Chen, Y.; Yu, H.; Wu, H.; Pan, Y.; Wang, K.; Jin, Y.; Zhang, C. Characterization and quantification by LC-MS/MS of the chemical components of the heating products of the flavonoids extract in *Pollen typhae* for transformation rule exploration. *Molecules* **2015**, *20*, 18352–18366. [CrossRef] [PubMed]
34. Geng, P.; Sun, J.; Zhang, M.; Li, X.; Harnly, J.M.; Chen, P. Comprehensive characterization of C-glycosyl flavones in wheat (*Triticum aestivum* L.) germ using UPLC-PDA-ESI/HRMSn and mass defect filtering. *J. Mass Spectrom.* **2016**, *51*, 914–930. [CrossRef] [PubMed]
35. Dokkedal, A.L.; Lavarda, F.; Dos Santos, L.C.; Vilegas, W. Xeractinol—A new flavanonol C-glucoside from *Paepalanthus argenteus* var. argenteus (Bongard) Hensold (Eriocaulaceae). *J. Braz. Chem. Soc.* **2007**, *18*, 437–439. [CrossRef]
36. Mbafor, J.T.; Fomum, Z.T.; Promsattha, R.; Sanson, D.R.; Tempesta, M.S. Isolation and characterization of taxifolin 6-c-glucoside from garcinia epunctata. *J. Nat. Prod.* **1989**, *52*, 417–419. [CrossRef] [PubMed]
37. Rawat, P.; Kumar, M.; Sharan, K.; Chattopadhyay, N.; Maurya, R. Ulmosides A and B: Flavonoid 6-C-glycosides from *Ulmuswallichiana*, stimulating osteoblast differentiation assessed by alkaline phosphatase. *Bioorg. Med. Chem. Lett.* **2009**, *19*, 4684–4687. [CrossRef] [PubMed]
38. Sokolová, R.; Nycz, J.E.; Ramešová, Š.; Fiedler, J.; Degano, I.; Szala, M.; Kolivoška, V.; Gál, M. Electrochemistry and spectroelectrochemistry of bioactive hydroxyquinolines: A mechanistic study. *J. Phys. Chem. B* **2015**, *119*, 6074–6080. [CrossRef]
39. Nonaka, G.-I.; Goto, Y.; Kinjo, J.-E.; Nohara, T.; Nishioka, I. Tannins and related compounds. LII Studies on the constituents of the leaves of *Thujopsisdolabrata* SIEB. et ZUCC. *Chem. Pharm. Bull.* **2011**, *35*, 1105–1108. [CrossRef]
40. Tofazzal Islam, M.; Tahara, S. Dihydroflavonols from *Lanneacoromandelica*. *Phytochemistry* **2000**, *54*, 901–907. [CrossRef]
41. Xiao, J.; Capanoglu, E.; Jassbi, A.R.; Miron, A. Advance on the Flavonoid *C-gly* cosides and Health Benefits. *Crit. Rev. Food Sci. Nutr.* **2016**, *56*, S29–S45. [CrossRef]
42. Gocer, H.; Topal, F.; Topal, M.; Küçük, M.; Teke, D.; Gülçin, I.; Alwasel, S.H.; Supuran, C.T. Acetylcholinesterase and carbonic anhydrase isoenzymes i and II inhibition profiles of taxifolin. *J. Enzyme Inhib. Med. Chem.* **2016**, *31*, 441–447. [CrossRef] [PubMed]
43. Kuang, H.; Tang, Z.; Zhang, C.; Wang, Z.; Li, W.; Yang, C.; Wang, Q.; Yang, B.; Kong, A.N. Taxifolin activates the Nrf2 anti-oxidative stress pathway in mouse skin epidermal JB6 P+ cells through epigenetic modifications. *Int. J. Mol. Sci.* **2017**, *18*, 1546. [CrossRef] [PubMed]
44. Saito, S.; Yamamoto, Y.; Maki, T.; Hattori, Y.; Ito, H.; Mizuno, K.; Harada-Shiba, M.; Kalaria, R.N.; Fukushima, M.; Takahashi, R.; et al. Taxifolin inhibits amyloid-β oligomer formation and fully restores vascular integrity and memory in cerebral amyloid angiopathy. *Acta Neuropathol. Commun.* **2017**, *5*, 26. [CrossRef] [PubMed]
45. Sun, X.; Chen, R.C.; Yang, Z.H.; Sun, G.B.; Wang, M.; Ma, X.J.; Yang, L.J.; Sun, X.B. Taxifolin prevents diabetic cardiomyopathy in vivo and in vitro by inhibition of oxidative stress and cell apoptosis. *Food Chem. Toxicol.* **2014**, *63*, 221–232. [CrossRef] [PubMed]
46. Gupta, P.; Singh, A.; Tiwari, S.; Mishra, A.; Maurya, R.; Singh, S. Ulmosides A: Flavonoid 6-C-glycosides from Ulmuswallichiana attenuates lipopolysacchride induced oxidative stress, apoptosis and neuronal death. *Neurotoxicology* **2019**, *73*, 100–111. [CrossRef] [PubMed]
47. Enzymatic C-Alkylation of Aromatic Compounds. In *Biocatalysis in Organic Synthesis*; hieme E-Books & E-Journals Partner: Stuttgart, Germany, 2016.

48. Ruela, H.S.; Leal, I.C.R.; de Almeida, M.R.A.; dos Santos, K.R.N.; Wessjohann, L.A.; Kuster, R.M. Antibacterial and antioxidant activities and acute toxicity of *Bumeliasartorum* Mart., Sapotaceae, a Brazilian medicinal plant. *Rev. Bras. Farmacogn.* **2011**, *21*, 86–91. [CrossRef]
49. Chemical Computing Group ULC. Molecular Operating Environment (MOE). Available online: https://www.chemcomp.com/ (accessed on 5 August 2019).
50. Halgren, T.A. MMFF VI. MMFF94s option for energy minimization studies. *J. Comput. Chem.* **1999**, *20*, 720–729. [CrossRef]
51. Becke, A.D. Density-functional exchange-energy approximation with correct asymptotic behavior. *Phys. Rev. A* **1988**, *38*, 3098. [CrossRef]
52. Perdew, J.P. Density-functional approximation for the correlation energy of the inhomogeneous electron gas. *Phys. Rev. B* **1986**, *33*, 8822. [CrossRef]
53. Karton, A.; Tarnopolsky, A.; Lamère, J.F.; Schatz, G.C.; Martin, J.M.L. Highly accurate first-principles benchmark data sets for the parametrization and validation of density functional and other approximate methods. Derivation of a robust, generally applicable, double-hybrid functional for thermochemistry and thermochemical. *J. Phys. Chem. A* **2008**, *112*, 12868–12886. [CrossRef]
54. Schäfer, A.; Horn, H.; Ahlrichs, R. Fully optimized contracted Gaussian basis sets for atoms Li to Kr. *J. Chem. Phys.* **1992**, *97*, 2571–2577. [CrossRef]
55. Weigend, F.; Ahlrichs, R. Balanced basis sets of split valence, triple zeta valence and quadruple zeta valence quality for H to Rn: Design and assessment of accuracy. *Phys. Chem. Chem. Phys.* **2005**, *7*, 3297–3305. [CrossRef] [PubMed]
56. Sinnecker, S.; Rajendran, A.; Klamt, A.; Diedenhofen, M.; Neese, F. Calculation of solvent shifts on electronic g-tensors with the conductor-like screening model (COSMO) and its self-consistent generalization to real solvents (direct COSMO-RS). *J. Phys. Chem. A* **2006**, *110*, 2235–2245. [CrossRef] [PubMed]
57. Bruhn, T.; Schaumlöffel, A.; Hemberger, Y.; Bringmann, G. SpecDis: Quantifying the comparison of calculated and experimental electronic circular dichroism spectra. *Chirality* **2013**, *25*, 243–249. [CrossRef] [PubMed]

10

Quality Assessment of Commercial Spagyric Tinctures of *Harpagophytum procumbens* and their Antioxidant Properties

Pinarosa Avato * and Maria Pia Argentieri

Dipartimento di Farmacia-Scienze del Farmaco, Università degli Studi di Bari Aldo Moro, via Orabona 4, 70125 Bari, Italy; mariapia.argentieri@uniba.it
* Correspondence: pinarosa.avato@uniba.it;

Abstract: Preparations from the dried tubers of *Harpagophytum procumbens* (Burch.) DC ex Meisn, commonly known as devil's claw, are mainly used in modern medicine to relieve joint pain and inflammation in patients suffering from rheumatic and arthritic disorders. This paper describes for the first time the chemical profile of a commercial spagyric tincture (named 019) prepared from the roots of the plant. For comparison purposes, a commercial not-spagyric devil's claw tincture (NST) was also analyzed. Chemical investigation of the content of specialized metabolites in the three samples indicated that harpagoside was the main compound, followed by the two isomers acteoside and isoacteoside. Compositional consistence over time was obtained by the chemical fingerprinting of another spagyric tincture (named 014) from the same producer that was already expired according to the recommendation on the label of the product. The two spagyric preparations did not show significant compositional differences as revealed by HPLC and MS analyses, except for a decrease in harpagide content in the expired 014 tincture. Moreover, their antioxidant capacities as assessed by 2,2′-di-phenyl-1-picrylhydrazyl (DPPH) and 2.2′-azin-bis (3-ethylbenzothiazoline-6-sulfonic acid) (ABTS) methods resulted in very similar IC50 values. The expired 014 tincture showed instead a lower IC50 value compared to the 019 and NST tinctures with the ferric reducing antioxidant potential (FRAP) assay, indicating a higher ferric-reducing antioxidant ability. Overall, these results indicated that the two preparations could generally maintain good stability and biological activity at least for the four years from the production to the expiration date.

Keywords: *Harpagophytum procumbens*; devil's claw; harpagoside; spagyric tincture; antioxidant activity

---

1. Introduction

Harpagophytum procumbens (Burch.) DC ex Meisn, commonly known as devil's claw, is a plant native to southern Africa, where it is traditionally used as a bitter tonic and a stomachic and also for the treatment of fever, gout, myalgia, and arthritis [1,2]. Accordingly, preparations from the dried tubers of the plant are mainly used in modern medicine and as health products to relieve joint pain and inflammation in patients suffering from rheumatic and arthritic disorders. Clinical studies have in fact shown that extracts from the roots of this plant are good therapeutic remedies for degenerative diseases of the musculoskeletal and locomotor systems [1,3]. In addition, the use of devil's claw secondary tubers is also approved in preparations for the relief of mild digestive disorders and for the temporary loss of appetite [4,5].

The European Medicines Agency (EMA) recommends preparations obtained by comminuting or powdering the roots of the plant. Liquid, soft, or dry extracts for oral use made in ethanol or water are also included in the recommendation [4,5]. Spagyric tinctures based on *H. procumbens* are also available on the market for articular and rheumatic complaints.

The manufacturing of a spagyric tincture is based on two main stages, namely maceration and fermentation of the drug in alcohol. Processing of the plant material is accomplished in dark thick-walled glass flasks hermetically closed and maintained in greenhouses under a controlled temperature of about 37 °C for 28 days. After this period, the tincture is decanted, and the drug residue is removed from the solution, completely dried, and burnt to ashes to recover the inorganic elements of the plant material. Ashes from the calcined drug are then dissolved in the alcoholic solution from maceration, and the final spagyric preparation is left to stand for 12 days before use.

The practice of "spagyria" dates back to Paracelsus (1493–1541), who first coined the term to mean "separate" (*spao*) and "combine" (*ageiro*), indicating that spagyric preparations are based on "separation", "extraction", and "recombination" of the active extractives, including mineral components [6].

The quality control of herbal products aims to assure their consistency, efficacy, and safety. The overall quality of botanicals depends on several factors, including the selection of raw plant materials, harvest time, seasonal changes, and post-harvest processing, and it also relies on extraction procedures and product preparations. All of these factors can primarily affect the plant/drug content of bioactive constituents and impair the efficacy of the final formulation.

The determination of chemical fingerprinting can be a powerful tool to verify the quality of botanicals [7–10]. Thus, the selection of specific chemical markers of a drug sample/preparation is considered to be crucial for the analysis of its quality. According to the EMA, chemical markers are of interest for quality control regardless of whether they possess any therapeutic or physiological activity, although ideal chemical markers should be unique metabolites that contribute to the biological efficacy of the drug or its preparation [11,12].

The use of fingerprinting in the analytical control of herbal preparation is now a widely accepted official method [7–10] to assess quality and stability over time and eventually disclose some variation in the chemical content that could reflect a decline in biological activity.

Bitter iridoid glucosides such as harpagoside and harpagide are widely regarded as the active constituents responsible for the pharmacological anti-inflammatory properties of *H. procumbens* [13–16]. Other components reported as present in the drug are the iridoid procumbide, 8-*O*-*p*-coumaroyl-harpagide, 6′-*O*-*p*-coumaroyl-procumbide, phenylethyl glycosides (such as acteoside and isoacteoside), polyphenolic acids, and flavonoids. All of these phytochemicals are considered to have antioxidant properties and to provide protection against lipid peroxidation [17]. According to the *European Pharmacopoeia* [18], roots from *H. procumbens* must contain ≥1.2% harpagoside. Therefore, a chromatographic profile based on the content of the above main components, taken as the reference chemical markers, should be used in the analytical control of preparations from the roots of *H. procumbens*.

The present manuscript aims to assess quality in terms of the quantitative and qualitative fingerprinting of selected chemical markers of a commercial spagyric preparation based on *H. procumbens*. Compositional data of specialized metabolites were compared to those from a commercial not-spagyric devil's claw tincture (NST) with June 2020 as the declared expiration date. In addition, an evaluation of possible deterioration of the chemical profile was carried out through chemical fingerprinting of an *H. procumbens* spagyric food supplement from the same manufacturer that was already expired according to the recommendation published on the label of the product. Finally, the antioxidant activity of the two spagyric preparations was determined and compared to possibly reveal any variation in activity due to the aging of the products and degradation of the bioactive phytochemicals.

2. Results

2.1. Chemical Analysis

As shown in Figure 1, the two spagyric tinctures 014 and 019 did not show significant compositional differences as revealed by thin layer chromatography-TLC. No substantial compositional differences were also observed when compared to the NST. As indicated, harpagoside, acteoside, and harpagide could be detected in all of the samples as the main specialized metabolites.

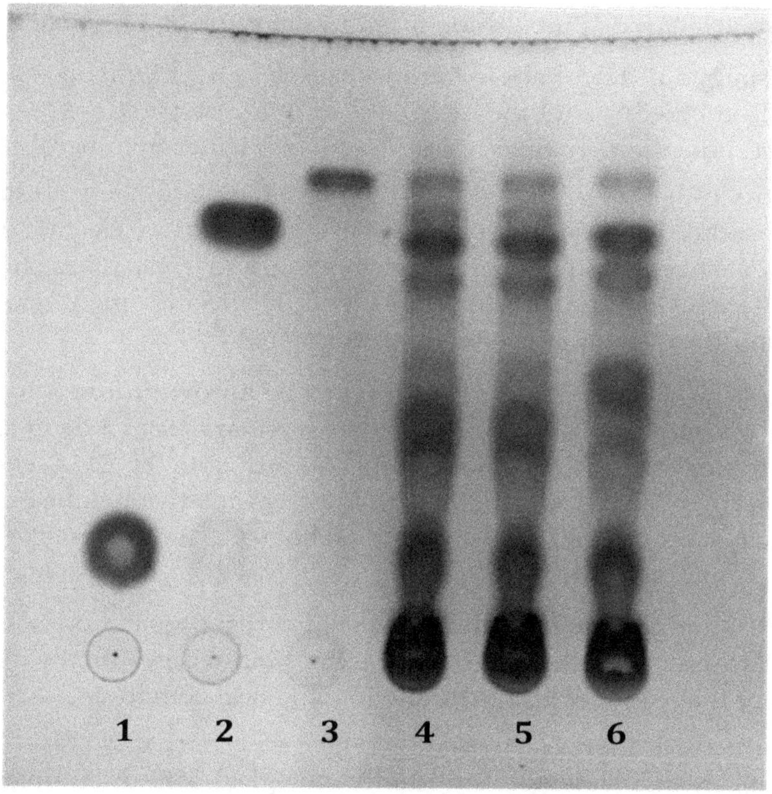

Figure 1. TLC analysis of the two spagyric tinctures, 014 and 019. Mobile phase: EtOAc/HCOOH/CH_3CO_2H/H_2O (100:11:11:26 *v*/*v*); visualization with AS (see Section 4.4). Harpagide, 1; harpagoside, 2; acteoside, 3; 014, 4; 019, 5; not-spagyric tincture (NST), 6.

In agreement with TLC analyses, a comparison of the HPLC-DAD (diode-array detector) chromatograms indicated that the three samples 019, 014, and NST did not differ in their general composition (Figure 2). Typical UV absorptions (Table 1) detecting around 217, 246–248, 290, and 325–330 nm for compounds **1** and **2** indicated the presence of phenylethanoid glycosides [19], while the detection of UV maxima at 217 and 280 nm were consistent with an iridoid enol ether system, including a cinnamoyl chromophore in compounds **5** and **6** [20]. In addition, UV absorptions at around 224 and 311 nm suggested the presence of *p*-coumaric acid moieties in compounds **3** and **4**.

Consistent with the above observations, the chemical profile investigated by combining HPLC-DAD and LC–MS/MS and through spiking it with available reference compounds confirmed that the main peak (t_R = 39.58 min) in both samples was represented by harpagoside (Figure 2, peak 5).

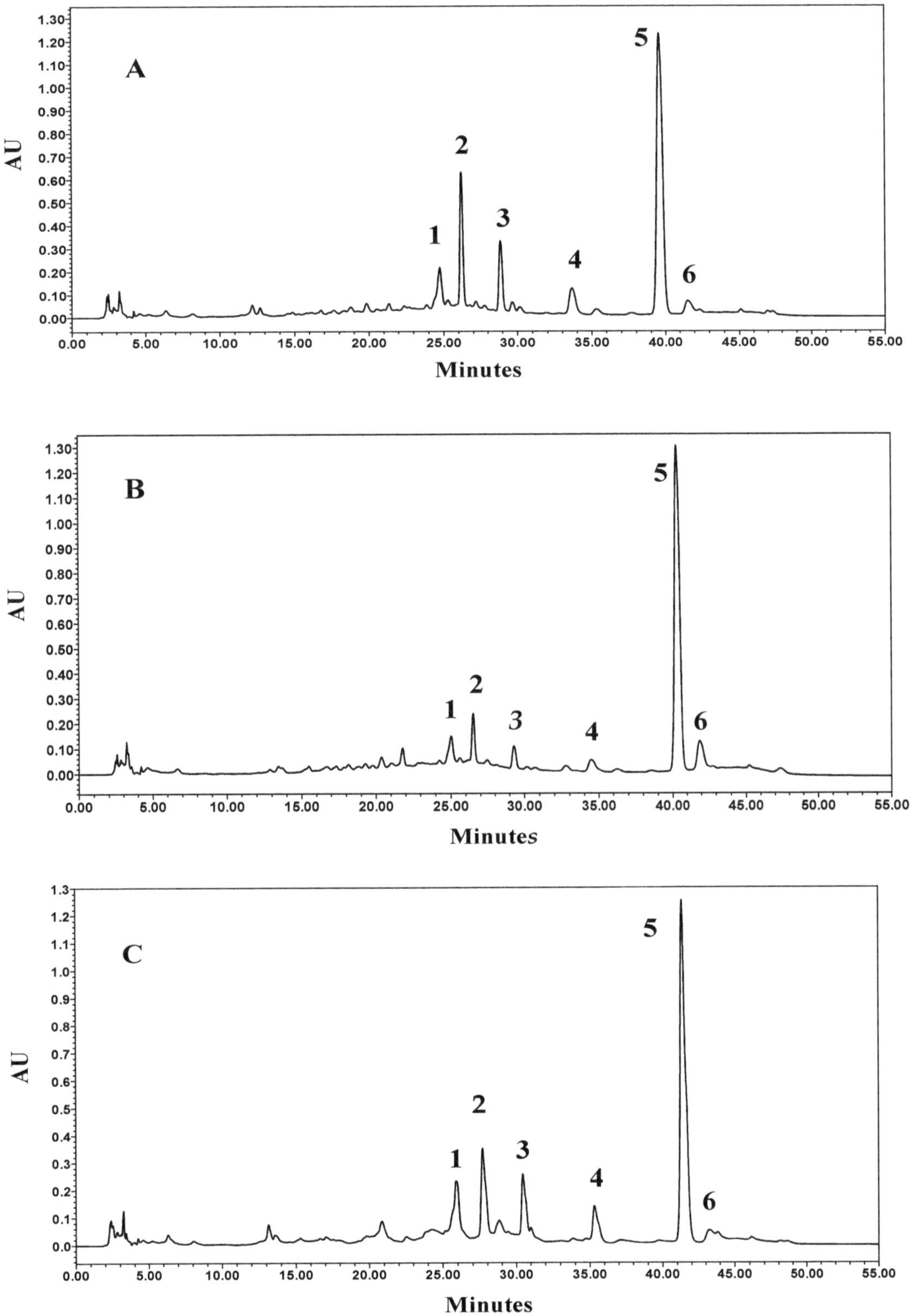

Figure 2. HPLC-DAD (270 nm) chromatograms of the tinctures 019 (**A**), 014 (**B**), and the NST (**C**). For peak naming, see Table 1.

Table 1. MS fragmentation and UV-VIS absorption data of compounds detected in the tinctures of Harpagophytum procumbens by HPLC-DAD (270 nm).

Number *	R_t (min)	Name	UV (λ max, nm)	ms1	ms2
				m/z (%)	
1	24.70	Acteoside	216.6, 246.5 sh, 290.5 sh, 325.7	623.0 (100) $[M-H]^-$	461.0 (100) $[(M-H)\text{-}162]^-$; 315.0 (4) $[(M-H)\text{-}162\text{-}146]^-$; 179.0 (2), $[\text{caffeoyl moiety}]^-$
2	26.20	Isoacteoside	217.7, 248.5 sh, 292.3 sh, 326.9	623.0 (100) $[M-H]^-$	461.0 (100) $[(M\text{-}H)\text{-}162]^-$; 315.0 (4) $[(M-H)\text{-}162\text{-}146]^-$; 179.0 (2), $[\text{caffeoyl moiety}]^-$
3	28.87	8-*O*-*p*-Coumaroyl-harpagide	224.8, 311.4	533.1 (100) $[M+Na]^+$	369.2 (100) $[(M+Na)\text{-}164]^+$; 351.0 (44) $[(M+Na)\text{-}164\text{-}18]^+$; 203.0 (6) $[\text{harpagide-162}]^+$
4	33.60	Pagoside	224.8, 311.4	491.0 (100) $[M-H]^-$	311.2 (100) $[(M-H)\text{-}162\text{-}18]^-$; 163.0 (31) $[\text{coumaric acid}]^-$
5	39.58	Harpagoside	217.7, 280.4	1011.5 (5) $[2M+Na]^+$ /517.2 (100) $[M+Na]^+$	369.2 (100) $[(M+Na)\text{-}148]^+$; 351.0 (44) $[(M+Na)\text{-}148\text{-}18]^+$; 203.0 (6) $[(M+Na)\text{-}148\text{-}166]^+$
6	41.64	8-Cinnamoylmyoporoside	217.7, 278.1	501.0 (100) $[M+Na]^+$	353.1 (100) $[(M+Na)\text{-}148]^+$; 335.2 (69) $[(M+Na)\text{-}148\text{-}18]^+$; 339.0 (41) $[(M+Na)\text{-}162]^+$; 203.0 (6) $\text{harpagide-162}]^+$

* For peak numbers, see text and Figure 2.

The UV spectrum showing two absorption bands at 217.7 and 280.4 (max) nm and the LC–MS/MS fragmentation pattern ([*m/z* 1011.5 (5) 2M + Na]$^+$, [*m/z* 517.2 (100) M + Na]$^+$, [*m/z* 369.2 (100) (M + Na)-148, cinnamic acid]$^+$, [*m/z* 351.0 (44) (M + Na)-148-18]$^+$, [*m/z* 203.0 (6) (M + Na)-148-166, harpagide]$^+$) were in fact unequivocally consistent with the identification of harpagoside [12,17]. The identity of harpagoside was also acquired by its isolation as a pure constituent through a fast and reliable solid-phase extraction (SPE) optimization method (see Section 4.4). The other major peaks (Figure 2) were respectively identified as peak 1, acteoside (verbascoside), (t_R = 24.70 min), UV 216.6, 246.5 (sh), 290.5 (sh), and 325.7 (max) nm, fragmentation pattern ([*m/z* 623.0 (100) M − H]$^-$, [*m/z* 461 (100) (M − H)-162, glucose]$^-$, [*m/z* 315.0 (4) (M − H)-162-146, rhamnose]$^-$, [*m/z* 179.0 (2), caffeoyl moiety]$^-$); peak 2, isoacteoside, (t_R = 26.20 min), UV 217.7, 248.5 (sh), 292.3 (sh), and 326.9 (max) nm, fragmentation pattern ([*m/z* 623.0 (100) M − H]$^-$, [*m/z* 461 (100) (M − H)-162, glucose]$^-$, [*m/z* 315.0 (4) (M − H)-162-146, rhamnose]$^-$, [*m/z* 179.0 (2), caffeoyl moiety]$^-$); peak 3, 8-p-coumaroyl-harpagide, (t_R = 28.87 min), UV 224.8, 311.4 (max) nm, fragmentation pattern ([*m/z* 533.1 (100) M + Na]$^+$, [*m/z* 369.2 (100) (M + Na)-164, coumaric acid]$^+$, [*m/z* 351.0 (44) (M + Na)-164-18]$^+$, [*m/z* 203.0 (6) harpagide-162, glucose]$^+$); peak 4, pagoside, (t_R = 33.60 min), UV 224.8 and 311.4 (max) nm, fragmentation pattern ([*m/z* 491.0 (100) M − H]$^-$, [*m/z* 311.2 (100) (M − H)-18-162, glucose]$^-$, [*m/z* 163.0 (31), coumaric acid]$^-$); peak 6, 8-cinnamoylmyoporoside (t_R = 41.64 min), UV 217.7 (max) and 278.1 nm, fragmentation pattern ([*m/z* 501.0 (100) M + Na]$^+$, [*m/z* 353.1 (100) (M + Na)-148, cinnamic acid]$^+$, [*m/z* 335.2 (69) (M + Na)-148-18]$^+$, [*m/z* 339.0 (41) (M + Na)-162, glucose]$^+$, [*m/z* 203.0 (6) harpagide-162, glucose]$^+$). The presence of harpagide (lacking absorbance at 270 nm), already detected by TLC, was confirmed by HPLC-ELSD (evaporative light scattering detector) analysis (Figures 1 and 3) and by coelution with an authentic compound, and it was in addition identified through its mass spectrum: ([*m/z* 365.0 (100) M + H]$^+$, [*m/z* 347.1 (36) (M + H)-18]$^+$, [*m/z* 305.1 (75) (M + H)-42-18]$^+$, [*m/z* 275.1 (41) (M + H)-90]$^+$, [*m/z* 203.0 (100) (M + H)-162]$^+$, [*m/z* 185.0 (68) (M + H)-162-18]$^+$). The identification of constituents of the two spagyric tinctures was also supported by the available literature [13,21–24].

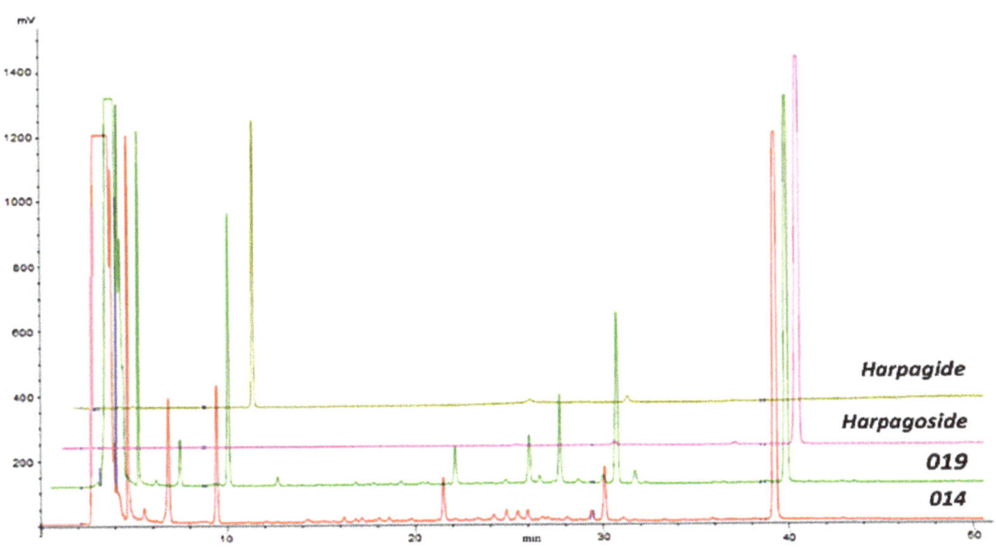

Figure 3. HPLC-ELSD chromatograms of the two spagyric tinctures, 014 and 019: Harpagoside and harpagide.

In addition to a similar chemical profile, the two spagyric tinctures also showed to a large extent a comparable quantitative composition (Table 2). A quantification of harpagoside as determined by HPLC-DAD against the calibration curve indicated that the compound was equally abundant in the two extracts, amounting respectively to 14.97 ± 0.09 μg/mg ext (59.47%) in the 019 sample and to 13.68 ± 0.19 μg/mg ext (69.68%) in the 014 sample. Other major metabolites were represented by acteoside (019: 1.99 ± 0.23 μg/mg ext, 7.90%; 014: 1.49 ± 0.02 μg/mg ext, 7.59%) and isoacteside (019:

3.94 ± 0.006 μg/mg ext, 15.65%; 014: 1.87 ± 0.14 μg/mg ext, 9.52%). A relatively higher amount of 8-*O*-*p*-coumaroyl-harpagide (019: 2.21 ± 0.0003 μg /mg ext, 8.78%; 014: 0.68 ± 0.006 μg/mg ext, 3.46%) and pagoside (019: 1.37 ± 0.01 μg/mg ext 5.44%; 014: 0.53 ± 0.009 μg/mg ext, 2.70%) was detected in the 019 sample, while 8-cinnamoylmyoporoside was more abundant in 014, 1.38 ± 0.009 μg/mg, 7.03%, versus 0.69 ± 0.008 μg/mg ext, 2.74%, in 019. The same specialized metabolites in the NST sample amounted, respectively, to acteoside, 1.35 ± 0.15 μg/mg ext, 7.39%; isoacteoside, 1.55 ± 0.04 μg/mg ext, 8.48%; 8-*O*-*p*-coumaroyl-harpagide, 0.95 ± 0.04 μg/mg ext, 5.20%; pagoside, 0.72 ± 0.02 μg/mg ext, 3.94%; harpagoside, 13.25 ± 0.07 μg/mg ext, 75.52%; 8-cinnamoylmyoporoside, 0.45 ± 0.005 μg/mg ext, 2.46% (Table 2).

Table 2. Specialized metabolites identified in 019, 014, and the NST.

Compound	014		019		NST	
	μg/mg ext	%	μg/mg ext	%	μg/mg ext	%
1	1.49 ± 0.02	7.59	1.99 ± 0.23	7.90	1.35 ± 0.15	7.39
2	1.87 ± 0.14	9.52	3.94 ± 0.006	15.65	1.55 ± 0.04	8.48
3	0.68 ± 0.006	3.46	2.21 ± 0.0003	8.78	0.95 ± 0.04	5.2
4	0.53 ± 0.009	2.70	1.37 ± 0.01	5.44	0.72 ± 0.02	3.94
5	13.68 ± 0.19	69.68	14.97 ± 0.09	59.47	13.25 ± 0.07	72.52
6	1.38 ± 0.009	7.03	0.69 ± 0.008	2.74	0.45 ± 0.005	2.46

For peak naming, see Table 1.

Due to the lack of a chromophore in the molecule, harpagide quantitation was achieved by HPLC-ELSD, which indicated that the content of this phytochemical was slightly higher in the 019 preparation (15.98 ± 0.23 μg/mg ext) compared to the 014 sample (8.50 ± 0.32 μg/mg ext). Similarly to the 019 tincture, harpagide extract accounted for 19.53 ± 0.17 μg/mg ext in the NST.

2.2. *Antioxidant Activity*

The antioxidant capacity of the two spagyric tinctures of *H. procumbens* was evaluated by in vitro DPPH, ABTS, and FRAP assays (see Sections 4.9–4.11) and compared to quercetin and acteoside. As shown in Figure 4, the free radical scavenging activity determined by the DPPH and ABTS methods and the ferric-reducing power calculated by the FRAP assay gave almost superimposable behaviors for the two samples, 019 and 014. They displayed a good dose-dependent inhibition of DPPH activity in the range of tested concentrations (up to 89–90% inhibition for 019 and 014, respectively) at 330 μg/mL and up to 98% inhibition of ABTS activity at 260 μg/mL. The ferric-reducing antioxidant power results were instead already high at lower concentrations (52–69% inhibition at 26 μg/mL and up to 76–83% at 60 μg/mL for 019 and 014, respectively).

With regard to the NST sample, its free radical scavenging activity and its ferric-reducing activity (determined by DPPH, ABTS, and FRAP assays) gave results almost superimposable on those obtained for the two spagyric tinctures, with a good dose versus % inhibition correlation.

However, compared to quercetin and acteoside, all three tinctures (019, 014, and the NST) displayed lower antioxidant activity (Figure 4). Both of these two compounds showed antiradical activity reaching 96–100% of DPPH inhibition at concentrations between 26 and 50 μg/mL for quercetin and acteoside. Similarly, quercetin and acteoside were very effective in scavenging the $ABTS^+$ radical cation, displaying 100% inhibition between 7 and 13 μg/mL. In addition, they showed discrete FRAP values amounting to 330 (quercetin) and 67 (acteoside) μg/mL to obtain 95% inhibition.

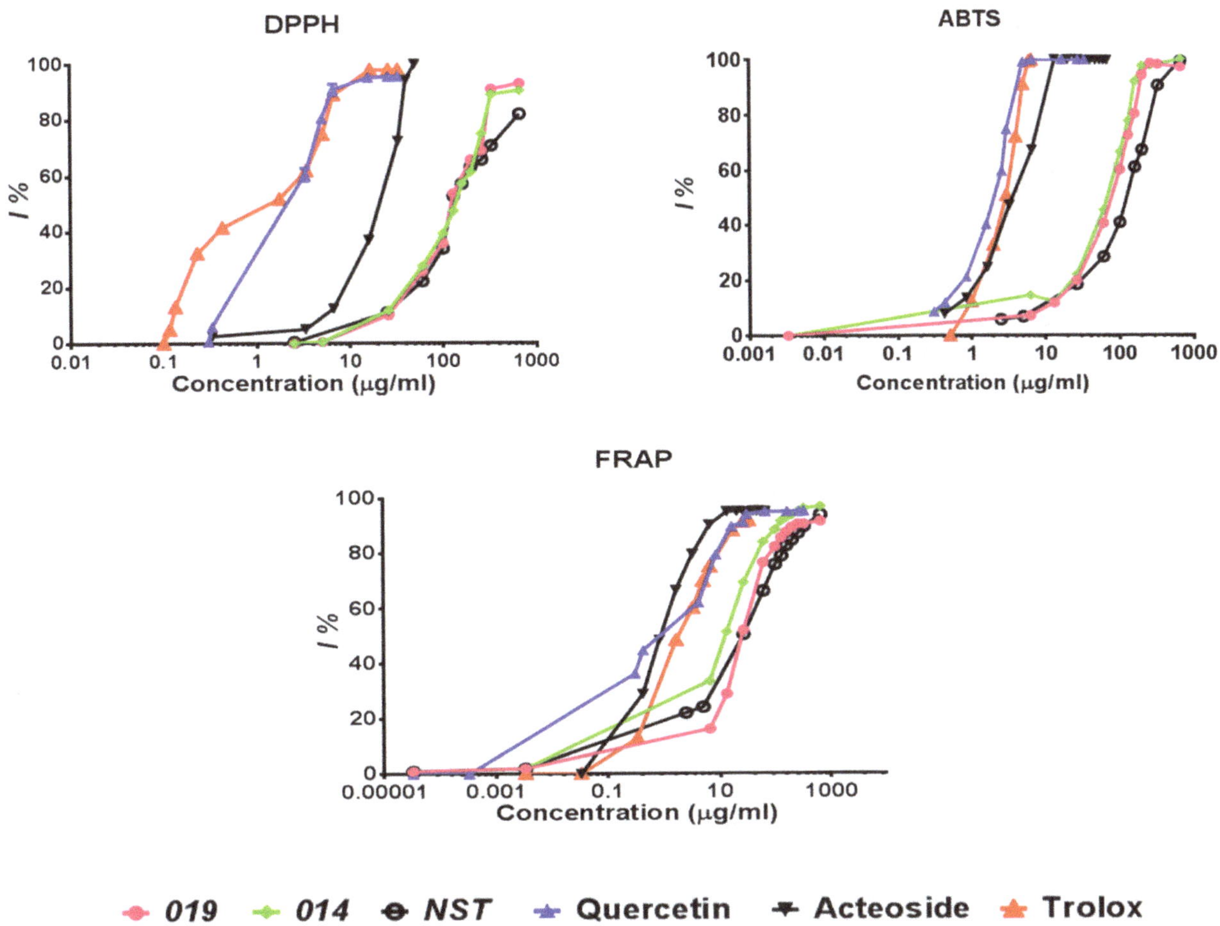

Figure 4. Antioxidant activity of spagyric tinctures 019 and 014, the NST, quercetin, acteoside, and Trolox as a positive control, as determined by DPPH, ABTS, and FRAP methods.

Values of their IC50 (concentration that gives half-maximal response), expressed as mEq of Trolox, are reported in Table 3. Both the 019 and 014 samples showed similar IC50 values of free radical scavenging activity in DPPH and ABTS, amounting to 92.53 ± 0.31 (019) and 93.33 ± 0.25 (014) mEq Trolox and 22.89 ± 0.19 (019) and 19.49 ± 0.13 (014) mEq Trolox, respectively. In contrast to the above, the expired 014 tincture showed a lower IC50 value compared to the 019 tincture in the FRAP method, indicating a higher ferric-reducing antioxidant ability. IC50 values obtained for the NST (Table 3) in the three assays (DPPH, ABTS, and FRAP) were very close to those detected for 019 and even slightly lower, indicating slightly higher antioxidant activity.

Table 3. Antioxidant activity (IC50) of the spagyric tinctures 019 and 014 and the NST of *H. procumbens*.

Sample	IC50 (mEq Trolox) ± SD		
	DPPH	ABTS	FRAP
019	92.53 ± 0.31	22.89 ± 0.19	14.11 ± 0.08
014	93.33 ± 0.25	19.49 ± 0.13	6.69 ± 0.07
NST	83.02 ± 0.28	17.78 ± 0.12	11.32 ± 0.08
Acteoside	13.83 ± 0.09	0.96 ± 0.05	0.44 ± 0.04
Quercetin	1.38 ± 0.01	0.60 ± 0.07	0.38 ± 0.02

The IC50 values of quercetin and acteoside were much lower than those of 019 and 014, indicating the better antioxidant capacity of these two pure reference compounds. Moreover, the IC50 values of quercetin and acteoside, as assessed by the ABTS and FRAP methods, were very similar, while quercetin displayed a more powerful capacity for DPPH reduction than acteoside did (Table 3).

The DPPH assay was also applied to harpagoside, the major iridoid present in the two samples: The IC50 result was higher than 330 ± 0.05 μg/mL, and therefore its antioxidant potency was not tested with the other methods, ABTS and FRAP.

3. Discussion

To the best of our knowledge, this is the first report on the phytochemical and biological characterization of spagyric preparations. In this study, we compared the compositional profile of two commercial food supplements (declared to be spagyric tinctures (019 and 014) and provided by the same producer company) with the aim of assessing the quality of the preparations in terms of chemical fingerprinting and biological activity. One of the two spagyric tinctures (014) was already expired according to the recommendation published on the label of the product, and therefore evaluation of the antioxidant activity (using three different methods) was important to display a correlation with the chemical profile and eventually with the aging of the preparation.

The major phytochemicals that have been detected in root extracts from *H. procumbens* include iridoids and phenolic glycosides [13,14,25]. Harpagoside, harpagide, and procumbide are regarded as the most representative iridoid glycosides isolated from the drug, along with the two phenylpropanoid glycosides acteoside and isoacteoside. Several other compounds have been isolated over time in different investigations [13,14,26], such as conjugated esters of iridoid glycosides (8-*O*-*p*-coumaroyl-harpagide, 6′-*O*-*p*-coumaroyl-procumbide, 8-*O*-feruloyl-harpagide, 8-cinnamoylmyoporoside).

As shown in Figure 2, the adopted HPLC analytical method provided a good separation of the phytochemical constituents of the commercial spagyric tinctures. In addition, the method fulfilled all of the validation criteria, showing good linearity of the calibration curve and good limit of detection (LoD) and limit of quantification (LoQ) values, including precision parameters, therefore showing validated repeatability and reproducibility. Compositional requirements in terms of specific chemical markers were also fulfilled in that the two spagyric tinctures, analyzed through TLC, HPLC, UV, and MS methods, displayed the expected phytochemical profile, with harpagoside as the main component along with harpagide, acteoside, and isoacteoside (Table 1).

In addition, the validation of the compositional requirements of both spagyric samples was also confirmed by the analysis of the NST sample, which showed a similar chemical profile, with harpagoside as the most abundant component, followed by acteoside and isoacteoside. Interestingly, the content of harpagide in the NST tincture was comparable (19.53 ± 0.17 μg/mg ext vs 15.98 ± 0.23 μg/mg ext) to that of 019, the tincture that was still not expired.

Spagyric preparations are not conventional herb preparations, but they are based on old alchemic procedures dating back to Paracelsus, who first developed this methodology and described it in his medical treatise *Opus Paramirum*. Our results indicated that the spagyric method allowed us to obtain preparations of good quality based on the presence of marker compounds.

In addition, considering that the two products differed by at least five years in their expiration date and presumably in their production date, fingerprinting analysis and the quantitative determination of the representative constituents in the expired spagyric preparation 014 allowed us to prove a general significant long-term stability of *H. procumbens* active metabolites. A significant decrease of harpagide content was, however, observed in the expired 014 tincture compared to 019 (Table 2).

Preparations based on devil's claw are mainly used to relieve pain and inflammation due to arthritis and other painful disorders, although the mechanism of action has not yet been fully elucidated. It is known that the generation of oxygen-free radicals is involved in the development of inflammation. Radicals freed from phagocytes are implicated in the activation of nuclear factors, which in turn induces the synthesis of cytokines. Then, a synergic action of oxygen-free radicals and cytokines promotes the synthesis of inflammatory mediators. Maintenance of an adequate antioxidant status may thus help to attenuate the symptoms of inflammation.

There are some indications that the antioxidant properties of some of the specialized metabolites also contribute to the anti-inflammatory effects of pharmaceutical preparations based on *H. procumbens* [14,15,25,27]. However, the antioxidant activity of devil's claw has not been extensively investigated, and there have been no previous investigations on the antioxidant bioactivity of spagyric preparations. Previous studies have only reported moderate antioxidant activity in methanolic root extracts of *H. procumbens*, while an aqueous extract containing 2.6% harpagoside was shown to have a good capacity to scavenge DPPH. In addition, intraperitoneal administration of a 53% ethanolic extract of devil's claw to male Wistar rats indicated antioxidant effects similar to those induced by selegiline [4,14,28].

Based on this, we evaluated the antioxidant potency of the two spagyric tinctures to eventually detect any variation in their bioactivity due to the aging of the product and possible degradation of the bioactive phytochemicals. A comparison of the chemicals in and the bioactivity of these two tinctures was also made with a commercial NST.

As for the chemical analysis, significant stability in bioactivity over the long term was also demonstrated by the almost identical antioxidant activity (as determined by the DPPH and ABTS methods (Figure 4)) and the relative IC50 values (Table 3) calculated for the two spagyric preparations, 019 and 014.

An unexpected exception was represented by the lower IC50 value (Table 3) calculated for the expired 014 tincture compared to the 019 tincture in the FRAP method, indicating a higher ferric-reducing antioxidant ability. Reasonably, this might have been due to some species (likely formed upon the aging of the product and not detectable in the used analytical conditions) that were present in the 014 sample and able to efficiently react with the ferric tripyridyltriazine complex.

For instance, it has been reported that the deglycosylation of harpagide gives a degradation product called H-harpagide (2-(formylmethyl)-2,3,5-trihydroxy-5-methylcyclopentane carbaldehyde) that is able to induce the inhibition of the COX-2 enzyme in vitro, in contrast to the parent molecule, which is instead completely inactive [29]. Due to its structure, this molecular species might also undergo oxidation and possibly be more powerful as a ferric-reducing agent. We can suggest that if such a reaction happened upon the aging of the 014 product, it could account for the lower IC50 observed with the FRAP method and the lower amount of harpagide detected in this sample.

Further support for this hypothesis might come from the observation that in the NST tincture, harpagide was present almost in the same amount as in 019 (19.53 ± 0.17 μg/mg ext vs 15.98 ± 0.23 μg/mg ext), and the IC50 values for the antioxidant activity of this sample were very similar to those obtained for the 019 tincture in the three bioassays, including the FRAP test. A deeper investigation should, however, be carried out to clarify this point.

As already reported [13,14,16,30], we also found that acteoside was a powerful antioxidant, while harpagoside did not display antioxidant capacity. Thus, acteoside might reasonably have a role in the antioxidant activity displayed by the two spagyric extracts.

In this study, an evaluation of the antioxidant activity (using three different methods) of the two spagyric tinctures aimed to show a correlation between the chemical profile and eventually the aging of the products. Thus, based on the obtained results, the two analyzed preparations should both be considered to have good biological activity, even when compared to an NST.

4. Materials and Methods

4.1. Solvents and Reagents

All solvents (HPLC grade and analytical grade) were obtained from Sigma/Aldrich, Italy. Phosphomolybdic acid spray reagent and anisaldehyde for TLC visualization were purchased from Sigma/Aldrich, Italy. Reagents used for the antioxidant bioassays, including DPPH (2,2′-di-phenyl-1-picrylhydrazyl), TPTZ (2,4,6-tripyridyl-*s*-triazine), Trolox (6-hydroxy-2,5,7,8-tetramethylchroman-2-ca rboxylic acid), and ABTS (2,2′-azino-bis (3-ethylbenzothiazoline-6-sulfonic acid) were all purchased from Sigma/Aldrich, Italy.

4.2. Samples

Two commercial samples of food supplements (kindly provided by Erbenobili, Italy) consisting of spagyric tinctures (40% ethanol) of *H. procumbens* roots were used in this study. The two samples differed in their shelf-life date: 2014 and 2019, respectively. That is, one of the two samples, conventionally named 014, was already expired when analyzed, while the other one, named 019, was still valid. For comparison purposes, a commercial NST (40% ethanol) was also analyzed.

4.3. Thin Layer Chromatography (TLC)

The composition of devil's claw extracts 019 and 014 was first investigated by TLC (precoated silica gel 60 F254 aluminum plates, Merck, Milan, Italy) eluted with $EtOAc/HCOOH/CH_3CO_2H/H_2O$ (100:11:11:26 *v/v*) or with $CHCl_3$/MeOH (90:10 *v/v*). Visualization of the components was obtained with phosphomolybdic acid reagent (10% EtOH) or alternatively with anisaldehyde-sulphuric acid reagent (0.5 mL anisaldehyde in 10 mL glacial acetic acid, 85 mL of MeOH in 5 mL of H_2SO_4) (AS). After spraying, TLC plates were heated at 110 °C for 5–10 min and observed under visible 254-nm or UV 366-nm light. For TLC and further analyses, the two spagyric tinctures 019 and 014 and the reference NST were died under vacuum and redissolved in 80% MeOH to obtain a 60-mg/mL solution.

4.4. Harpagoside Isolation

Harpagoside purification from the two tinctures 019 and 014 was achieved by solid-phase extraction (SPE) on Waters Sep-Pak Vac 1 cc C18 cartridges by using an SPE Extraction Manifold-20 position (Waters, Italy). Cartridges were first conditioned with 5 mL of MeOH and with 10 mL of H_2O in that order. Then, 1 mL from each of the two samples 019 and 014 was dried under vacuum, redissolved in 80% MeOH, and loaded onto the SPE cartridge. Harpagoside elution was obtained by flushing the cartridge with H_2O (5 × 1 mL), followed by subsequent elutions with MeOHaq 10% (5 × 1 mL), MeOHaq 50% (5 × 1 mL), and finally MeOHaq 70% (5 × 1 mL). All of the fractions were analyzed by TLC and HPLC. Pure harpagoside was obtained in fractions eluted with MeOHaq 70%.

4.5. HPLC-DAD-ELSD

HPLC-DAD-ELSD analyses were performed with a Waters HPLC 600 Liquid Chromatograph equipped with a diode array detector, DAD 2998 Waters, and an evaporative light scattering detector, ELSD 2424 Waters. Data were processed with EmpowerTM 2 Waters Software (Waters S.p:A, Sesto San Giovanni, Milan, Italy). Nitrogen was used as the driving gas for nebulization at 60 psi. Helium was used as the degassing solvent. Extracts were separated with a Gemini C18 (Phenomenex) column (250 × 4.60 mm, 5-µm particle size) equipped with a Security Guard C18 Cartridge (4 × 3 mm, Phenomenex). The following elution system was used with DAD detection: Solvent A, H_2O; solvent B, CH_3CN. The elution gradient was 5% B in A increasing to reach 25% B at 20 min and 40% B at 40 min. UV spectra of each extract were conventionally recorded at 210, 270, 310, and 350 nm. The presence of harpagide in the two samples was monitored by acquiring the HPLC-DAD trace at 210 nm. Alternatively, the presence of harpagide was detected by ELSD at the following parameters: Drift tube temperature, 55 °C; gain, 1000. Nitrogen was used as the driving gas for nebulization at 60 psi. Helium was used as the degassing solvent. Reference harpagoside and harpagide were analyzed in the same analytical conditions. All of the HPLC analyses were run in triplicate.

4.6. Validation

The quantification of iridoid components in the tinctures under investigation was made by HPLC-DAD against a calibration curve obtained with harpagoside (Phytolab) at six different concentrations in the linear range of 1000–31 μg/mL in MeOHaq 80%. The correlation coefficient (r^2) of the standard curve in the linear plot was $r^2 = 0.9999$ ($y = 4E + 07x + 391{,}135$), indicating good linearity between peak areas and concentrations within the used concentration range. The quantitation of harpagide was made by HPLC-ELSD against a calibration curve obtained with harpagide at six different concentrations in the linear range of 2000–62.5 μg/mL. The correlation coefficient (r^2) of the standard curve in the linear plot of log-transformed data was $r^2 = 0.9992$ ($y = 1.7569x - 1.7101$), indicating good linearity between the log-transformed areas and log-transformed concentrations within the tested concentration range.

The limit of detection (LoD) and limit of quantification (LoQ) were calculated according to conventional guidelines [31,32] on the basis of signal-to-noise ratios (S/Ns) of 3:1 and 10:1, respectively, by injecting a series of dilute solutions of known concentrations of harpagoside in the range of 31–0.061 μg/mL. The LoD for harpagoside in the adopted analytical conditions was 0.061 μg/mL, while the LoQ was 0.210 μg/mL.

The precision of the analytical HPLC method was assessed by calculating intraday repeatability and interday intermediate precision [33]. Multiple injections of harpagoside solutions (0.03125 μg/mL) were performed within the same day for intraday precision, while for interday precision, analyses were run in triplicate over three consecutive days. Precision was expressed as the percent relative standard deviation (RSD%) of retention times and peak areas resulting from the analysis of the spagyric tinctures. The intraday and interday variabilities of harpagoside in the two spagyric tinctures 019 and 014 were also calculated with the same procedure. Intraday precision of the chromatographic method for harpagoside was observed in the range of 0.25–0.59% for retention times and between 0.87% and 0.90% for peak areas. Interday RSD values were 0.28% and 0.95% for retention times and peak areas, respectively. The intraday RSD values of retention times and peak areas for the 6 major analytes in the spagyric tinctures were in the range of 0.10–1.10% and 0.50–3.00%, respectively. Percent RSD values of retention times and peak areas for interday evaluation were in the range of 0.21–3.47% and 0.17–3.55%, respectively. Overall, the results obtained indicated that the method applied for the compositional analysis was precise and accurate.

4.7. LC-ESI-MS/MS

Flow injection LC-ESI-MS/MS analyses were performed on a 1100 Series Agilent LC/MSD Trap-System VL (Agilent Technologies Italia SpA, Cernusco sul Naviglio, Milan, Italy). The chromatographic conditions were as described above for the HPLC-DAD analyses. An Agilent Chemstation (LC/MSD TrapSoftware 4.1, (Agilent Technologies Italia SpA, Cernusco sul Naviglio, Milan, Italy) was used for the acquisition and processing of the data. The mass spectrometer operated in the positive and negative ion mode under the following settings: Capillary voltage, 47 V; nebulizer gas (N_2), 5 psi; drying gas (N_2), heated at 220 °C and introduced at a flow rate of 10 μL/mL. Data were acquired in the MS scanning mode over the range of 150–1500 *m*/*z* with a scan time of 13000 *m*/*z*/s. Automated MS/MS was performed by isolating the base peaks (pseudomolecular ions) using an isolation width of 4.0 *m*/*z*, a fragmentation amplitude of 1.0 V, the threshold set at 100, and the ion charge control on, with the maximum acquire time set at 300 ms. Samples were dissolved in MeOHaq 80% and injected at a flow rate of 0.2 mL/min.

4.8. Antioxidant Activity

Antioxidant activity of the three tinctures of *H. procumbens* (019, 014, and NST) was determined by different methods: DPPH, ferric-reducing antioxidant power (FRAP) assay, and Trolox/ABTS equivalent antioxidant capacity [34–36]. For comparative purposes, the antioxidant activity of quercetin (Sigma/Aldrich, Italy), harpagoside (Phytolab, Germany), and acteoside (Sigma-Aldrich S.r.l., Milan, Italy) were also determined with the same procedures. Determinations were carried out in triplicate.

4.9. DPPH

The scavenging activity for DPPH (Sigma, Milan, Italy) free radicals was measured according to Brand–Williams (1995), with some modifications. To 2.9 mL of a 10×10^{-5}-M solution of DPPH in MeOH, 0.1 mL of a properly diluted MeOH sample test solution was added and vortexed, that is, different dilutions of each test sample (019, 014) were prepared to determine the actual IC50 values. After 30 min of incubation in the dark at room temperature, the UV absorbance (Perkin-Elmer Lambda Bio 20 Spectrophotometer) of each sample was recorded at 515 nm against the blank (reagent solution without the test sample). All determinations were carried out in triplicate. The inhibition percentage (I%) of DPPH radicals in the test samples was calculated with the following equation: $I\% = [(A_{blank} - A_{sample})/A_{blank}] \times 100$, where A_{blank} is the absorbance of the blank solution at $t = 0$, and A_{sample} is the absorbance of the test sample at $t = 30$ min. The IC50 concentration is the amount of drug necessary to give 50% inhibition of the DPPH radicals. Acteoside, quercetin, and harpagoside were used as reference compounds.

4.10. FRAP

The following stock solutions were prepared for the bioassay according to Benzie and Strain (1996): a) a 300-mM acetate buffer solution, pH 3.6; b) a 10-mM TPTZ (2,4,6-tripyridyl-s-triazine) solution in MeOH; and c) a 20-mM $FeCl_3 \cdot 6\,H_2O$ solution. The FRAP working solution was prepared by mixing TPTZ and $FeCl_3 \cdot 6\,H_2O$ and acetate buffer in a ratio of 1:1:10. Test samples and reference compounds (100 μL) were added to 2.6 mL of FRAP reagent, along with 300 μL of H_2O, and allowed to react for 30 min at 37 °C in dark conditions. Absorbance readings (ferrous tripyridyltriazine complex) were taken at 595 nm. A blank solution consisted of FRAP solutions above and in water. The standard curve was ($r^2 = 0.9992$; $y = 0.0005x + 0.0005$) using a concentration range of $FeSO_4$ between 0.42 μg/mL and 20 μg/mL.

4.11. Trolox/ABTS

Radical scavenging capacity was also studied based on the reduction of ABTS+· radicals by the test samples. An ABTS+· radical cation was obtained by mixing an ABTS stock solution (7 mM in H_2O) with 2.5 mM of potassium persulfate, $K_2S_2O_8$. This solution was allowed to stand at room temperature in the dark for 12–16 h before use. For the analyses, the ABTS+· solution was diluted with water to an absorbance of 0.7 (±0.02) at 734 nm. For the UV determinations, 2.9 mL of the ABTS+· solution and 100 μL of each of the test samples were mixed, and an absorbance reading was taken at 734 nm, 2–6 min after mixing. Appropriate ABTS blanks were run in each assay. All solutions were freshly prepared for the daily experiments. The scavenging activity of each test sample was compared to that of Trolox (6-hydroxy-2,5,7,8-tetramethylchroman-2-carboxylic acid) as the positive control. A linear calibration curve ($r^2 = 0.9970$; $y = 0.0005x + 0.0005$) was constructed using Trolox in a range from 4 μM to 26 μM.

4.12. Statistical Analysis

The quantitative results for each analysis and bioassay were expressed as the mean ± standard deviation (SD) of at least three replicates for each experiment. Microsoft Office Excel 2017 was used for processing the data.

Author Contributions: P.A. conceived of and designed the experiments; M.P.A. performed the experiments; P.A. and M.P.A. analyzed the data; P.A. wrote the paper.

Acknowledgments: The authors thank Erbenobili s.r.l. for supplying the spagyric tinctures.

References

1. Stewart, K.M.; Cole, D. The commercial harvest of devil's claw (*Harpagophytum* spp.) in southern Africa: The devil's in the details. *J. Ethnopharmacol.* **2005**, *100*, 225–236. [CrossRef] [PubMed]
2. van Wyk, B.-E. A broad review of commercially important southern African medicinal plants. *J. Ethnopharmacol.* **2008**, *119*, 342–355. [CrossRef] [PubMed]
3. Wegener, T.; Lüpke, N.-P. Treatment of patients with artrosis of hip and knee with an aqueous extract of devil's claw (*Harpagophytum procumbens* D.C.). *Phytother. Res.* **2003**, *17*, 1165–1172. [CrossRef] [PubMed]
4. *European Union Herbal Monograph on Harpagophytum Procumbens DC. and/or Harpagophytum zeyheri Decne., Radix*; EMA/HMPC/627057/2015; European Medicines Agency: Amsterdam, The Netherlands, 2016; pp. 2–8.
5. *Devil's Claw Root-Harpagophytum Procumbens DC. and/or Harpagophytum zeyheri Decne., radix*; EMA/571858/2016; European Medicines Agency: Amsterdam, The Netherlands, 2016; pp. 1–2.
6. Moritz, S. Alchemy and contemporary spagyric medicine: A historical and socio-scientific approach. *Interdiscip. Sci. Rev.* **2016**, *41*, 13–27. [CrossRef]
7. Li, S.; Han, Q.; Qiao, C.; Song, J.; Cheng, C.L.; Xu, H. Chemical markers for the quality control of herbal medicines: An overview. *Chinese Med.* **2008**, 1–16. [CrossRef]
8. Zhang, Y.; Sun, S.; Dai, J.; Wang, W.; Cao, H.; Wu, J.; Gou, X. Quality control method for herbal medicine–Chemical fingerprinting analysis. In *Quality Control of Herbal Medicines and Related Areas*; Shoyama, Y., Ed.; InTech: Rijeka, Croatia, 2011; pp. 171–194. [CrossRef]
9. Donno, D.; Boggia, R.; Zunin, P.; Cerutti, A.K.; Guido, M.; Mellano, M.G.; Prgomet, Z.; Beccaro, G.L. Phytochemical fingerprinting and chemometrics for natural food preparation pattern recognition: An innovative technique in food supplement quality control. *J. Food Sci. Technol.* **2016**, *53*, 1071–1083. [CrossRef]
10. Xie, P.; Chen, S.; Liang, Y.; Wang, X.; Tian, R.; Upton, R. Chromatographic fingerprint analysis—A rational approach for quality assessment of traditional Chinese herbal medicine. *J. Chromatog. A* **2006**, *1112*, 171–180. [CrossRef]
11. *Reflection Paper on Markers Used for Quantitative and Qualitative Analysis of Herbal Medicinal Products and Traditional Herbal Medicinal Products*; EMEA/HMPC/253629/2007; European Medicines Agency: Amsterdam, The Netherlands, 2008; pp. 1–6.
12. *Guideline on Quality of Herbal Medicinal Products/Traditional Herbal Medicinal Products. Final*; European Medicines Agency: Amsterdam, The Netherlands, 2011; pp. 1–13.
13. Boje, K.; Lechtenberg, M.; Nahrstedt, A. New and known iridoid- and phenylethanoid glycosides from *Harpagophytum procumbens* and their in vitro inhibition of human leukocyte elastase. *Planta Med.* **2003**, *69*, 820–825.
14. Mncwangi, N.; Chen, W.; Vermaak, I.; Viljoen, A.M.; Gericke, N. Devil's claw–A review of the ethnobotany, phytochemistry and biological activity of *Harpagophytum procumbens*. *J. Ethnopharmacol.* **2012**, *143*, 755–771. [CrossRef]
15. Viljioen, A.; Mncwangi, N.; Vermaak, I. Anti-inflammatory iridoids of botanical origin. *Curr. Med. Chem.* **2012**, *19*, 2104–2127. [CrossRef]
16. Ahmed, B.; Al-Rehaily, A.J.; Al-Howiriny, T.A.; El-Sayed, K.A.; Ahmad, M.S. Scropoloside D_2 and harpagoside–B: Two new iridoid glycosides from *Scrophularia deserti* and their antidiabetic and anti-inflammatory activity. *Biol. Pharm. Bull.* **2003**, *26*, 462–467. [CrossRef] [PubMed]
17. Schaffer, L.F.; Peroza, L.R.; Boligon, A.A.; Althayde, M.L.; Alves, S.H.; Faschinetto, R.; Wagner, C. *Harpagophytum procumbens* prevents oxidative stress and loss of cell viability in vitro. *Neurochem. Res.* **2013**, *38*, 2256–2267. [CrossRef] [PubMed]
18. European Pharmacopoeia (Ph. Eur.) 9th Edition. Available online: https://www.edqm.eu/en/european-pharmacopoeia-ph-eur-9th-edition (accessed on 26 February 2019).
19. Li, L.; Tsao, R.; Liu, Z.; Liu, S.; Yang, R.; Young, J.C.; Zhu, H.; Deng, Z.; Xie, M.; Fu, Z. Isolation and purification of acteoside and isoacteoside from *Plantago psyllium* L. by high-speed counter-current chromatography. *J. Chromatogr. A* **2005**, *1063*, 161–169. [CrossRef] [PubMed]
20. Nguyen, A.-T.; Fontaine, J.; Malonne, H.; Clayes, M.; Luhmer, M.; Duez, P. A sugar ester and an iridoid glycoside from *Scrophularia ningpoensis*. *Phytochemistry* **2005**, *66*, 1186–1191. [CrossRef] [PubMed]

21. Clarkson, C.; Staerk, D.; Hansen, S.H.; Smith, P.J.; Jaroszewski, J.W. Identification of major and minor constituents of *Harpagophytum procumbens* (Devil's claw) using HPLC-SPE-NMR and HPLC-ESIMS/APCIMS. *J. Nat. Prod.* **2006**, *69*, 1280–1288. [CrossRef] [PubMed]
22. Wu, Q.; Yuan, Q.; Liu, E.-H.; Qi, L.-W.; Bi, Z.-M.; Li, P. Fragmentation study of iridoid glycosides and phenylpropanoid glycosides in *Radix scrophulariae* by rapid-resolution liquid chromatography with diode-array detection and electrospray ionization time-of-flight mass spectrometry. *Biomed. Chromatogr.* **2010**, *24*, 808–819. [CrossRef] [PubMed]
23. Karioti, A.; Fani, E.; Vincieri, F.F.; Bilia, A.R. Analysis and stability of the constituents of *Curcuma longa* and *Harpagophytum procumbens* tinctures by HPLC-DAD and HPLC-ESI.MS. *J. Pharm. Biomed. Anal.* **2011**, *55*, 479–486. [CrossRef] [PubMed]
24. Qi, J.; Chen, J.-J.; Cheng, Z.-H.; Zhou, J.-H.; Yu, B.-Y.; Qiu, S.X. Iridoid glycosides from *Harpagophytum procumbens* DC. (devil's claw). *Phytochemistry* **2006**, *67*, 1372–1377. [CrossRef] [PubMed]
25. Georgiev, M.I.; Ivanovska, N.; Alipieva, K.; Dimitrova, P.; Veerporte, R. Harpagoside: From Kalahari desert to pharmacy shelf. *Phytochemistry* **2013**, *92*, 8–15. [CrossRef]
26. Kikuchi, T.; Matsuda, S.; Kubo, Y.; Namba, T. New iridoids glucoisdes from *Harpagophytum procumbens* DC. *Chem. Pharm. Bull.* **1983**, *31*, 2296–2301. [CrossRef]
27. Schopohl, P.; Grüneberg, P.; Melzig, M.F. The influence of harpagoside and harpagide on TNFα-secretion and cell adhesion molecule mRNA-expression in IFNγ/LPS-stimulated THP-1 cells. *Fitoterapia* **2016**, *110*, 157–165. [CrossRef] [PubMed]
28. Barnes, J.; Anderson, L.A.; Phillipson, J.D. *Herbal Medicines*, 3rd ed.; Pharmaceutical Press: London, UK, 2007; pp. 207–214.
29. Zhang, L.; Fenbg, L.-F.; Jia, Q.; Xu, J.; Wang, R.; Wang, Z.; Wu, Y.; Li, Y. Effects of ß-glucisidase hydrolyzed products of harpagide and harpagoside on cyclooxygenase-2 (COX-2) in vitro. *Biorg. Med. Chem.* **2011**, *19*, 4882–4886. [CrossRef] [PubMed]
30. Arthur, H.; Joubert, E.; De Beer, D.; Malherbe, C.J.; Witthuhn, R.C. Phenylethanoid glycosides as major antioxidants in *Lippia multiflora* herbal infusion and their stability during steam pasteurization of plant material. *Food Chem.* **2011**, *127*, 581–588. [CrossRef] [PubMed]
31. Jenke, D.R. Chromatographic method validation: A review of current practices and procedures. II. Guidelines for primary validation parameters. *J. Liq. Chromatogr. Relat. Technol.* **1996**, *19*, 737–757. [CrossRef]
32. Vial, J.; Jardy, A. Experimental comparison of the different approaches to estimate LOD and LOQ for an HPLC method. *Anal. Chem.* **1999**, *71*, 2672–2677. [CrossRef]
33. Carbonara, T.; Pascale, R.; Argentieri, M.P.; Papadia, P.; Fanizzi, F.P.; Villanova, L.; Avato, P. Phytochemical analysis of a herbal tea from *Artemisia annua* L. *J. Pharm. Biomed. Anal.* **2012**, *62*, 79–86. [CrossRef] [PubMed]
34. Thaipong, K.; Boonprakob, U.; Crosby, K.; Cisneros-Zevallos, L.; Byrne, D.H. Comparison of ABTS, DPPH, FRAP and ORAC assays for estimating antioxidant activity from guava fruit extracts. *J. Food Compo. Anal.* **2006**, *19*, 669–6775. [CrossRef]
35. Brand-Williams, W.; Cuvelier, M.E.; Berset, C. Use of a free radical method to evaluate antioxidant activity. *Lebensm. Wiss. Technol.* **1995**, *28*, 25–30. [CrossRef]
36. Benzie, I.F.F.; Strain, J.J. The ferric reducing ability of plasma (FRAP) as a measure of "antioxidant power": The FRAP assay. *Anal. Biochem.* **1996**, *239*, 70–76. [CrossRef]

11

Flavonoids as Putative Epi-Modulators: Insight into their Binding Mode with BRD4 Bromodomains Using Molecular Docking and Dynamics

Fernando D. Prieto-Martínez * and José L. Medina-Franco *

Facultad de Química, Departamento de Farmacia, Universidad Nacional Autónoma de México, Avenida Universidad 3000, Mexico City 04510, Mexico

* Correspondence: fprieto@comunidad.unam.mx (F.D.P.-M.); medinajl@unam.com.mx (J.L.M.-F.);

Abstract: Flavonoids are widely recognized as natural polydrugs, given their anti-inflammatory, antioxidant, sedative, and antineoplastic activities. Recently, different studies showed that flavonoids have the potential to inhibit bromodomain and extraterminal (BET) bromodomains. Previous reports suggested that flavonoids bind between the Z and A loops of the bromodomain (ZA channel) due to their orientation and interactions with P86, V87, L92, L94, and N140. Herein, a comprehensive characterization of the binding modes of fisetin and the biflavonoid, amentoflavone, is discussed. To this end, both compounds were docked with BET bromodomain 4 (BRD4) using four docking programs. The results were post-processed with protein–ligand interaction fingerprints. To gain further insight into the binding mode of the two natural products, the docking results were further analyzed with molecular dynamics simulations. The results showed that amentoflavone makes numerous contacts in the ZA channel, as previously described for flavonoids and kinase inhibitors. It was also found that amentoflavone can potentially make contacts with non-canonical residues for BET inhibition. Most of these contacts were not observed with fisetin. Based on these results, amentoflavone was experimentally tested for BRD4 inhibition, showing activity in the micromolar range. This work may serve as the basis for scaffold optimization and the further characterization of flavonoids as BET inhibitors.

Keywords: docking; epigenetics; epi-informatics; molecular interactions; molecular dynamics; natural products; flavonoids

1. Introduction

Epigenetics has arisen as the missing link in the biogenesis of disease. Histone modifications have a significant effect on the fate of certain genes. Current research is primarily focused on the writing and erasing mechanisms of the epigenome. There are many examples of this in the literature [1], one of the most prominent being histone acetylation. Acetylation is regulated by two main systems: histone acetyl transferases (HATs) and histone deacetylases (HDACs) [2]. Histone deacetylases have been studied thoroughly by means of pharmacophore modeling [3], molecular docking [4], and molecular dynamics (MD) [5]. These efforts contributed to the identification and development of two FDA-approved HDAC inhibitors, the most notable being a natural product, romidepsin [6].

Readers are epi-enzymes whose function is to recognize certain modifications and their patterns on histones [7]. Therefore, reader enzymes are interesting molecular targets for a better understanding of epigenetics. Bromodomains are 120-residue proteins that were first discovered on the brahma (*brm*) gene of the *Drosophila* genus [8]. Later, it was confirmed as a common motif in most eukaryotic organisms. As of today, 62 isoforms were identified and are classified in eight families [9]. Family II, known as the bromodomain and extraterminal domain (BET), is extensively studied, as shown in Figure 1. This family includes bromodomain 2 (BRD2), BRD3, BRD4, and bromodomain testis-specific (BRDT) isoforms, each with their respective first and second domains (BD1 and BD2). Figure 2 shows the active site of bromodomains, which comprises three main hotspots: the WPF shelf, a region exclusive to BET bromodomains, a hydrophobic triad comprised by tryptophan, proline and phenylalanine (residues 80 to 83), and the ZA channel, located between the Z and A loops (residues 85 through 96), often seen as a frontier region with mixed contacts (mainly hydrophobic). The third hotspot is the Ac-binding pocket, responsible for reading histones and their ε-*N*-acetylated lysine residues (Kac). This hotspot is defined by a "tandem checkpoint" made by N140 and Y97 [10].

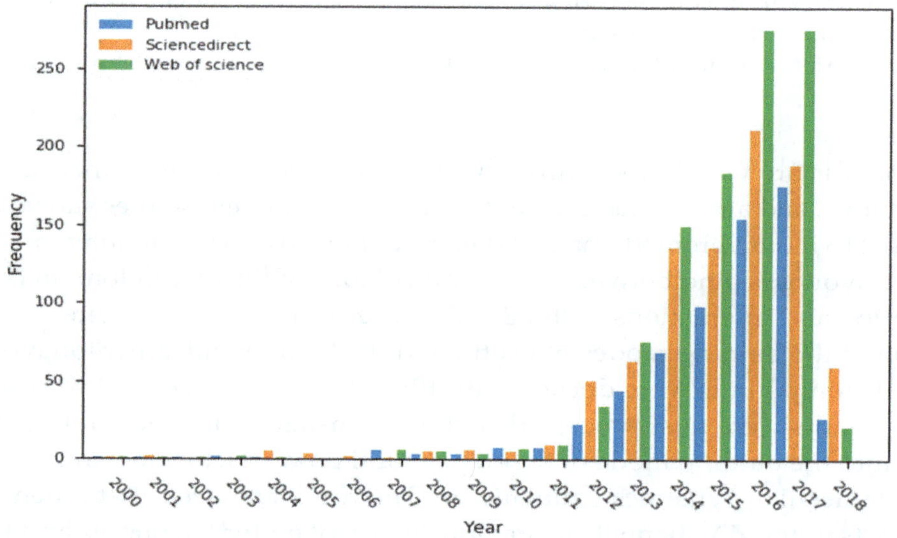

Figure 1. Frequency of the "bromodomain" keyword in three major search engines during the past 18 years.

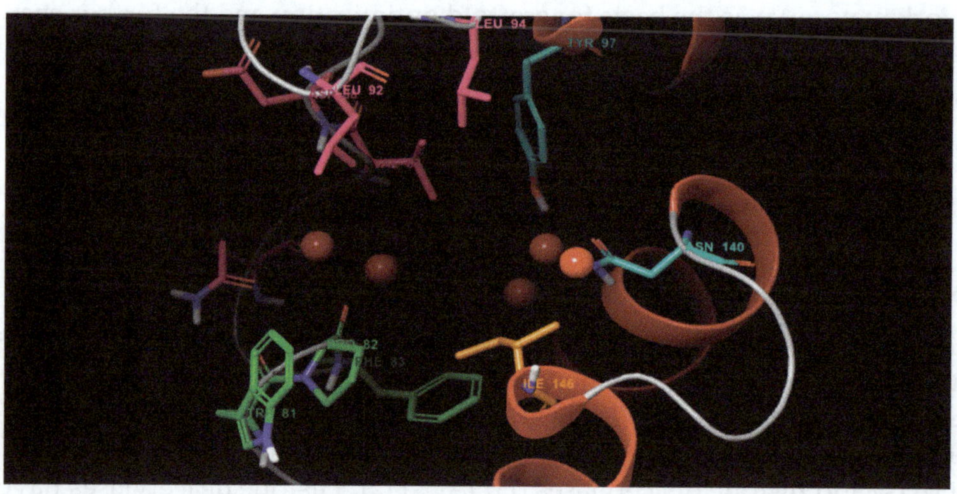

Figure 2. Binding pocket of bromodomain and extraterminal domain (BET) bromomains. The main structural features are the WPF shelf (green), ZA channel (pink), an Ac-pocket (cyan), and the gatekeeper (orange). Red spheres represent structural waters found with BET isoforms.

Additionally, evidence of structural water molecules was shown on a double bridge with ligands and Y97 [11]. Generally speaking, the role of water in binding is a dividing issue for drug design [12]. For example, structure-based design often ignores it or recognizes few instances of its importance [13]. Because of this, early approaches to ligand design followed a water-displacement strategy [14]. Nonetheless, a slow but steady paradigm shift came with increasing evidence of water-based stabilization in binding kinetics [15] and target selectivity [16]. One of the main problems in this approach is the increased difficulty of modeling of such phenomena, i.e., identifying "crucial waters" [17,18]. For bromodomains, recent studies showed that the network of structural waters in the ZA channel plays a significant role in binding [19,20] and this topic served as a case study for the development of novel methods in the field [21].

Bromodomain inhibition is currently at an impasse [22], as chemotypes are not diverse enough to make more robust models and approaches toward their pharmacology. Hence, current efforts are focused on the synthesis and identification of plausible and novel inhibitors [23]. As part of this effort, quinazolones were proposed as novel inhibitors of BETs. An interesting property of these ligands is their selectivity toward BD2 [24]. Later, it was found that some kinase inhibitors can bind to bromodomains [25], e.g., flavopiridol. Figure 3a illustrates the quintessential BRD inhibitors. These results led to the hypothesis of flavonoids as putative modulators of bromodomains; nonetheless, this possibility was only explored in recent studies [26].

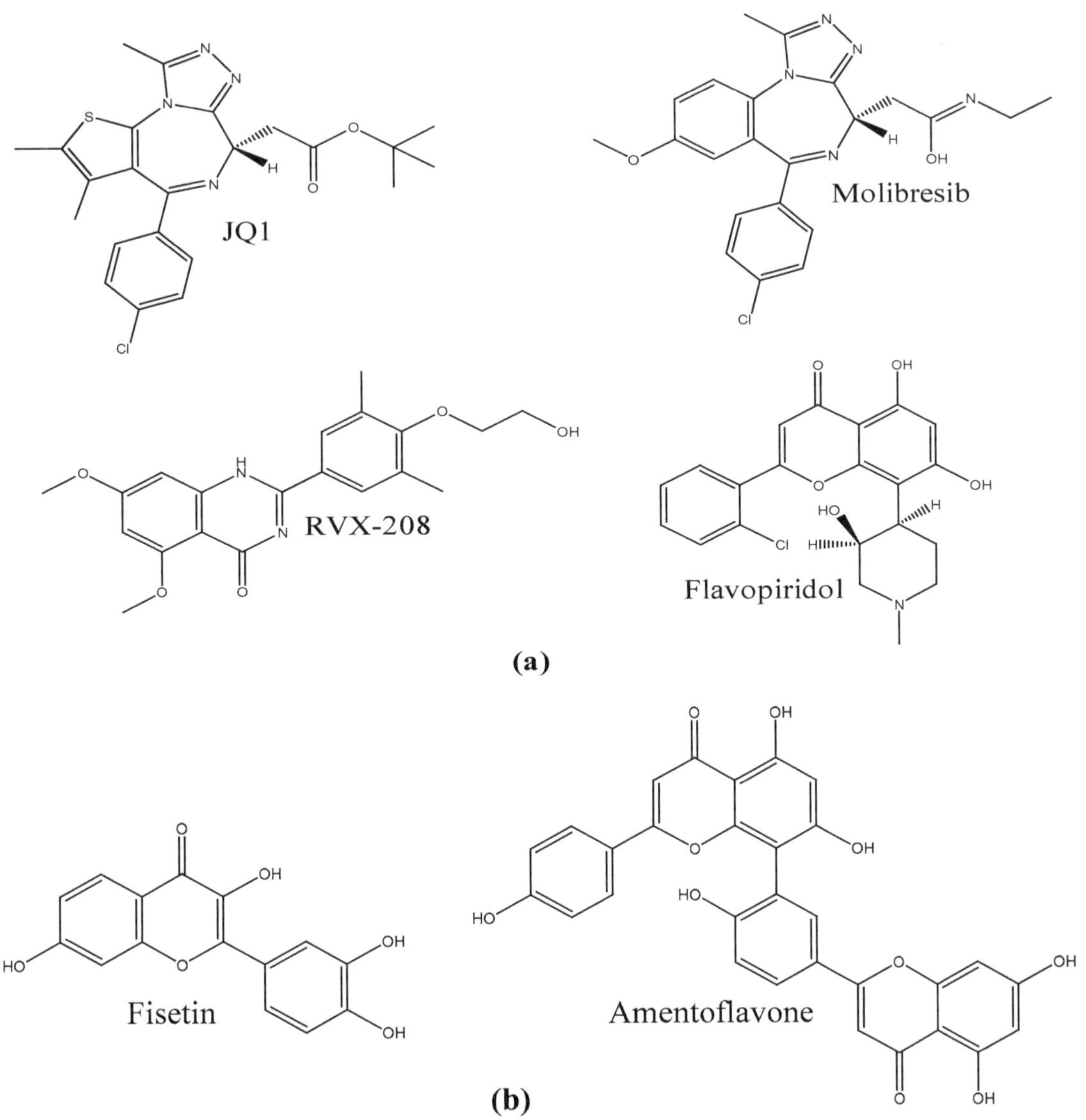

Figure 3. Chemical structures of (**a**) reference ligands for BET inhibition, and (**b**) flavonoids studied in this work.

Flavonoids are one of the most well-known natural products, often regarded as major scaffolds in medicinal chemistry [27]. Flavonoids showed antioxidant [28], anti-inflammatory [29], and sedative [30] effects in various studies. Moreover, flavonoid scaffolds present the outstanding potential of being chemoprotective agents toward cancer [31]. Consequently, flavonoids are often seen as quintessential nutraceuticals; e.g., the average intake of flavonoids in the United States is around 1 g/day [32]. Finally, it was suggested that flavonoids may interact significantly with the epigenome; however, as of today, this is limited to writing and eraser epi-enzymes [33].

Fisetin, shown in Figure 3b, is a dietary flavonoid found in a broad array of vegetables such as strawberry, apple, grape, onion, and cucumber [34], and is considered a health-promoting compound [35]. Studies showed that fisetin is capable of blocking cell proliferation on many cancer lines [36]. One of the most interesting aspects of its pharmacology is its capacity to modulate nuclear factor kappa B (NF-κB) [37]. Fisetin is capable of doing this through the mitogen-activated protein kinase (MAPK) pathway and tumor necrosis factor (TNF)-blocking, downregulating pro-inflammatory genes [38]. Of note, recent studies showed the role of BRD4 in the recruitment of NF-κβ [39]. Thus, bromodomains were also studied for their role in chronic diseases like diabetes [40] and psoriasis [41]. Amentoflavone (Figure 3b) is a biflavonoid produced from two apigenin units. It is commonly found in *Ginko biloba*, *Hypericum perforatum*, *Biophytum sensitivum*, and *Nandina domestica* [42]. Like fisetin, amentoflavone was also identified as an NF-κβ modulator [43], thus giving rise to its capacity to reduce inflammation.

Computational methods are valuable approaches to solving chemical problems. Molecular docking, for example, allows the simulation of protein–ligand binding. Despite its simplifications and limitations, docking yields significant results used for binding-mode predictions [44]. Molecular dynamics is gaining increasing attention with regards to the elucidation of ligand binding and protein behavior [45].

Since amentoflavone and fisetin were identified as putative ligands of BRD4 in two independent studies [46,47], a comprehensive characterization of the putative binding profile of both flavonoids with BRD4 is presented herein. The binding profile was carried out with consensus docking and molecular dynamics. Based on the computational results, amentoflavone was experimentally tested for activity as BRD4 inhibitor, showing activity in the micromolar range. These results further support the activity of flavonoids as putative epi-modulators.

2. Materials and Methods

2.1. Protein Preparation

An ensemble of 14 structures for the BET isoform, BRD4, was selected from the Protein Data Bank (PBD). Full details are presented in Table S1 of the Supplementary Materials. Selection criteria were based on their resolutions (<1.8 Å) and *R*-values (<0.25). Additional criteria were the structural similarity between the co-crystal ligand and the flavonoid scaffold, and the ability of the ligand to form hydrogen bonds with the binding pocket. All protein–ligand complexes were prepared with the Quickprep module of the MOE software [48]. Energy minimization was carried with the Amber 14: EHT force field (using Amber 14 forcefield [49] for protein parametrization and Extended Hückel Theory for ligands [50]). Complexes were visually inspected to ensure that key interactions were kept.

2.2. Molecular Docking

Docking was carried out using four programs: Autodock Vina [51], LeDock [52], MOE (v.2018.01), and PLANTS [53]. The rationale for selecting these programs was their performance and different scoring functions for consensus (vide infra). Protein inputs were kept from the preparation step and were validated with their respective native ligands. Details are provided in Table S2 of the Supplementary Materials. Amentoflavone and fisetin were parameterized with the Amber 14: EHT force field for the MOE software, and a charge reassignment was done with the LeDock, Vina, and PLANTS programs. The charge used for these programs was calculated with the MOPAC 2016 software [54] using PM6-D3H4X, as this correction was shown to enhance docking performance [55]. The docking poses were post-processed using protein–ligand interaction fingerprints (PLIF) as available in the MOE software. Docking poses were analyzed for clustering, based on the most common interactions found across the four programs.

2.3. Molecular Dynamics

Molecular dynamics simulations were carried out using Desmond [56] for both BRD4 (see Supplementary Materials, Figures S2, S3, and S6, and Table S12) and BRD4–ligand complexes. The complex used was the top ranked pose from the MOE software with consensus interactions. Complexes were then submitted to the System Builder utility in Maestro to assign a buffered 10 Å × 10 Å × 10 Å orthorhombic box using the transferable intermolecular potential with 3 points (TIP3P) water model and the OPLS_2005 force field. The system was neutralized, and a 0.15 M concentration of NaCl was added. Further details can be found in the Supplementary Materials, Figure S1. The production time for MD was set at 100 ns. The simulation was repeated three times. Electrostatics were computed using the Particle Mesh Ewald algorithm with a 9 Å cut-off, and constraints were enforced by the M-SHAKE algorithm [57]. Integration was done every 1.2 fs, with the recording interval set to 50 ps. The trajectories were then analyzed using the Simulation Interaction Diagram, Simulation Event Analysis, and Simulation Quality Analysis utilities in Maestro.

2.4. Experimental Testing of Amentoflavone

Amentoflavone was purchased from Sigma-Aldrich (St. Louis, MO, USA), and was tested for BRD4 tandem (BD1 + BD2) binding by means of AlphaScreen [58], using an H4 peptide (1–21) K5/8/12/16 Ac. Experimental work was performed by the Reaction Biology Corp., providing 2-mg samples to obtain duplicate dose-response curves beginning at a 100-μM concentration, following a three-fold dilution. The positive control for the test was the JQ-1 compound. The half maximal inhibitory concentration (IC_{50}) values were obtained from the curves, and the Hill slope for amentoflavone was calculated.

3. Results

3.1. Molecular Docking

Table 1 summarizes the docking scores for amentoflavone and fisetin as computed with the four docking programs (the raw docking scores for each protein used are reported in the Supplementary Materials, Tables S4–S11). Figure 4 shows the consensus PLIF found for both compounds.

Table 1. Summary statistics of docking scores for the programs used.

Molecule	Summary Stats *	Autodock VINA (kcal/mol)	LeDock (kcal/mol)	MOE (kcal/mol)	PLANTS
Amentoflavone	Min	−10.5	−7.9	−9.0	−102.1
	1Q	−9.5	−7.3	−7.9	−89.4
	Avg	−9.2	−7.0	−7.6	−86.9
	3Q	−9.0	−6.8	−7.2	−84.0
	Max	−8.2	−6.3	−6.4	−77.4
	SD	0.46	0.34	0.54	4.6
Fisetin	Min	−8.6	−6.0	−7.4	−79.6
	1Q	−8.2	−5.6	−6.5	−73.2
	Avg	−7.9	−5.4	−6.2	−71.0
	3Q	−7.7	−5.3	−6.0	−68.9
	Max	−7.1	−4.7	−5.6	−65.0
	SD	0.31	0.24	0.39	2.94

* Min: Minimum; 1Q: First quartile; Avg: Average; 3Q: Third quartile; Max: Maximum; and SD: Standard deviation values.

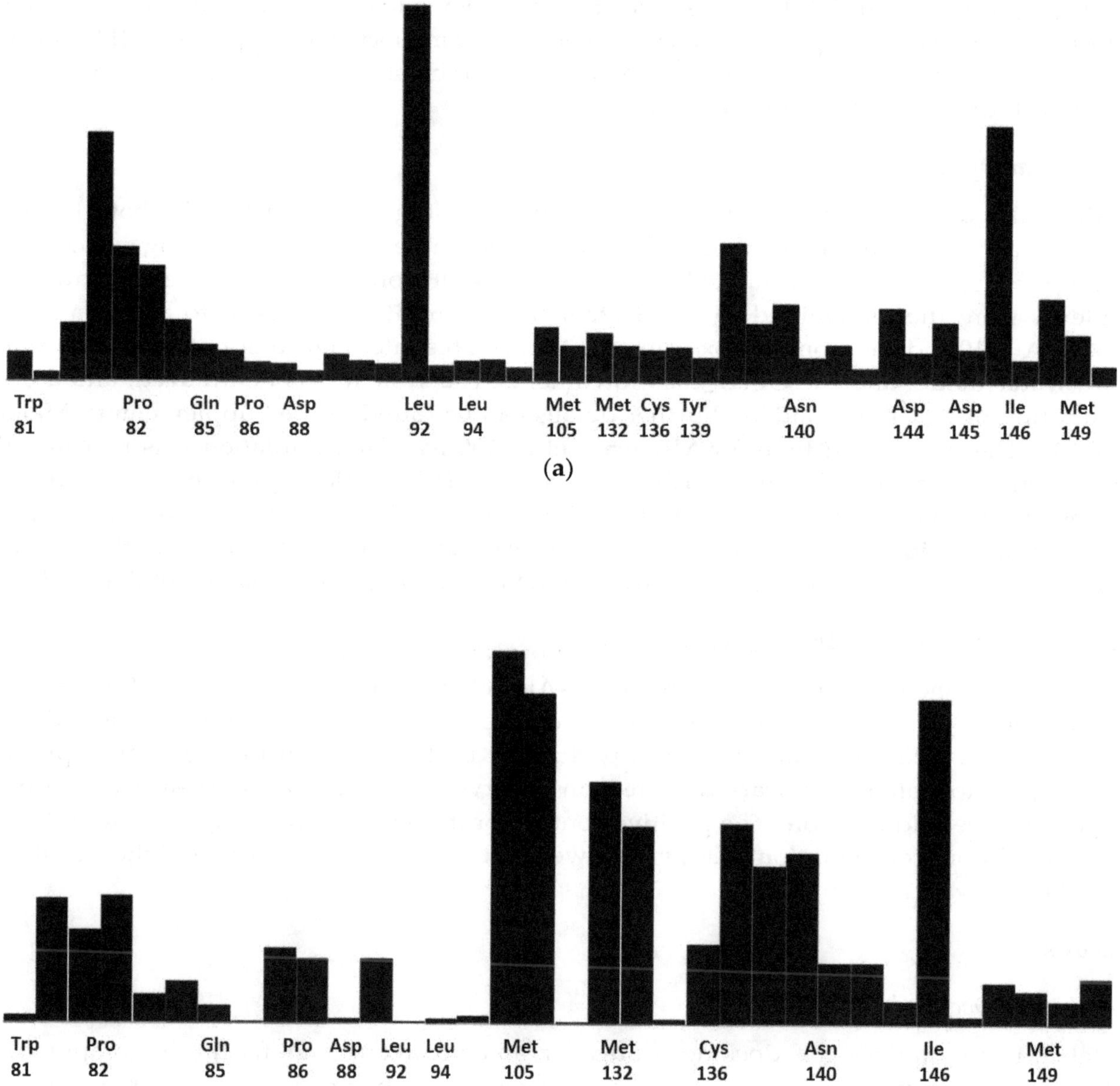

Figure 4. Consensus protein–ligand interaction fingerprint obtained from a consensus analysis of the docking with the Autodock Vina, LeDock, MOE, and PLANTS programs. (**a**) Amentoflavone; (**b**) Fisetin.

3.2. Molecular Dynamics

The overall quality of the MD simulations was measured with the corresponding utilities in Maestro. Energy, potential energy, temperature, pressure, and volume values were computed (results are shown in Figures S4 and S5, and Tables S13 and S14 in the Supplementary Materials). Once complex stability was assessed, the root-mean-square deviation (RMSD) values for backbone, Cα, side chains, and ligand were computed, as shown in Figure 5a,b. This measure shows the global deviation of atoms to a reference status (frame 0); usually, values below 5.0 Å can be considered as valid [59].

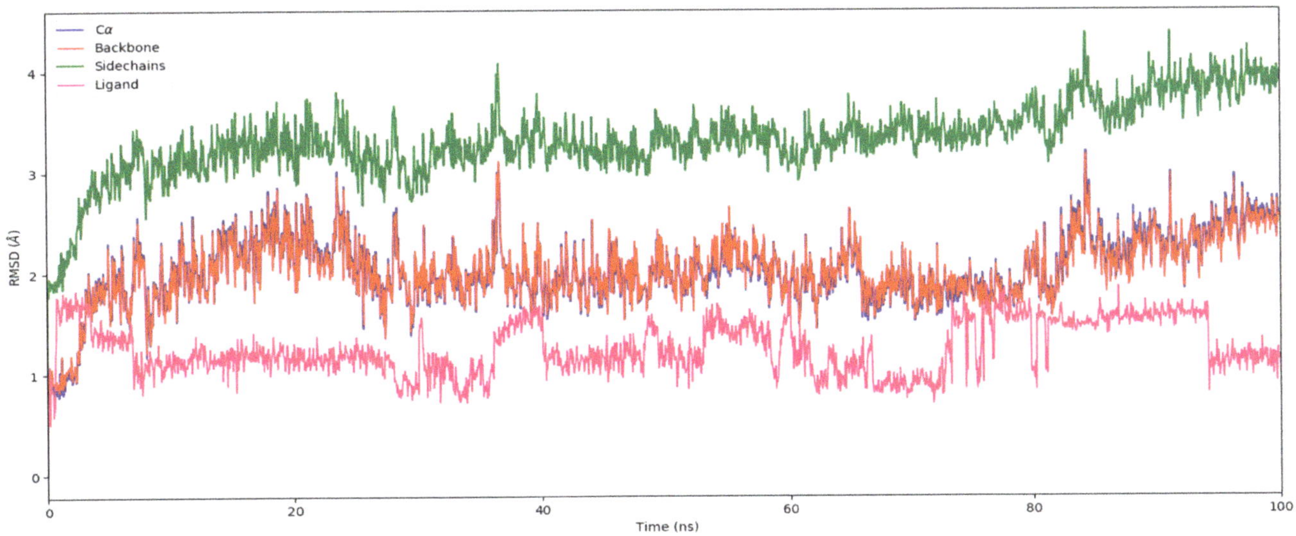

(a)

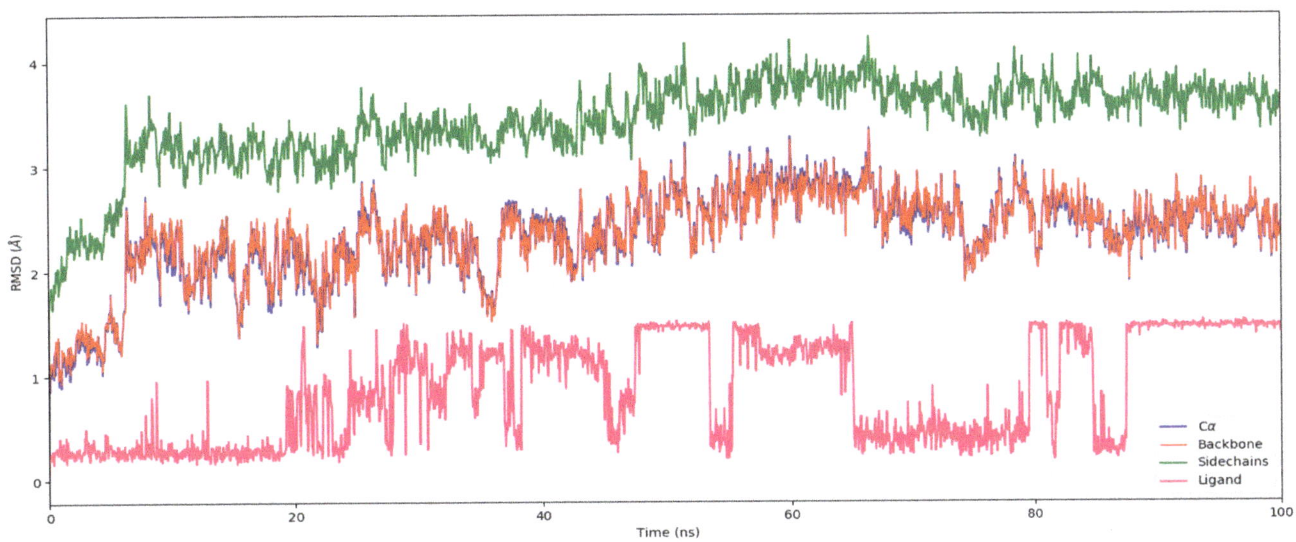

(b)

Figure 5. Root-mean-square deviation (RMSD) values for the protein backbone, alpha carbons, side chains, and ligand. (**a**) Amentoflavone; (**b**) Fisetin.

Root-mean-square fluctuation (RMSF) was also calculated, as shown in Figure 6a,b. These values show the general movement of each residue across the total simulation time. In this figure, the ligand contacts are shown as green lines matching the residue index, while the orange lines indicate protein secondary structures (helices, in this case). See Figure S6 in the Supplementary Materials for further details.

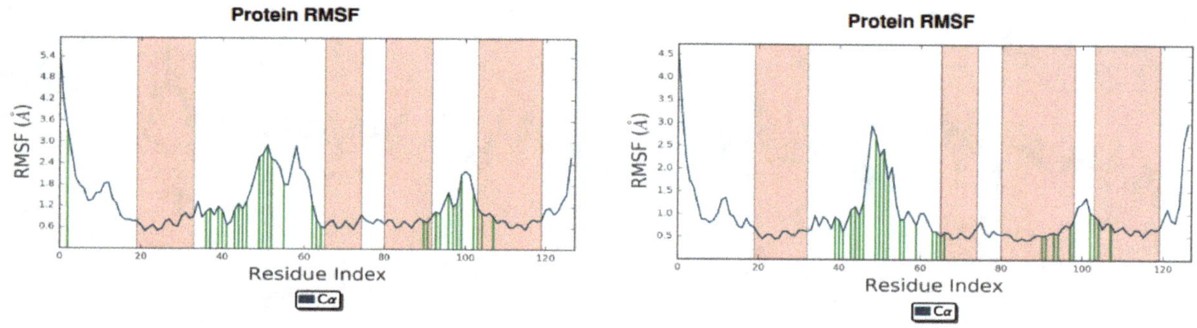

(a) (b)

Figure 6. Root-mean-square fluctuation (RMSF) values based on alpha carbons; ligand contacts are presented in green, and protein helices in orange. (**a**) Amentoflavone; (**b**) Fisetin.

Figures 7 and 8 show the protein–ligand contact analysis for the MD simulations. Protein–ligand contacts can be interpreted as "dynamic PLIFs", showing the population of contacts during the simulation. Plots at the bottom of both figures represent the number of contacts and their density, i.e., a darker shade of orange indicates more than one contact in that frame. These plots also show the type of contact mapped to the structure of the ligand.

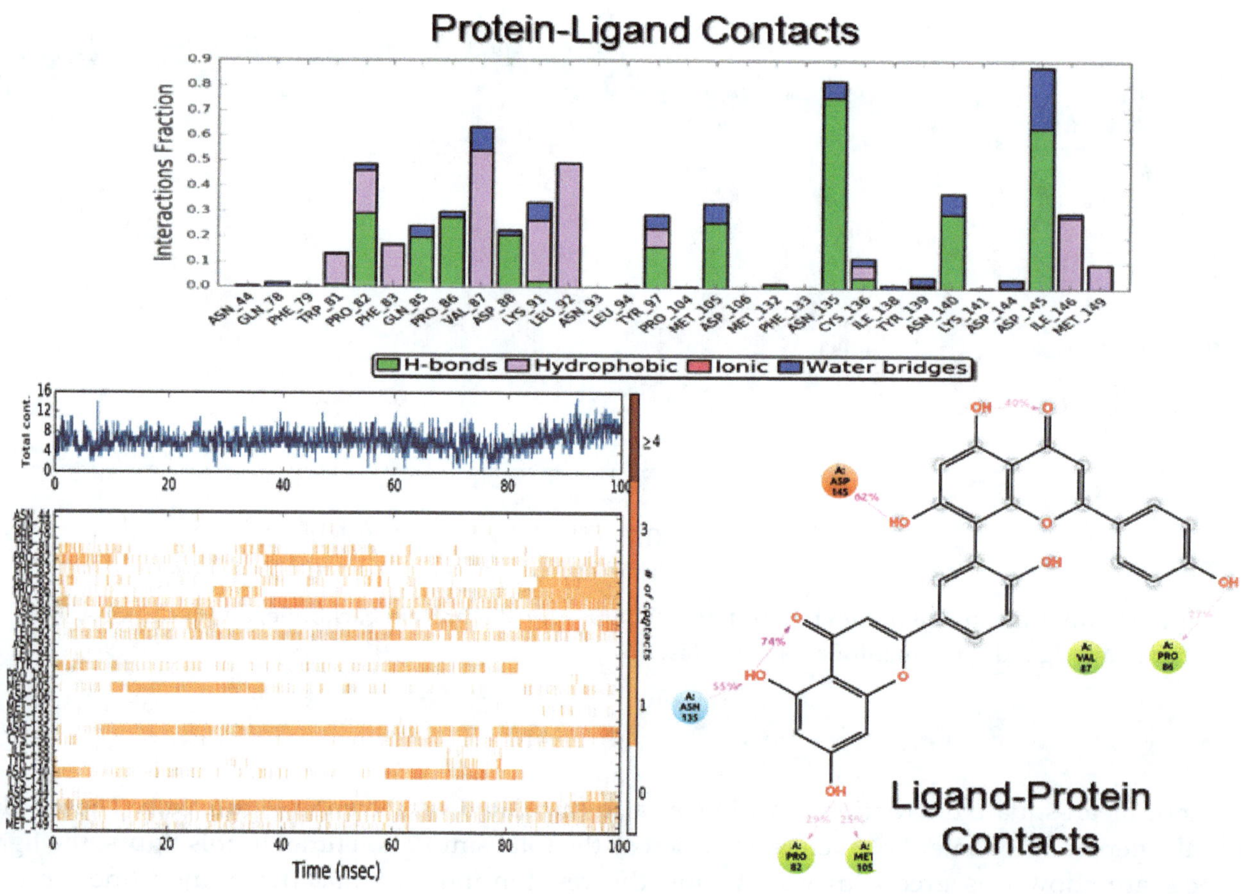

Figure 7. Protein–ligand contact analysis for amentoflavone during the molecular dynamics (MD) simulation.

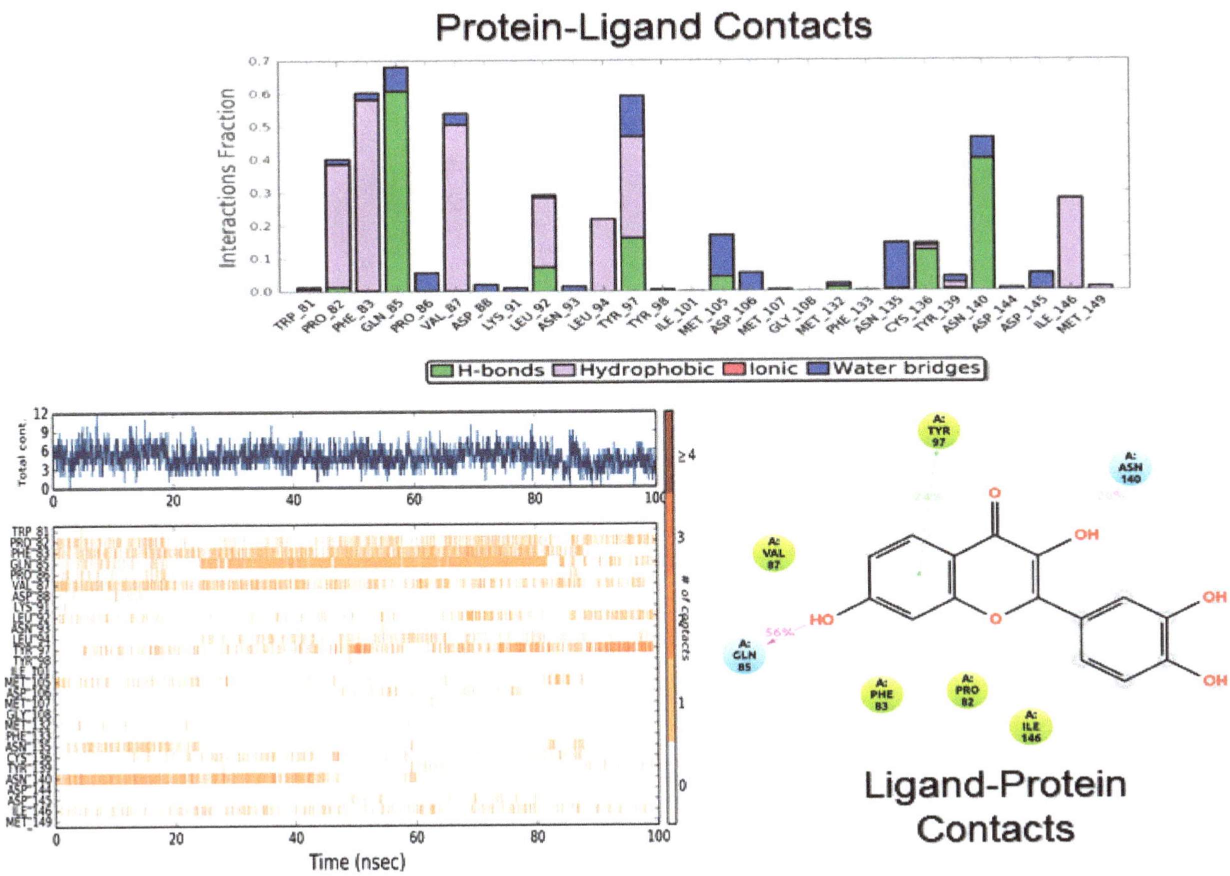

Figure 8. Protein–ligand contact analysis for fisetin during the MD simulation.

Figure 9a,b show other ligand properties during the MD simulations. These include the radius of gyration, intramolecular hydrogen bonding, van der Waals (VdW) surface area, solvent-accessible surface area, and polar surface area. Of note, if a ligand is not capable of intramolecular hydrogen bonding, this plot appears empty.

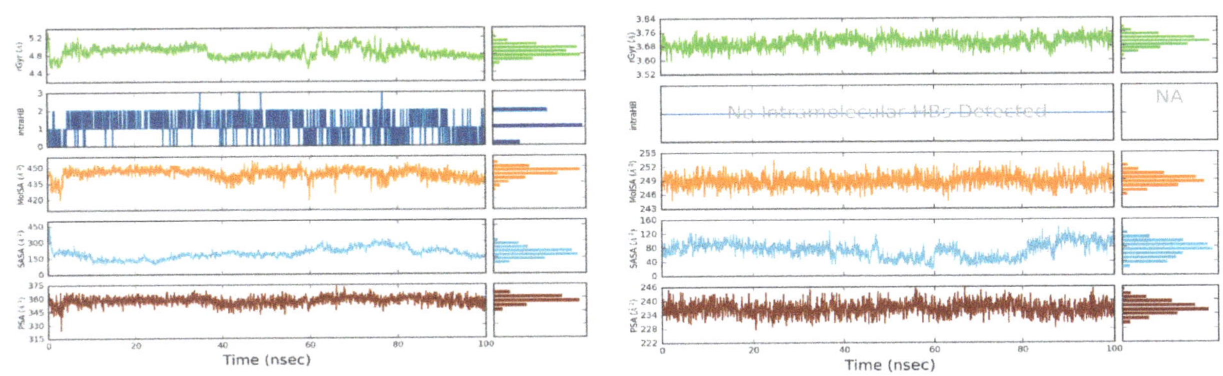

(a) (b)

Figure 9. Ligand properties during the 100-ns simulations. (**a**) Amentoflavone; (**b**) Fisetin.

Figure 10a,b show the energy values for dihedral angles (line plot), which account for torsional analysis. The histogram shows the density of probability of that torsion, while the dial on the left shows the rotation of that bond during the simulation (the beginning is marked by the center). The plots in Figure 10 allow determining whether or not a given ligand undergoes torsional strain during binding.

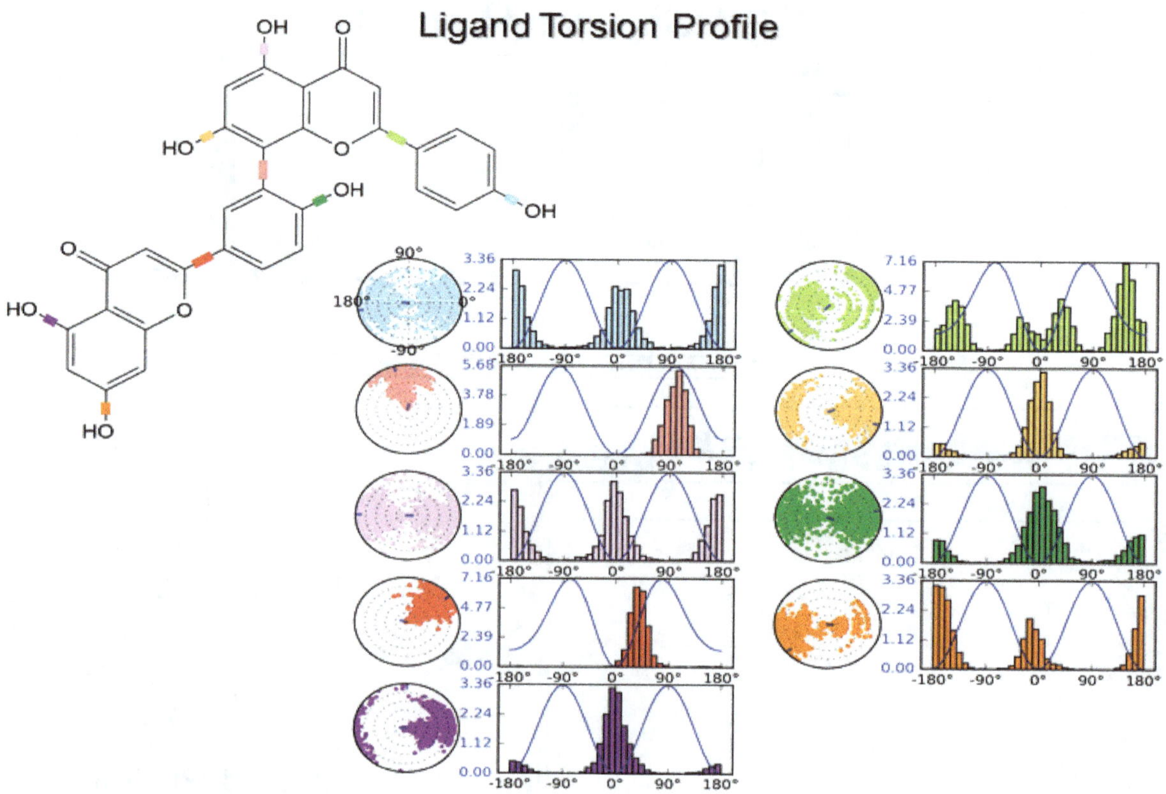

(a)

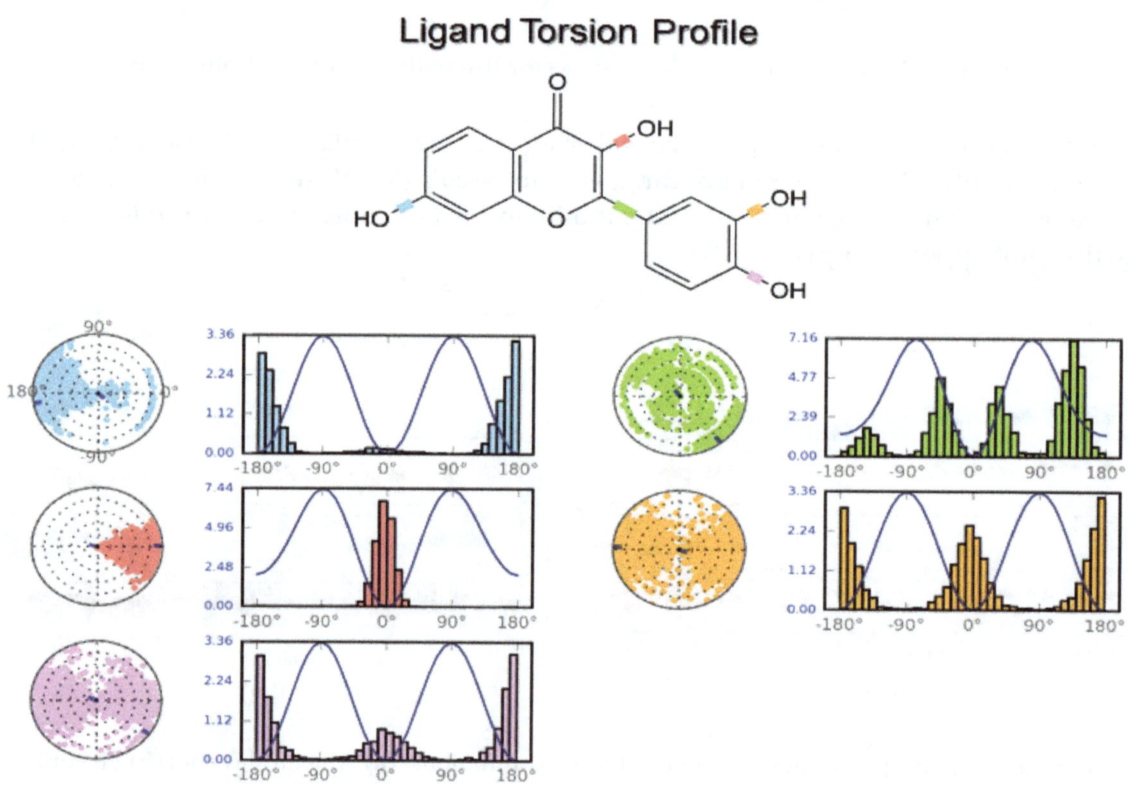

(b)

Figure 10. Torsional analysis of ligand conformations during the 100-ns simulations. (**a**) Amentoflavone; (**b**) Fisetin. The colors represent the different rotatable bonds of the ligands. Values on the Y-axis are in kcal/mol.

3.3. Binding Assay of Amentoflavone

Table 2 summarizes the experimentally determined activity of amentoflavone.

Table 2. Values for the half maximal inhibitory concentration (IC_{50}) and the Hill slope of amentoflavone, as obtained using AlphaScreen † against the bromodomain 4 (BRD4) tandem.

	DATA 1	DATA 2
IC_{50} (μM)	36.1	30.4
Hill slope	−2.5	−1.9

† As mentioned in the Methods section, experimental characterization was performed with the Reaction Biology application using the AlphaScreen assay.

4. Discussion

4.1. Molecular Docking

Bromodomain inhibitors may be classified into two broad categories: KAc-mimicking and non-mimicking, the former being the most prominent [60]. Flavonoids belong to this category as their carbonyl groups are their main anchor toward Asn140 and Tyr97 [46]. Nonetheless, as shown in Figure 4, these interactions are not as populated as might be expected. Certainly, this may seem negative, as the Ac-pocket is the main anchor for bromodomain inhibition. Nonetheless, the exclusion of molecules based solely on this criterion was questioned [61].

Because of this, an integral approach based on ensemble docking and consensus scoring was conducted, as a means of correctly assessing the probability of a given interaction. Ensemble docking is a common technique used to account for protein flexibility [62], and was applied successfully to several workflows [63]. Consensus scoring, on the other hand, significantly increases the rate of hit identification [64]. However, the rate of success has a strong dependence on the selected programs for consensus. Consequently, a naïve choice leads to an overestimation of weighted terms if similar parameters in scoring functions are used [65]. Hence, we selected the docking software based on searching-algorithm capabilities and scoring-function diversity. Briefly, the rationale for each selection is presented hereunder.

- Autodock VINA: It has a well-established performance against several protein families; additionally, its empirical scoring function has a significant correlation with experimental values [66]. Finally, its hybrid search algorithm optimized by local search allows a better sampling of the free-energy landscape [67].
- LeDock: Its search algorithm based on simulated annealing provides a significant clustering of poses. In addition, it was implemented successfully in virtual screening campaigns for BET bromodomains [52].
- MOE: Its docking algorithm allows for induced-fit search. Furthermore, its force-field-based scoring function (using AMBER parameters with generalized Born/volume integral (GB/VI) solvation) considers the solvation contributions to ligand binding [68].
- PLANTS: It provides a notable sampling of side-chain flexibility. Also, its searching algorithm (based on metaheuristics) and its empirical scoring function have a well-established performance [69].

Additionally, knowledge-based filtering was used to improve consensus results. This method takes advantage of PLIFs to identify trends in binding while selecting poses with "canonical" interactions [47]. Of note, the interactions of both flavonoids with Asn140 show a similar shift in MD simulations, which suggests a good sampling of our ensemble, and a notable performance of the protocol presented herein.

Based on the docking scores, both amentoflavone and fisetin are comparable to currently known inhibitors (see Supplementary Materials, Table S3). To the best of our knowledge, there are no studies or data showing a correlation of docking scores with experimental binding energies of bromodomain inhibitors. While such analysis goes beyond the scope of this work, we provided reference values obtained from the literature (see Supplementary Materials, Table S2).

Notably, docking scores calculated with LeDock were lower when compared to the scores computed with other programs. Nevertheless, this same trend was observed for reference inhibitors. This result was mostly due to the scoring function, as it was shown that, while accurate for identifying correct binding poses, energy values assigned to them are often underestimated [70].

Additionally, the difference in score values for both compounds is significant. Roughly, these values suggest that amentoflavone could be three times more potent than fisetin. Arguably, this may be due to the bigger size of amentoflavone and the higher number of hydroxyl groups giving it more anchors toward BRD4. However, average scoring values rank them with a virtual IC_{50} of around 1–5 μM, based on scaffold similarity and reference values.

Amentoflavone showed mainly hydrophobic contacts with the WPF shelf (Pro81) and the ZA channel (Leu92). Fisetin on the other hand, showed more contacts with residues Met105 and Met132. Previous reports of docking indicate that flavonoids have a notable preference toward these residues [26]; in the case of fisetin, affinity for Cys136 was also observed [46]. This hints to flavonoids having a significant affinity toward different residues beyond the Ac-pocket, while their aromatic characteristics gives them selectivity for the WPF shelf.

Interestingly, the consensus PLIF (Figure 4) shows that amentoflavone made fewer contacts than fisetin. Moreover, the population of Asn140 bonding was significantly reduced for amentoflavone. In contrast, the MD simulations of both compounds showed a similar interaction profile, whereby the fraction is higher for amentoflavone (0.9 vs. 0.7). The Asn140-interaction fraction was similar for both flavonoids (around 0.4). Tyr97 on the other hand, made a stronger and more lasting interaction with fisetin by means of pi stacking and hydrogen bonding. This may be due to the size of amentoflavone and its orientation in the protein cavity, evidenced by the contacts with "non-canonical" residues. An example of this was Asp145, a contact with amentoflavone with a rather small population. However, this contact was identified as significant, as it provides ligand stabilization and water-network interactions [71].

4.2. *Molecular Dynamics*

As stated, MD simulations were conducted to contrast docking results, and to provide further insight into the binding mode of flavonoids. Based on the protein RMSD values, BRD4 remained stable enough during the simulation with both flavonoids. The ligand RMSD values, on the other hand, showed higher deviations at times. This could suggest that both ligands underwent conformational changes during the simulation, i.e., they had two binding modes.

Therefore, torsional profiling plots assisted in this interpretation (Figure 10), as these provided the spatial and energetic distributions of bond torsions during the simulation, showing that both flavonoids were mostly strained in two main conformations. This could imply that fisetin changes its conformation more quickly than amentoflavone, due to a rotation of its catechol ring. However, this observation differs from a previous report [37], which suggested that fisetin keeps a restrained conformation when bound to BRD4. The main reason for this may be related to the use of different force fields (OPLS_2005 vs. OPLS3). On this matter, it is noteworthy that other ligand properties (Figure 9) showed similar trend values for fisetin to those in the previous study.

Amentoflavone, on the other hand, kept a restrained conformation of its shared phenol ring. This behavior can be related to atropisomerism features present on the biflavonoid. Based on these results, it can be hypothesized that amentoflavone activity on BETs is mediated by atropisomerism. Of course, stability studies of amentoflavone and its atropisomers are required to confirm this hypothesis. However, such techniques and focus were beyond the aims of this work. It suffices to say that, even though such phenomena may be common in bioflavonoids, their recognition in medicinal chemistry is often overlooked [72]. Moreover, the interest in atropisomerism is recently increasing [73]. Thus, we believe that knowledge of this feature could improve novel ligand designs, giving a paradigm shift mostly needed for these targets.

The RMSF plots (Figure 6) also showed that the protein–ligand complexes remained consistently stable, and the main secondary structures were four α-helices, which confirms a correct sampling of the system. These plots also showed that the main contacts in both flavonoids were with the ZA channel, with high fluctuations of these residues during the simulation. Interestingly, when these protein–ligand contacts were analyzed, different interaction profiles arose for both flavonoids.

Amentoflavone clearly made more contacts with the ZA channel as the MD simulation went on. Also, its presence in the cavity made a significant impact on the secondary structure of the protein, increasing the helical portion of this region (Figure S6 in the Supporting Materials). As stated above, this may be related to the bigger size of the structure. However, based on the "contact mixture" this could also be related to the strained conformation of the molecule, allowing a more favorable angle toward hydrogen bonding and the hydrophobic interactions.

Again, the contact with Asp145 is remarkable; in this case, it was the most populated contact in the MD simulations with amentoflavone. Also, the presence of water bridges with this residue proved significant, a feature recently observed by other groups [71]. Furthermore, this residue is present only in BRD4 BD1, providing specific contact with histone H3 via hydrogen bonding, an interaction not present with inhibitors such as JQ-1 [74]. This would suggest that amentoflavone can be selective for the first domain of BRD4. This is noteworthy, considering molecular similarity toward RVX-208 would suggest selectivity for BRD4 BD2.

4.3. *Experimental Evaluation*

Based on the results of molecular docking and dynamics, it was decided to acquire a sample, and to experimentally test amentoflavone as a BRD4 inhibitor. Fisetin was not considered for testing due to a previous report of quercetin showing an IC_{50} of 38 µM [58]. With this value as reference, our efforts focused on the biflavonoid scaffold. It is very positive that amentoflavone showed significant binding for BRD4, with an IC_{50} in the micromolar range. Indeed, it was more potent when compared to a flavonoid monomer (38 vs. 30 µM). Additionally, its Hill slope value could indicate that amentoflavone is indeed selective for one domain of BRD4. However, more testing is required, i.e., binding assays for separate domains of BRD4.

Furthermore, this experimental confirmation provides further evidence of flavonoids as general chemoprotective agents. One of the main concerns about the use of flavonoids as nutraceutics is their putative toxicity, as fisetin and other flavonoid monomers inhibit DNA topoisomerases [75] and actin polymerization [36]. Biflavonoids, on the other hand, do not present this feature; however, they were reported as potentially mutagenic [76]. Nonetheless, such negative effects are only present at concentrations between 100 and 250 µM [77,78]. As such, based on the IC_{50} values of both quercetin and amentoflavone, flavonoids have significant potential as epi-nutraceutics.

Summarizing, the work presented here serves as a remarkable proof of concept for both the flavonoids as epi-modulators and the computational methods used herein. Putting the results together, amentoflavone showed the characteristic contacts previously reported for flavonoids, i.e., strong contacts with the ZA region, in addition to novel predicted interactions with Asp145 and the water network. Biological tests supported the hypothesis of binding and the plausible selectivity.

Despite the fact that flavonoids have small room for optimization and break Lipinski's rule of five, their true potential is as chemoprotective agents. As previously mentioned, this finding further advances the field of nutriepigenomics. Moreover, it is remarkable that these natural products provide pharmacophoric templates for novel inhibitors of an epigenetic target.

5. Conclusions

Amentoflavone is a natural product with several associated biological effects. Its ability to block NF-κβ is the key for its anti-inflammatory potential. BETs were identified as NF-κβ promoters, with JQ-1 being highly effective in psoriasis models. Previously, a similar effect was reported for amentoflavone. Based on these results and other reports, we conducted a binding characterization of this ligand, and compared it to fisetin, another flavonoid with reports of putative activity. We presented a consensus docking methodology which allowed binding characterization and hit selection. Certainly, such an approach is impractical for large virtual-screening campaigns. However, based on the performance and results presented, it provides a powerful tool for pose selection, as supported by the MD results.

The simulations conducted herein indicated that amentoflavone can make numerous contacts in the ZA channel, as previously described for flavonoids and kinase inhibitors. It was also determined that amentoflavone can potentially make contacts with "non-canonical" residues for BET inhibition, e.g., Met105, Asn135, Cys136, and Asp145. Most of these contacts were not observed with fisetin (except for Cys136). Based on the analysis of torsional values, it is plausible that this behavior was due to the atropisomerism present in the molecule. As a first step toward testing this hypothesis, the in vitro inhibition of BRD4 was evaluated. The experimental evaluation showed that amentoflavone was indeed active in the micromolar range, with plausible selectivity against one domain in the BRD4 tandem.

Perspectives of this work include the experimental testing of fisetin and the contrast of its result with molecular modeling predictions. Additionally, for amentoflavone, specific tests for BD1 and BD2 are required to confirm its selectivity. Finally, we consider that these results, while preliminary, offer a new paradigm for inhibitor design, as well as characteristics for novel modulation of BETs.

Supplementary Materials
Figure S1: Relaxation protocol and MD workflow used in this work, Table S1: BRD4 PDBIDs used for cross-docking studies Figure S2: Simulation Quality parameters for the BRD4 protein for 100 ns, Table S2: IC_{50} and experimental binding energy values and of reference ligands for BRD4 inhibition as reported on the literature, Figure S3: RMSD values for BRD4 protein for 100ns, Table S3: Scoring values for reference ligands as obtained by the docking software used herein, Figure S4: Simulation Quality parameters for the BRD4 protein with fisetine for 100 ns, Table S4: Scoring values obtained with LeDock for amentoflavone per protein-ligand complex of the ensemble, Figure S5: Simulation Quality parameters for the BRD4 protein with amentoflavone for 100 ns, Table S5: Scoring values obtained with MOE for amentoflavone per protein-ligand complex of the ensemble, Figure S6: Secondary structure of BRD4 as observed for 100 ns. A) BRD4 without ligand. B) amentoflavone. C) fisetin., Table S6: Scoring values obtained with PLANTS for amentoflavone per protein-ligand complex of the ensemble, Table S7: Scoring values obtained with Vina for amentoflavone per protein-ligand complex of the ensemble, Table S8: Scoring values obtained with LeDock for fisetin per protein-ligand complex of the ensemble, Table S9: Scoring values obtained with MOE for fisetin per protein-ligand complex of the ensemble, Table S10: Scoring values obtained with PLANTS for fisetin per protein-ligand complex of the ensemble, Table S11: Scoring values obtained with Vina for fisetin per protein-ligand complex of the ensemble, Table S12: Summary values for quality measures for the BRD4 protein, Table S13: Summary values for quality measures BRD4 protein with fisetine, Table S14: Summary values for quality measures BRD4 protein with amentoflavone.

Author Contributions: Conceptualization, F.D.P.-M. Methodology, F.D.P.-M. Formal analysis, F.D.P.-M. Investigation, F.D.P.-M. and J.L.M.-F. Resources, J.L.M.-F. Writing—original draft preparation, F.D.P.-M. Writing—review and editing, J.L.M.-F. Supervision, J.L.M.-F. Project administration, J.L.M.-F. Funding acquisition, J.L.M.-F.

Acknowledgments: F.D.P.-M. acknowledges the PhD scholarship from CONACyT No. 660465/576637. The authors would like to thank Joaquín Barroso-Flores (Centro Conjunto de Investigación en Química Sustentable, Instituto de Química, UNAM) and Durbis Castillo-Pazos (Universidad Nacional Autónoma del Estado de México) for the suggestion of software used for MD. Additionally, discussions with Marcelino Arciniega (Instituto de Fisiología Celular, UNAM) were highly valuable to this work. The authors are grateful for the support given by the Programa de Apoyo a la Investigación y el Posgrado (PAIP) grant 5000–9163, Facultad de Química, UNAM; and by the Programa de Apoyo a Proyectos de Investigación e Innovación Tecnológica (PAPIIT) grant IA203718, UNAM. The authors are grateful for the computational resources granted by the Dirección General de Cómputo y de Tecnologías de Información y Comunicación (DGTIC), project grant LANCAD-UNAM-DGTIC-335 that allowed the use of the Miztli supercomputer at UNAM. We also thank the Programa de Nuevas Alternativas de Tratamiento para Enfermedades Infecciosas (NUATEI-IIB-UNAM).

References

1. Cabaye, A.; Nguyen, K.T.; Liu, L.; Pande, V.; Schapira, M. Structural diversity of the epigenetics pocketome. *Proteins Struct. Funct. Bioinform.* **2015**, *83*, 1316–1326. [CrossRef] [PubMed]
2. Eberharter, A.; Becker, P.B. Histone acetylation: A switch between repressive and permissive chromatin. Second in review on chromatin dynamics. *EMBO Rep.* **2002**, *3*, 224–229. [CrossRef] [PubMed]
3. Kalyaanamoorthy, S.; Chen, Y.P.P. Energy based pharmacophore mapping of HDAC inhibitors against class i HDAC enzymes. *Biochim. Biophys. Acta Proteins Proteomics* **2013**, *1834*, 317–328. [CrossRef]
4. Ortore, G.; Colo, F.D.; Martinelli, A. Docking of Hydroxamic Acids into HDAC1 and HDAC8: A Rationalization of Activity Trends and Selectivities. *J. Chem. Inf. Model.* **2009**, *49*, 2774–2785. [CrossRef] [PubMed]
5. Hassanzadeh, M.; Bagherzadeh, K.; Amanlou, M. A comparative study based on docking and molecular dynamics simulations over HDAC-tubulin dual inhibitors. *J. Mol. Graph. Model.* **2016**, *70*, 170–180. [CrossRef] [PubMed]
6. VanderMolen, K.M.; McCulloch, W.; Pearce, C.J.; Oberlies, N.H. Romidepsin (Istodax, NSC 630176, FR901228, FK228, depsipeptide): A natural product recently approved for cutaneous T-cell lymphoma. *J. Antibiot. (Tokyo)* **2011**, *64*, 525–531. [CrossRef] [PubMed]
7. Arrowsmith, C.H.; Bountra, C.; Fish, P.V.; Lee, K.; Schapira, M. Epigenetic protein families: a new frontier for drug discovery. *Nat. Rev. Drug Discov.* **2012**, *11*, 384–400. [CrossRef] [PubMed]
8. Berkovits, B.D.; Wolgemuth, D.J. The Role of the Double Bromodomain-Containing BET Genes During Mammalian Spermatogenesis. *Curr. Top. Dev. Biol.* **2013**, *102*, 293–326. [CrossRef] [PubMed]
9. Hewings, D.S.; Rooney, T.P.C.; Jennings, L.E.; Hay, D.A.; Schofield, C.J.; Brennan, P.E.; Knapp, S.; Conway, S.J. Progress in the Development and Application of Small Molecule Inhibitors of Bromodomain–Acetyl-lysine Interactions. *J. Med. Chem.* **2012**, *55*, 9393–9413. [CrossRef] [PubMed]
10. Ferri, E.; Petosa, C.; McKenna, C.E. Bromodomains: Structure, function and pharmacology of inhibition. *Biochem. Pharmacol.* **2016**, *106*, 1–18. [CrossRef] [PubMed]
11. Brand, M.; Measures, A.M.; Wilson, B.G.; Cortopassi, W.A.; Alexander, R.; Höss, M.; Hewings, D.S.; Rooney, T.P.C.; Paton, R.S.; Conway, S.J. Small Molecule Inhibitors of Bromodomain–Acetyl-lysine Interactions. *ACS Chem. Biol.* **2015**, *10*, 22–39. [CrossRef] [PubMed]
12. Ladbury, J.E. Just add water! The effect of water on the specificity of protein-ligand binding sites and its potential application to drug design. *Chem. Biol.* **1996**, *3*, 973–980. [CrossRef]
13. Plumridge, T.H.; Waigh, R.D. Water structure theory and some implications for drug design. *J. Pharm. Pharmacol.* **2002**, *54*, 1155–1179. [CrossRef] [PubMed]
14. Crawford, T.D.; Tsui, V.; Flynn, E.M.; Wang, S.; Taylor, A.M.; Côté, A.; Audia, J.E.; Beresini, M.H.; Burdick, D.J.; Cummings, R.; et al. Diving into the Water: Inducible Binding Conformations for BRD4, TAF1(2), BRD9, and CECR2 Bromodomains. *J. Med. Chem.* **2016**, *59*, 5391–5402. [CrossRef] [PubMed]
15. Pan, A.C.; Borhani, D.W.; Dror, R.O.; Shaw, D.E. Molecular determinants of drug-receptor binding kinetics. *Drug Discov. Today* **2013**, *18*, 667–673. [CrossRef] [PubMed]
16. Huggins, D.J.; Sherman, W.; Tidor, B. Rational approaches to improving selectivity in drug design. *J. Med. Chem.* **2012**, *55*, 1424–1444. [CrossRef] [PubMed]
17. Ross, G.A.; Morris, G.M.; Biggin, P.C. Rapid and accurate prediction and scoring of water molecules in protein binding sites. *PLoS ONE* **2012**, *7*, e32036. [CrossRef] [PubMed]
18. García-Sosa, A.T.; Firth-Clark, S.; Mancera, R.L. Including tightly-bound water molecules in de novo drug design. exemplification through the in silico generation of poly(ADP-ribose)polymerase ligands. *J. Chem. Inf. Model.* **2005**, *45*, 624–633. [CrossRef] [PubMed]

19. Shadrick, W.R.; Slavish, P.J.; Chai, S.C.; Waddell, B.; Connelly, M.; Low, J.A.; Tallant, C.; Young, B.M.; Bharatham, N.; Knapp, S.; et al. Exploiting a water network to achieve enthalpy-driven, bromodomain-selective BET inhibitors. *Bioorgan. Med. Chem.* **2018**, *26*, 25–36. [CrossRef] [PubMed]
20. Bharatham, N.; Slavish, P.J.; Young, B.M.; Shelat, A.A. The role of ZA channel water-mediated interactions in the design of bromodomain-selective BET inhibitors. *J. Mol. Graph. Model.* **2018**, *81*, 197–210. [CrossRef] [PubMed]
21. Geist, L.; Mayer, M.; Cockcroft, X.L.; Wolkerstorfer, B.; Kessler, D.; Engelhardt, H.; McConnell, D.B.; Konrat, R. Direct NMR Probing of Hydration Shells of Protein Ligand Interfaces and Its Application to Drug Design. *J. Med. Chem.* **2017**, *60*, 8708–8715. [CrossRef] [PubMed]
22. Prieto-Martínez, F.D.; Fernandez-de Gortari, E.; Méndez-Lucio, O.; Medina-Franco, J.L. A chemical space odyssey of inhibitors of histone deacetylases and bromodomains. *RSC Adv.* **2016**, *6*, 56225–56239. [CrossRef]
23. Galdeano, C.; Ciulli, A. Selectivity on-target of bromodomain chemical probes by structure-guided medicinal chemistry and chemical biology. *Future Med. Chem.* **2016**, *8*, 1655–1680. [CrossRef] [PubMed]
24. Kharenko, O.A.; Gesner, E.M.; Patel, R.G.; Norek, K.; White, A.; Fontano, E.; Suto, R.K.; Young, P.R.; McLure, K.G.; Hansen, H.C. RVX-297-a novel BD2 selective inhibitor of BET bromodomains. *Biochem. Biophys. Res. Commun.* **2016**, *477*, 62–67. [CrossRef] [PubMed]
25. Ember, S.W.J.; Zhu, J.Y.; Olesen, S.H.; Martin, M.P.; Becker, A.; Berndt, N.; Georg, G.I.; Schonbrunn, E. Acetyl-lysine binding site of bromodomain-containing protein 4 (BRD4) interacts with diverse kinase inhibitors. *ACS Chem. Biol.* **2014**, *9*, 1160–1171. [CrossRef] [PubMed]
26. Dhananjayan, K. Molecular Docking Study Characterization of Rare Flavonoids at the Nac-Binding Site of the First Bromodomain of BRD4 (BRD4 BD1). *J. Cancer Res.* **2015**, *2015*, 1–15. [CrossRef]
27. Singh, M.; Kaur, M.; Silakari, O. Flavones: An important scaffold for medicinal chemistry. *Eur. J. Med. Chem.* **2014**, *84*, 206–239. [CrossRef] [PubMed]
28. Perry, N.S.L.; Bollen, C.; Perry, E.K.; Ballard, C. Salvia for dementia therapy: Review of pharmacological activity and pilot tolerability clinical trial. *Pharmacol. Biochem. Behav.* **2003**, *75*, 651–659. [CrossRef]
29. Hwang, S.-L.; Shih, P.-H.; Yen, G.-C. Citrus Flavonoids and Effects in Dementia and Age-Related Cognitive Decline. In *Diet and Nutrition in Dementia and Cognitive Decline*; Elsevier: Cambridge, MA, USA, 2015; pp. 869–878, ISBN 9780124079397.
30. Fernández, S.P.; Wasowski, C.; Paladini, A.C.; Marder, M. Synergistic interaction between hesperidin, a natural flavonoid, and diazepam. *Eur. J. Pharmacol.* **2005**, *512*, 189–198. [CrossRef] [PubMed]
31. Thilakarathna, W.W.; Langille, M.G.; Rupasinghe, H.V. Polyphenol-based prebiotics and synbiotics: potential for cancer chemoprevention. *Curr. Opin. Food Sci.* **2018**, *20*, 51–57. [CrossRef]
32. Khan, N.; Syed, D.N.; Ahmad, N.; Mukhtar, H. Fisetin: A Dietary Antioxidant for Health Promotion. *Antioxid. Redox Signal.* **2013**, *19*, 151–162. [CrossRef] [PubMed]
33. Vasantha Rupasinghe, H.P.; Nair, S.V.G.; Robinson, R.A. *Chemopreventive Properties of Fruit Phenolic Compounds and Their Possible Mode of Actions*, 1st ed.; Elsevier: Amsterdam, The Netherlands, 2014; Volume 42, ISBN 9780444632814.
34. Sung, B.; Pandey, M.K.; Aggarwal, B.B. Fisetin, an Inhibitor of Cyclin-Dependent Kinase 6, Down-Regulates Nuclear Factor-B-Regulated Cell Proliferation, Antiapoptotic and Metastatic Gene Products through the Suppression of TAK-1 and Receptor-Interacting Protein-Regulated IκBα Kinase Activation. *Mol. Pharmacol.* **2007**, *71*, 1703–1714. [CrossRef] [PubMed]
35. Syed, D.N.; Adhami, V.M.; Khan, N.; Khan, M.I.; Mukhtar, H. Exploring the molecular targets of dietary flavonoid fisetin in cancer. *Semin. Cancer Biol.* **2016**, *40–41*, 130–140. [CrossRef] [PubMed]
36. Sundarraj, K.; Raghunath, A.; Perumal, E. A review on the chemotherapeutic potential of fisetin: In vitro evidences. *Biomed. Pharmacother.* **2018**, *97*, 928–940. [CrossRef] [PubMed]
37. Kashyap, D.; Sharma, A.; Sak, K.; Tuli, H.S.; Buttar, H.S.; Bishayee, A. Fisetin: A bioactive phytochemical with potential for cancer prevention and pharmacotherapy. *Life Sci.* **2018**, *194*, 75–87. [CrossRef] [PubMed]
38. Rengarajan, T.; Yaacob, N.S. The flavonoid fisetin as an anticancer agent targeting the growth signaling pathways. *Eur. J. Pharmacol.* **2016**, *789*, 8–16. [CrossRef] [PubMed]
39. Nadeem, A.; Al-Harbi, N.O.; Al-Harbi, M.M.; El-Sherbeeny, A.M.; Ahmad, S.F.; Siddiqui, N.; Ansari, M.A.; Zoheir, K.M.A.; Attia, S.M.; Al-Hosaini, K.A.; et al. Imiquimod-induced psoriasis-like skin inflammation is suppressed by BET bromodomain inhibitor in mice through RORC/IL-17A pathway modulation. *Pharmacol. Res.* **2015**, *99*, 248–257. [CrossRef] [PubMed]

40. Coletta, D.K. Genetic and Epigenetics of Type 2 Diabetes. In *Pathobiology of Human Disease*; Elsevier: Amsterdam, The Netherlands, 2014; pp. 467–476, ISBN 9780123864567.
41. Mele, D.A.; Salmeron, A.; Ghosh, S.; Huang, H.-R.; Bryant, B.M.; Lora, J.M. BET bromodomain inhibition suppresses TH17-mediated pathology. *J. Exp. Med.* **2013**, *210*, 2181–2190. [CrossRef] [PubMed]
42. Burkard, M.; Leischner, C.; Lauer, U.M.; Busch, C.; Venturelli, S.; Frank, J. Dietary flavonoids and modulation of natural killer cells: implications in malignant and viral diseases. *J. Nutr. Biochem.* **2017**, *46*, 1–12. [CrossRef] [PubMed]
43. Catarino, M.D.; Talhi, O.; Rabahi, A.; Silva, A.M.S.; Cardoso, S.M. The Antiinflammatory Potential of Flavonoids. In *Studies in Natural Products Chemistry*; Elsevier: Amsterdam, The Netherlands, 2016; Volume 48, pp. 65–99, ISBN 9780444636027.
44. Onawole, A.T.; Sulaiman, K.O.; Adegoke, R.O.; Kolapo, T.U. Identification of potential inhibitors against the Zika virus using consensus scoring. *J. Mol. Graph. Model.* **2017**, *73*, 54–61. [CrossRef] [PubMed]
45. Śledź, P.; Caflisch, A. Protein structure-based drug design: from docking to molecular dynamics. *Curr. Opin. Struct. Biol.* **2018**, *48*, 93–102. [CrossRef] [PubMed]
46. Raj, U.; Kumar, H.; Varadwaj, P.K. Molecular docking and dynamics simulation study of flavonoids as BET bromodomain inhibitors. *J. Biomol. Struct. Dyn.* **2016**, *1102*, 1–12. [CrossRef] [PubMed]
47. Prieto-Martínez, F.D.; Medina-Franco, J.L. Charting the Bromodomain BRD4: Towards the Identification of Novel Inhibitors with Molecular Similarity and Receptor Mapping. *Lett. Drug Des. Discov.* **2018**, *15*, 1–10. [CrossRef]
48. *Molecular Operating Environment (MOE), 2013.08*; Chemical Computing Group ULC: Montreal, QC, Canada, 2018.
49. Case, D.A.; Babin, V.; Berryman, J.; Betz, R.; Cai, Q.; Cerutti, D.S.; Cheatham, T.; Darden, T.; Duke, R.; Gohlke, H.; et al. *AMBER 14*, University of California: San Francisco, CA, USA, 2014.
50. Gerber, P.R.; Müller, K. MAB, a generally applicable molecular force field for structure modelling in medicinal chemistry. *J. Comput. Aided. Mol. Des.* **1995**, *9*, 251–268. [CrossRef] [PubMed]
51. Trott, O.; Olson, A.J. AutoDock Vina: Improving the speed and accuracy of docking with a new scoring function, efficient optimization, and multithreading. *J. Comput. Chem.* **2009**, *31*. [CrossRef] [PubMed]
52. Unzue, A.; Zhao, H.; Lolli, G.; Dong, J.; Zhu, J.; Zechner, M.; Dolbois, A.; Caflisch, A.; Nevado, C. The "gatekeeper" Residue Influences the Mode of Binding of Acetyl Indoles to Bromodomains. *J. Med. Chem.* **2016**, *59*, 3087–3097. [CrossRef] [PubMed]
53. Korb, O.; Stützle, T.; Exner, T.E. Empirical scoring functions for advanced Protein-Ligand docking with PLANTS. *J. Chem. Inf. Model.* **2009**, *49*, 84–96. [CrossRef] [PubMed]
54. Stewart, J.J.P. Application of the PM6 method to modeling the solid state. *J. Mol. Model.* **2008**, *14*, 499–535. [CrossRef] [PubMed]
55. Hostaš, J.; Řezáč, J.; Hobza, P. On the performance of the semiempirical quantum mechanical PM6 and PM7 methods for noncovalent interactions. *Chem. Phys. Lett.* **2013**, *568–569*, 161–166. [CrossRef]
56. Bowers, K.; Chow, E.; Xu, H.; Dror, R.; Eastwood, M.; Gregersen, B.; Klepeis, J.; Kolossvary, I.; Moraes, M.; Sacerdoti, F.; et al. Scalable Algorithms for Molecular Dynamics Simulations on Commodity Clusters. In Proceedings of the 2006 ACM/IEEE SC Conference on Supercomputing (SC'06), Tampa, FL, USA, 11–17 November 2006.
57. Kräutler, V.; van Gusteren, W.F.; Hünenberger, P.H. A fast SHAKE algorithm to solve distance constraints for small molecules in molecular dynamics simulations. *J. Comput. Chem.* **2001**, *22*, 501–508. [CrossRef]
58. Andrews, F.H.; Singh, A.R.; Joshi, S.; Smith, C.A.; Morales, G.A.; Garlich, J.R.; Durden, D.L.; Kutateladze, T.G. Dual-activity PI3K–BRD4 inhibitor for the orthogonal inhibition of MYC to block tumor growth and metastasis. *Proc. Natl. Acad. Sci. USA* **2017**, *114*, E1072–E1080. [CrossRef] [PubMed]
59. Sargsyan, K.; Grauffel, C.; Lim, C. How Molecular Size Impacts RMSD Applications in Molecular Dynamics Simulations. *J. Chem. Theory Comput.* **2017**, *13*, 1518–1524. [CrossRef] [PubMed]
60. Romero, F.A.; Taylor, A.M.; Crawford, T.D.; Tsui, V.; Côté, A.; Magnuson, S. Disrupting Acetyl-Lysine Recognition: Progress in the Development of Bromodomain Inhibitors. *J. Med. Chem.* **2016**, *59*, 1271–1298. [CrossRef] [PubMed]
61. Ran, T.; Zhang, Z.; Liu, K.; Lu, Y.; Li, H.; Xu, J.; Xiong, X.; Zhang, Y.; Xu, A.; Lu, S.; et al. Insight into the key interactions of bromodomain inhibitors based on molecular docking, interaction fingerprinting, molecular dynamics and binding free energy calculation. *Mol. Biosyst.* **2015**, *11*, 1295–1304. [CrossRef] [PubMed]

62. Korb, O.; Olsson, T.S.G.; Bowden, S.J.; Hall, R.J.; Verdonk, M.L.; Liebeschuetz, J.W.; Cole, J.C. Potential and Limitations of Ensemble Docking. *J. Chem. Inf. Model.* **2012**, 1262–1274. [CrossRef] [PubMed]
63. Evangelista, W.; Weir, R.L.; Ellingson, S.R.; Harris, J.B.; Kapoor, K.; Smith, J.C.; Baudry, J. Ensemble-based docking: From hit discovery to metabolism and toxicity predictions. *Bioorganic Med. Chem.* **2016**, *24*, 4928–4935. [CrossRef] [PubMed]
64. Tuccinardi, T.; Poli, G.; Romboli, V.; Giordano, A.; Martinelli, A. Extensive consensus docking evaluation for ligand pose prediction and virtual screening studies. *J. Chem. Inf. Model.* **2014**, *54*, 2980–2986. [CrossRef] [PubMed]
65. Kitchen, D.B.; Decornez, H.; Furr, J.R.; Bajorath, J. Docking and scoring in virtual screening for drug discovery: methods and applications. *Nat. Rev. Drug Discov.* **2004**, *3*, 935–949. [CrossRef] [PubMed]
66. Palestro, P.H.; Gavernet, L.; Estiu, G.L.; Bruno Blanch, L.E. Docking Applied to the Prediction of the Affinity of Compounds to P-Glycoprotein. *Biomed Res. Int.* **2014**, *2014*, 1–10. [CrossRef] [PubMed]
67. Ferreira, L.; dos Santos, R.; Oliva, G.; Andricopulo, A. Molecular Docking and Structure-Based Drug Design Strategies. *Molecules* **2015**, *20*, 13384–13421. [CrossRef] [PubMed]
68. Naïm, M.; Bhat, S.; Rankin, K.N.; Dennis, S.; Chowdhury, S.F.; Siddiqi, I.; Drabik, P.; Sulea, T.; Bayly, C.I.; Jakalian, A.; et al. Solvated Interaction Energy (SIE) for scoring protein-ligand binding affinities. 1. Exploring the parameter space. *J. Chem. Inf. Model.* **2007**, *47*, 122–133. [CrossRef] [PubMed]
69. Richter, L.; de Graaf, C.; Sieghart, W.; Varagic, Z.; Mörzinger, M.; de Esch, I.J.P.; Ecker, G.F.; Ernst, M. Diazepam-bound GABAA receptor models identify new benzodiazepine binding-site ligands. *Nat. Chem. Biol.* **2012**, *8*, 455–464. [CrossRef] [PubMed]
70. Wang, Z.; Sun, H.; Yao, X.; Li, D.; Xu, L.; Li, Y.; Tian, S.; Hou, T. Comprehensive evaluation of ten docking programs on a diverse set of protein-ligand complexes: The prediction accuracy of sampling power and scoring power. *Phys. Chem. Chem. Phys.* **2016**, *18*, 12964–12975. [CrossRef] [PubMed]
71. Hoffer, L.; Voitovich, Y.V.; Raux, B.; Carrasco, K.; Muller, C.; Fedorov, A.Y.; Derviaux, C.; Amouric, A.; Betzi, S.; Horvath, D.; et al. Integrated Strategy for Lead Optimization Based on Fragment Growing: The Diversity-Oriented-Target-Focused-Synthesis Approach. *J. Med. Chem.* **2018**. [CrossRef]
72. Waterman, M.J.; Nugraha, A.S.; Hendra, R.; Ball, G.E.; Robinson, S.A.; Keller, P.A. Antarctic Moss Biflavonoids Show High Antioxidant and Ultraviolet-Screening Activity. *J. Nat. Prod.* **2017**, *80*, 2224–2231. [CrossRef] [PubMed]
73. Glunz, P.W. Recent encounters with atropisomerism in drug discovery. *Bioorgan. Med. Chem. Lett.* **2018**, *28*, 53–60. [CrossRef] [PubMed]
74. Jung, M.; Philpott, M.; Müller, S.; Schulze, J.; Badock, V.; Eberspächer, U.; Moosmayer, D.; Bader, B.; Schmees, N.; Fernández-Montalván, A.; Haendler, B. Affinity map of bromodomain protein 4 (BRD4) interactions with the histone H4 tail and the small molecule inhibitor JQ1. *J. Biol. Chem.* **2014**, *289*, 9304–9319. [CrossRef] [PubMed]
75. Scotti, L.; Bezerra Mendonca, F.J.; Ribeiro, F.F.; Tavares, J.F.; da Silva, M.S.; Barbosa Filho, J.M.; Scotti, M.T. Natural Product Inhibitors of Topoisomerases: Review and Docking Study. *Curr. Protein Pept. Sci.* **2018**, *19*, 275–291. [CrossRef] [PubMed]
76. Cardoso, C.R.P.; de Syllos Cólus, I.M.; Bernardi, C.C.; Sannomiya, M.; Vilegas, W.; Varanda, E.A. Mutagenic activity promoted by amentoflavone and methanolic extract of Byrsonima crassa Niedenzu. *Toxicology* **2006**, *225*, 55–63. [CrossRef] [PubMed]
77. Lee, E.-J.; Shin, S.-Y.; Lee, J.-Y.; Lee, S.-J.; Kim, J.-K.; Yoon, D.-Y.; Woo, E.-R.; Kim, Y.-M. Cytotoxic Activities of Amentoflavone against Human Breast and Cervical Cancers are Mediated by Increasing of PTEN Expression Levels due to Peroxisome Proliferator-Activated Receptor γ Activation. *Bull. Korean Chem. Soc.* **2012**, *33*, 2219–2223. [CrossRef]
78. Grynberg, N.F.; Carvalho, M.G.; Velandia, J.R.; Oliveira, M.C.; Moreira, I.C.; Braz- Filho, R.; Echevarria, A. DNA topoisomerase inhibitors: Biflavonoids from Ouratea species. *Braz. J. Med. Biol. Res.* **2002**, *35*, 819–822. [CrossRef] [PubMed]

Marine Organisms as Potential Sources of Bioactive Peptides that Inhibit the Activity of Angiotensin I-Converting Enzyme

Dwi Yuli Pujiastuti [1,*], Muhamad Nur Ghoyatul Amin [1], Mochammad Amin Alamsjah [1,*] and Jue-Liang Hsu [2,3]

1 Department of Marine, Faculty of Fisheries and Marine, Universitas Airlangga, Surabaya 60115, Indonesia
2 Department of Biological Science and Technology, National Pingtung University of Science and Technology, Pingtung 91201, Taiwan
3 Research Center for Austronesian Medicine and Agriculture, National Pingtung University of Science and Technology, Pingtung 91201, Taiwan
* Correspondence: dwiyp@fpk.unair.ac.id (D.Y.P.); alamsjah@fpk.unair.ac.id (M.A.A.);

Abstract: Angiotensin I-converting enzyme (ACE) is a paramount therapeutic target to treat hypertension. ACE inhibitory peptides derived from food protein sources are regarded as safer alternatives to synthetic antihypertensive drugs for treating hypertension. Recently, marine organisms have started being pursued as sources of potential ACE inhibitory peptides. Marine organisms such as fish, shellfish, seaweed, microalgae, molluscs, crustaceans, and cephalopods are rich sources of bioactive compounds because of their high-value metabolites with specific activities and promising health benefits. This review aims to summarize the studies on peptides from different marine organisms and focus on the potential ability of these peptides to inhibit ACE activity.

Keywords: ACE inhibitory peptide; antihypertensive; bioactive peptides; hypertension; marine resources

1. Introduction

Hypertension or high blood pressure is generally caused by behavioral risk factors, ageing, and population growth. It emerged in upper-middle income countries among adults aged >25 years. Hypertension causes 9.4 million deaths each year worldwide [1]. Currently, hypertension is one of the leading causes of morbidity and mortality globally, followed by metabolic disorder [2]. It is a key risk factor for cardiovascular disease, heart attack, stroke, and arteriosclerosis. The common examination used to diagnose hypertension is the measurement of blood pressure; a systolic blood pressure (SBP) and diastolic blood pressure (DBP) higher than 140 mm Hg and 90 mm Hg, respectively, indicates hypertension. To mitigate the aberrations in blood pressure and restore normal physiological function, functional molecules derived from food have been widely pursued.

The renin angiotensin aldosterone system (RAAS) plays a significant role in the maintenance of arterial blood pressure and fluid balance and is regarded as the major target to combat hypertension [3]. In RAAS, angiotensinogen is cleaved by renin, producing angiotensin I. Angiotensin I is then converted to angiotensin II, a strong vasoconstrictor, by angiotensin I-converting enzyme (ACE). In addition, ACE inactivates the vasodilator bradykinin, which acts as a mediator of inflammation, a natriuretic peptide, and a potent stimulator of vasodilator prostaglandins, and is involved in nitric oxide synthesis [4]. Because the production of angiotensin II increases blood pressure [5,6], the inhibition of ACE is a reliable strategy to control hypertension [7]. ACE inhibitors decrease ACE activity and indirectly reduce the angiotensin II level, thereby exerting a vasorelaxation effect on blood vessels [8]. Captopril, enalapril, lisinopril, and benazepril are commonly used as effective synthetic ACE inhibitors and have been developed for treating hypertension. However, synthetic drugs usually cause undesirable side effects [9,10]. To reduce these side effects, food-derived ACE inhibitory peptides are preferred over synthetic drugs to combat hypertension. ACE inhibitory peptides are considered as potent antihypertensive drugs, and they do not have any undesirable side effects. ACE inhibitors are more effective than other hypertensive drugs in retarding the progression of renal damage and reducing proteinuria. Two health organization, namely the international society of hypertension-world health organization (ISHWHO) and the Canadian society of hypertension recommend ACE inhibitors as the first line of treatment for hypertension [11].

Proteins are an important macronutrient as they provide the necessary energy and amino acids essential for growth and the maintenance of normal bodily functions. Many physiological and functional properties of proteins are attributed to bioactive peptides [8]. Bioactive peptides derived from food protein have been growing attractive because of awareness of their health-boosting properties. Bioactive peptides from several natural and processed foods have now been isolated and characterized. They function as potential physiological modulators in the process of metabolism during intestinal digestion and are liberated depending on their structure, composition, and amino acid sequence. Some bioactive peptides have been identified to possess nutraceutical potential and promote overall human health [12], with the potential of being used as candidates for treating conditions, such as hypertension [13].

Bioactive peptides are usually isolated from milk and cheese. They are also isolated from other animal sources, such as meat, gelatin, eggs, and various fish species (salmon, sardine, tuna, and herring), and plant sources, such as mushroom, wheat, pumpkin, and sorghum [14]. For example, ACE inhibitory peptides derived from fish have been shown to have a favorable effect on blood pressure [7,15,16]. Unlike many synthetic ACE inhibitors, which cause dry cough and angioedema, natural peptide-inhibitors have no side effects and are considered to be safer and healthier [17]. In recent years, ACE inhibitors have been derived from food proteins, such as milk [18,19], corn [20,21], ovalbumin [22], legume [23,24], Chinese soft-shelled turtle eggs [25,26], bitter melon seeds [27], cheese [28,29], chicken eggs [30–33], casein [34–36], fish [37–39], and algae [40,41].

Oceans cover >70% of the earth's surface and are a rich resource for humans. There is increasing interest in marine organisms as new sources of natural products. Several compounds with unique biological activities have been isolated from marine organisms. The marine environment is rich in biological as well as chemical diversity; compounds isolated from marine organisms have been used as pharmaceuticals, nutraceuticals, cosmeceuticals, molecular probes, fine chemicals, and agrochemicals. Macro-and microorganisms in marine habitats possess a wide array of secondary metabolites, including terpenes, steroids, polyketides, peptides, alkaloids, polysaccharides, proteins, and porphyrins. Because the environment surrounding marine organisms is extreme, aggressive, and competitive, these organisms produce several secondary metabolites with a promising potential for use as drugs, nutritional supplements, and therapeutic agents [42–44]. Marine organisms, such as fish, shellfish, seaweed, microalgae, molluscs, crustaceans, and cephalopods, are rich sources of several functional compounds, such as bioactive peptides, enzymes, polyunsaturated fatty acids, vitamins, minerals, phenolic phlorotannins, and polysaccharides. Moreover, as some marine organisms, especially fish, are particularly rich sources of protein, they are ideal for generating protein-derived bioactive peptides [45,46]. Marine bioactive peptides have gained significant attention for their health promoting effects, such as antihypertensive, antioxidant, anticoagulant, antimicrobial, antithrombotic, and hypocholesterolemic properties [47]. Furthermore, compounds isolated from marine organisms have been commercially distributed in health markets [48]. In this review, we discuss the ACE inhibitory peptides derived from marine resources and provide information on their production, characterization, and potential health benefits. We also review the future prospects of ACE inhibitory peptides derived from marine organisms as therapeutic drugs to combat hypertension.

2. ACE Inhibitory Peptides Derived from Marine Organisms

Zinc ion (Zn^{2+})-dependent dipeptidyl carboxypeptidase, also known as ACE (EC 3.4.15.1), plays a pivotal role in the regulation of blood pressure because of its action in RAAS [49]. ACE is present in biological fluids, such as plasma and semen, and in many tissues, such as testis, intestinal epithelial cells, proximal renal tubular cells, brain, lungs, stimulated macrophages, vascular endothelium, and the medial and adventitial layers of blood vessel walls [4]. In humans, ACE exists in two isoforms: somatic ACE (sACE) and germinal ACE (gACE). sACE is distributed in many types of endothelial and epithelial cells, whereas gACE occurs in germinal cells in the testis, and is therefore also known as testicular ACE [6]. In RAAS, ACE cleaves the decapeptide angiotensin I (Asp-Arg-Val-Tyr-Ile-His-Pro-Phe-His-Leu) into the octapeptide angiotensin II (Asp-Arg-Val-Tyr-Ile-His-Pro-Phe) by removing the C-terminal dipeptide His-Leu. Angiotensin II stimulates the release of aldosterone and antidiuretic hormone or vasopressin, consequently increasing the retention of sodium and water; it also acts as a potent vasoconstrictor (Figure 1). These phenomena act in concert to directly increase the blood pressure [6]. Substrates of ACE include not only angiotensin I in RAAS and bradykinin in the kinin–kallikrein system, but also the haemoregulatory peptide *N*-acetyl-Ser-Asp-Lys-Pro, which is a putative bone marrow suppressor. It contributes to haemopoietic cell differentiation, regulating tissue and blood levels of the vasoactive hormones angiotensin II and bradykinin [50]. In addition, ACE shows endopeptidase activity against a wide range of substrates, such as cholecystokinin, substance P, and luliberin. The inhibition of ACE enzymatic activity on angiotensin I is one of the major challenges to combat hypertension-related disorders [51].

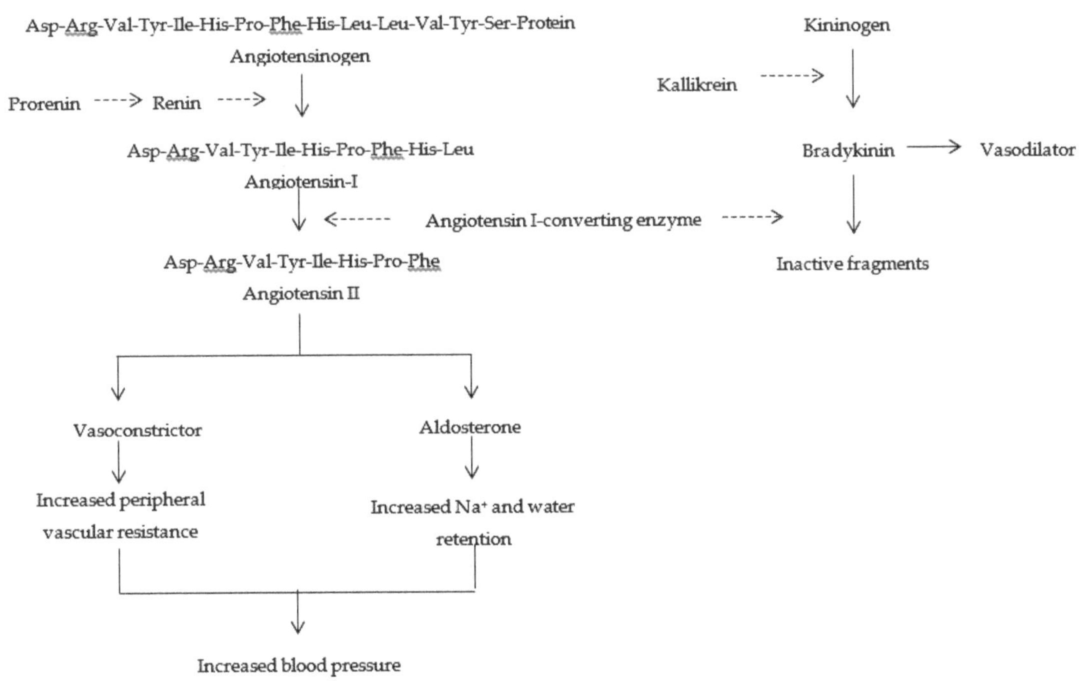

Figure 1. Role of angiotensin I-converting enzyme in the renin angiotensin aldosterone system and the kinin–kallikrein system [15].

Recently, natural marine products have been investigated as alternative synthetic drugs; they have been the topic of interest for many researchers due to their numerous beneficial effects, and some novel ACE-inhibitory compounds have been isolated from algae [52,53]. Marine proteins, such as Heshiko, a fermented mackerel product [38], sardine muscle [9], shark meat [54], Alaska pollock skin [55], marine shrimp [56], and chum salmon [57], exhibit ACE inhibitory activity. ACE inhibitory peptides usually contains 2–12 amino acid residues [10,58,59]. However, some studies have identified up to 27 amino acid residues in ACE inhibitory peptides [60,61]. Proteases, such as pepsin, chymotrypsin, alcalase, and trypsin, are frequently used in hydrolysis for generating ACE inhibitory peptides [9,10,55]. List of identified peptides derived from marine resources; origin, sequence peptides, and IC_{50} value, can be seen in Table 1.

Table 1. List of identified peptides derived from marine resources; origin, sequence peptides, and IC_{50} value.

Origin	Enzyme	Sequence Peptide	IC_{50} (μM)	Reference
	Fish			
Sea bream	Alkaline Protease	GY VY GF VIY	265 16 708 7.5	[62]
Lizard fish	Neutral Protease	MKCAF RVCLP	45.7 175	[63] [64]
Alaska pollock (*Theragra chalcogramma*)	Alcalase, Pronase E and Collagenase	GPL GPM	2.6 17.3	[55]
Grass carp	Alcalase	VAP	19.9	[10]
Atlantic salmon (*Salmo salar* L.)	Alcalase and Papain	AP VR	356.9 1301.1	[65]
Skipjack (*Katsuwonus pelamis*)	Alcalase	DLDLRKDLYAN MCYPAST MLVFAV	67.4 58.7 3.07	[66]
Yellowfin sole (*Limanda aspera*)	Chymotrypsin	MIFPGAGGPEL	268.3	[67]
Pacific cod	Pepsin	GASSGMPG LAYA	6.9 14.5	[68]
Paralichthys alivaceus	Pepsin	MEVFVP VSQLTR	79 105	[69]
Channa striatus	Thermolysin	VPAAPPK NGTWFEPP	0.45 0.63	[70]
	Microalgae			
Chlorella vulgaris	Pepsin	IVVE FAL AEL VVPPA AFL	315 26.3 57.1 79.5 63.8	[40]
Chlorella ellipsoidea	Alcalase	VEGY	128.4	[71]
Spirulina platensis	Pepsin	IAE IAPG VAF	34.7 11.4 35.8	[40]
	Molluscs			
Sea cucumber (*Acaudina molpadioidea*)	Bromelain and Alcalase	MEGAQEAQGD	15.9	[72]
Cuttlefish (*Sepia officinalis*)	Cuttlefish hepatopancreas	VYAP VIIF MAW	6.1 8.7 16.32	[73]
		GIHETTY EKSYELP VELYP	25.66 14.41 5.22	[74]
Squid (*Dosidicus gigas*) skin collagen	Esperase	GRGSVPAPGP	47.78	[75]
Corbicula fluminea	Protamex + Flavourzyme	VKP	3.7	[76]
		VKK	1045	

The potency of peptides derived from marine organisms is expressed as the half maximal inhibitory concentration (IC_{50}), which indicates the ACE inhibitor concentration that leads to 50% inhibition of ACE activity. Moreover, Lineweaver–Burk plots are usually used to determine the inhibition mode of

ACE inhibitory peptides. Most of the reported peptides act as competitive inhibitors of ACE. In the competitive inhibition mode, the inhibitor competes with the substrate and binds to the active site of ACE. In the non-competitive inhibition mode, the inhibitor binds to a site other than the active site. The binding of inhibitor to ACE alters the conformation of ACE, which prevents the substrate from binding to the active site of ACE. The enzyme, substrate, and inhibitor cannot form a complex; thus, the enzyme–substrate complex or enzyme–inhibitor complex is formed. In the uncompetitive inhibition mode, the inhibitor binds to only the substrate–enzyme complex. The C-terminal end of the inhibitory peptide associates with the active site pockets of ACE. ACE harbors three sub-sites: antepenultimate position (S1), penultimate position (S1′), and ultimate position (S2′). In the substrate, the amino acids Pro, Ala, Val, and Leu are the most favorable for S1; Ile is the most favorable for S1′; and Pro and Leu are the most favorable for S2′ [77]. The S1 sub-site includes Ala354, Glu384, and Tyr523 residues; S1′ pocket contains Glu162; and S2′ pocket includes Gln281, His353, His513, Lys511, and Tyr520 [78,79]. Many studies have shown that peptides with high ACE inhibitory activity contain Trp, Phe, Tyr, or Pro at the C-terminus and branched aliphatic amino acids at the N-terminus [49].

In China, soft-shelled turtle eggs have been used as a tonic food for a long time. Low-molecular weight peptides (<3 kDa) have been isolated from soft-shelled turtle egg by ultrafiltration and fractionated by reversed-phase high-performance liquid chromatography (RP-HPLC). In vitro screening of the resulting fractions for ACE inhibitory activity has revealed an IC_{50} value of 4.39 μM for the peptide IVRDPNGMGAW isolated from soft-shelled turtle egg white. This peptide has been identified as a competitive inhibitor of ACE [26]. The peptide AKLPSW, isolated from soft-shelled turtle egg yolk, has also been shown to exhibit potent ACE inhibitory activity, with an IC_{50} value of 15.3 μM, and inhibition kinetics has indicated that this peptide is a non-competitive inhibitor of ACE. The AKLPSW peptide significantly reduces the systolic blood pressure by approximately 13 mm Hg after 6 h of oral administration, thus confirming its antihypertensive effect [25]. In another study, Sardinella protein hydrolysates (SPHs) were obtained from fermentation with *Bacillus subtilis* (SPH-A26) and *Bacillus amyloliquefaciens* (SPH-An6). Approximately 800 peptides have been identified in SPH-A26 and SPH-An6 using nano electrospray ionization liquid chromatography tandem mass spectrometry. Of these 800 peptides, eight isolated from SPH-A26 and seven from SPH-An6 have been selected based on homologies with previously characterized peptides (Biopep data bank), as well as peptide length. Among the synthesized peptides, NVPVYEGY and ITALAPSTM show ACE inhibitory activity with IC_{50} values of 210 and 229 μM, respectively. Fermented SPHs have a potential for use as hypotensive nutraceutical ingredients [80]. The popular freshwater tilapia also reported the potential antihypertensive peptides from hydrolysate by using papain, bromelain, and pepsin. In order to enhance the activity, the hydrolysate was fractionated into four fractions (<1 kDa, 1–3 kDa, 3–5 kDa, and 5–10 kDa). The pepsin-hydrolyzed FPH (FPHPe) with the highest DH (23%) possessed the strongest ACE-inhibitory activity (IC_{50} of 0.57 mg/mL). Its <1 kDa ultrafiltration fraction (FPHPe1) suppressed both ACE (IC_{50} of 0.41 mg/mL). In addition, FPHPe1 significantly reduced SBP (maximum −33 mmHg), DBP (maximum −24 mmHg), mean arterial pressure (MAP) (maximum −28 mmHg), and hearth rates (HR) (maximum −58 beats) in SHRs [81].

The production of peptides with ACE inhibitory activity must consider the amino acid composition and molecular weight of hydrolysates. Purification is carried out to obtain a single peptide with a specific amino acid residues which is in accordance with characterized sequence of bioactive peptide inhibiting ACE. The pure peptide could be easily observed its activity and stability, as well as the dosage of peptide administration in the patients with hypertension symptom would be validly determined. Total hydrolysates with high molecular weight revealed lower activity for inhibiting the ACE rather than single peptide. The shorter amino acid residues is more visible to reach the target site when through the digestive tract and they can be absorbed easily. Then, lower-molecular weight peptides also have a higher probability of passing through the intestinal barrier and exerting biological function [65]. The C-terminal residue in tripeptides or dipeptides plays an important role in binding to sub-sites S1, S1′, and S2′ sub-sites within the active site of ACE [82]. Aromatic or hydrophobic amino acid residues, such as Trp, Phe, Tyr, and Pro, are more active if present at positions in the C-terminal end that bind to each of the three sub-sites of ACE. In addition, tripeptides or dipeptides with a branched aliphatic amino acid at the N-terminus show potent ACE inhibition. Basic amino acid residues, such as Lys and Arg, at the C-terminus also contribute to potent inhibition against ACE [83]. Many studies have shown that the C-terminal residue of potent ACE inhibitory peptides is usually a hydrophobic amino acid [39,70,74,84,85].

There is no correlation between competitive inhibitor with high ACE inhibitory activity. Several non-competitive inhibitors show high ACE inhibitory activity. The peptide Ala-Lys-Leu-Pro-Ser-Trp derived from soft-shelled turtle egg yolk exhibits a low IC_{50} value of 13.7 μM [25], whereas the peptide Val-Glu-Leu-Tyr-Pro isolated from cuttlefish muscle protein exhibits an even lower IC_{50} value of 5.22 μM [74]; both these peptides are considered non-competitive inhibitors. Moreover, some peptides inhibit ACE activity by the uncompetitive mode of inhibition. For example, the peptides Ile-Trp and Phe-Tyr have been ientified as uncompetitive inhibitors [86]; similarly, the peptides Tyr-Ley-Tyr-Glu-Ile-Ala and Tyr-Leu-Tyr-Glu-Ile-Ala-Arg-Arg have been identified as uncompetitive inhibitors [87]. Depending on the results of pre-incubation of the peptide with ACE, the ACE inhibitory peptides are divided into three categories: true inhibitors, prodrugs, and real substrates. A true inhibitor shows no significant difference in the IC_{50} value before and after pre-incubation with ACE, whereas a prodrug shows dramatic reduction in the IC_{50} value after pre-incubation with ACE. On the other hand, a real substrate shows an increase in the IC_{50} value after pre-incubation with ACE, suggesting a reduction in its inhibitory activity against ACE. Generally, the prodrug- and true inhibitor-type peptides are expected to exhibit long-lasting antihypertensive activity in spontaneously hypertensive rats used as a model to study hypertension in humans [88,89].

3. Generation of Bioactive Peptides

Protein hydrolysates have an excellent amino acid balance, are readily digestible, show rapid uptake, and contain bioactive peptides [90]. Bioactive peptides act as therapeutic agents and are characterized by high biological specificity, low toxicity, high structural diversity, high and wide spectrum of activity, and small size, which implies that they have a low likelihood of triggering undesirable immune responses [91]. Bioactive peptides are defined as protein fragments with beneficial effects on bodily functions and human health. Peptides isolated from food sources are structurally similar to endogenous peptides and therefore interact with the same receptors and play a prominent role as immune regulators, growth factors, and modifiers of food intake [92]. Depending on the sequence of amino acids, these peptides can exhibit diverse activities, including antimicrobial [93], antioxidant [94], antithrombotic [95], and antihypertensive [25].

Bioactive peptides are generally produced via enzymatic hydrolysis using digestive enzymes, fermentation using proteolytic starter cultures, or proteolysis using microorganism-or plant-derived enzymes. To generate short-chain functional peptides, enzymatic hydrolysis is used in combination with fermentation or proteolysis [96]. During growth, microorganisms release the protease enzyme into the extracellular medium, leading to proteolysis and peptide generation. Microorganisms are typically used for fermentation for several hours to several days, depending on the desired peptide and the type of fermentation [97]. During fermentation, microorganisms break down complex compounds into smaller molecules with various physiological functions [98]. Fermented marine food products are rich sources of bioactive compounds, including amino acids and peptides [99]. Digestive enzymes, such as trypsin, chymotrypsin, and pepsin, release the bioactive peptides for gastrointestinal digestion in vivo. To stimulate gastrointestinal digestion, several proteolytic enzymes, such as alcalase and thermolysin, engage with trypsin and pepsin. In addition, recombinant DNA technology and chemical synthesis have been used to produce bioactive peptides [92]. The physicochemical properties, such as molecular weight, isoelectric point, and hydrophilic or hydrophobic indices of the resulting peptides, change after enzymatic hydrolysis. Prominent amino acids, such as Pro and Val, play key roles in most antihypertensive peptides [91].

In the digestive system, bioactive peptides are absorbed through the intestine and enter the blood stream to exert systemic effects or local effects in the gastrointestinal tract. Dipeptides and tripeptides are easily absorbed in the intestine. To exert antihypertensive effects, bioactive peptides must reach the target cells after absorption through the intestine. Common bioactive peptides with antihypertensive effects include Val-Pro-Pro (VPP) and Ile-Pro-Pro (IPP); they are produced via fermentation using *Lactobacillus helveticus* and *Saccharomyces cerevisiae*. These two peptides have been detected in the aortal tissue using HPLC, and their effect on ACE activity was lower in the aorta in the study group than in the control group (saline) [14].

4. Screening Approach

The search for peptides capable of inhibiting ACE activity has been intensified. The pursue of ACE inhibitory peptides from marine, as well as other sources, has been substantiated. A reliable assay to determine the ability of peptides to inhibit ACE activity is of paramount concern. In vitro determination of ACE inhibitory peptides is preceded by enzymatic digestion or microbial fermentation, followed by the analysis of structure and chemical synthesis of active peptides. Most assays evaluating the ACE inhibitory activity of peptides have been performed as described previously [100]. The technique used to evaluate the ACE inhibitory activity of peptides must be simple, sensitive, and reliable. Several such methods have been developed, such as spectrophotometry, HPLC, fluorometric capillary electrophoresis, and radiochemistry. Among these, spectrophotometry is the most commonly used method to measure ACE inhibitory activity. This method involves the hydrolysis of hippuryl-histidyl-leucine (HHL) by ACE to hippuric acid (HA). The amount of HA produced from HHL is directly correlated with ACE activity [101]. The amount of HA formed is determined by measuring the absorbance at 228 nm (absorption maximum of HA) [102]. Although the spectrophotometry is useful, it is time consuming, complicated, and is unable to detect trace amounts of the sample.

In practice, results of different assays may vary because of the use of different substrates, such as the synthetic peptides HHL and furanacryloyl-L-phenylalanylglycyl-glycine (FAPGG), which are the most commonly used substrates, and the fluorescent molecule o-aminobenzoylglycyl-p-nitrophenylalanylproline for specific detection and quantification [103]. Results may also vary within the same assay because of the use of different test conditions or the use of ACE from different origins. Thus, ACE activity levels must be carefully controlled to obtain comparable and reproducible results [83,104].

HPLC is a common method to determine ACE inhibitory activity of peptides as it generates reproducible results. Although HPLC has been used for decades, it requires the extraction of the product from the reaction mixture using an organic solvent, which limits the number of samples that can be analyzed per day and is also a source of error [105]. Moreover, HPLC analysis shows peculiar results from samples with added inhibitor, which exhibit high HA release than samples without the added inhibitor. This occurs if the enzyme or the substrate (HHL) is unstable in solution. The evaluation of ACE inhibition is depends on the comparison between the concentration of HA in the presence or absence of an inhibitor (inhibitor blank). The occurrence of autolysis of HHL to give HA was evaluated by a reaction blank, i.e., a sample with the higher inhibitor concentration and without the enzyme [24]. Another substrate, FAPGG, has also been used for HPLC [106,107]; FAPGG releases 2-furylacryloyl-L-phenylalanine (FAP) as a product. This method is used to quantitate the levels and can be used a model of inhibition according to the sigmoid character of the response curve. The slope of the curve, describing absorbance versus time, is thus a direct measure of ACE activity. It is based on the combination of enzymatic reaction with HPLC detection of the inhibition of enzyme activity by measuring the levels of the substrate and product formed. The amount of FAP formed is determined by measuring the absorbance at 305 nm. This method is beneficial, as it does not require sophisticated equipment or radiolabelled compounds [108]. Because the price of the two substrates, HHL and FAPGG, is similar, the HPLC method is advantageous over spectrophotometry, as it requires less labor and has a higher throughput than spectrophotometry [103].

The determination of ACE activity also utilizes fluorescent tripeptides, such as *o*-aminobenzoylglycyl-*p*-nitro-L-phenylalanyl-L-proline [Abz-Gly-Phe(NO_2)-Pro]. The hydrolysis of this substrate by ACE generates o-aminobenzoylglycine (Abz-Gly) as a product, which is easily quantified fluorometrically using appropriate excitation and emission wavelengths. Fluorescence detection of the reaction products is highly sensitive and precise. Moreover, commercial availability of all reagents is a major advantage, allowing easy introduction of the assay in laboratories [109].

To obtain ACE inhibitory peptides, slight modification of the assay is crucial. Orthogonal bioassay-guided fractionation is considered as a potential method to obtain ACE inhibitory peptides. This method involves the separation of the potential peptides using two ways of fractionation: Strong cation exchange (SCX) and RP-HPLC (Figure 2). SCX separates peptides based on their charge, whereas RP-HPLC separates peptides based on their hydrophobicity [110]. Although both SCX and RP-HPLC separate peptides using different mechanisms, peptides are regarded as potential ACE inhibitors because they remain in the most active fraction using both methods. Pujiastuti et al. [25] revealed the identification of overlapping peptides using SCX and RP-HPLC.

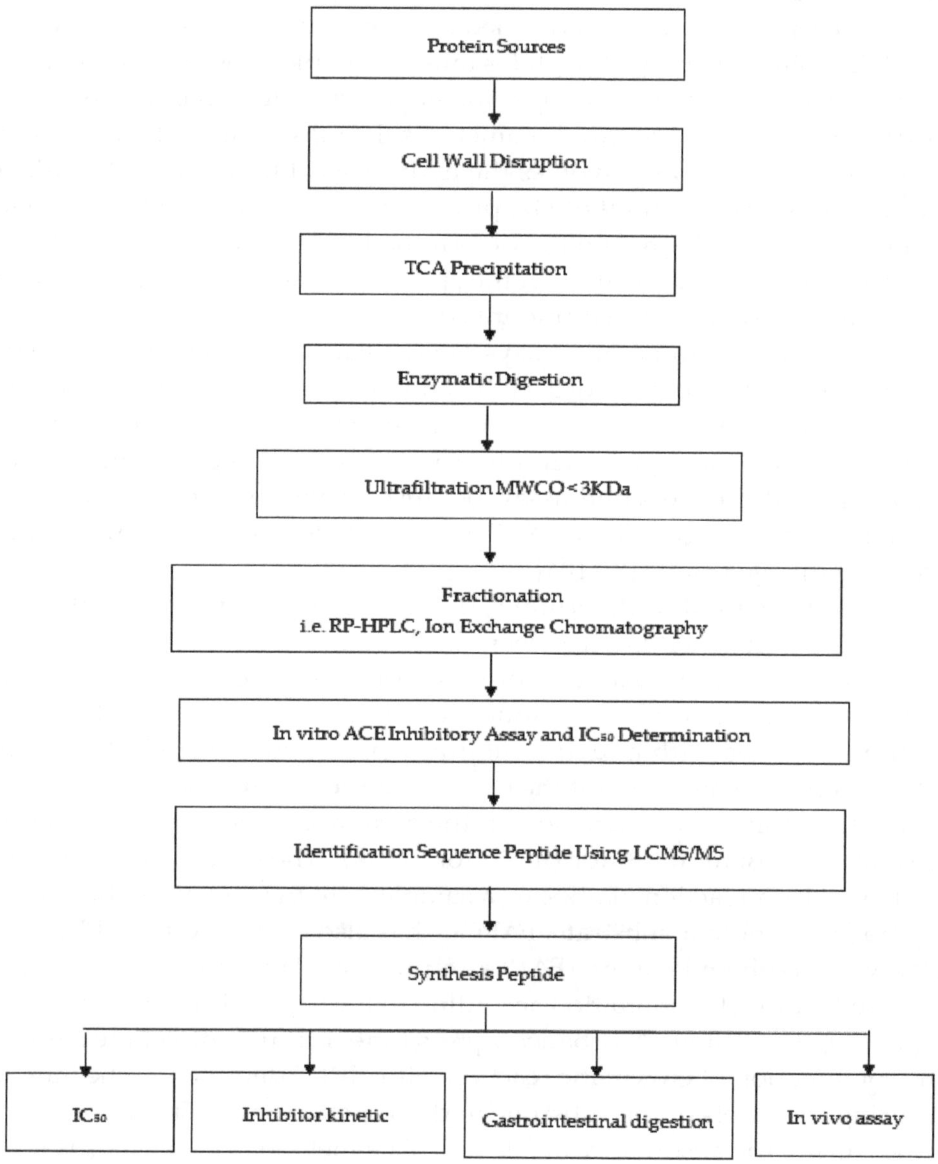

Figure 2. Flowchart showing the production of bioactive peptides for angiotensin I-converting enzyme (ACE) inhibitory assay [25].

A new method used to measure ACE activity is ultra-performance liquid chromatography (UPLC). The UPLC-mass spectrometry method has been developed to determine ACE activity using HHL as the substrate and purified rabbit ACE. This method is rapid, accurate, and reproducible, and is used to determine trace amounts of compounds. In addition, this method requires a short analysis time and small reaction volume and is highly selective compared to conventional methods. It is also suitable for high-throughput screening of potential ACE inhibitors and candidate compounds isolated from herbal medicines [111].

The in vitro gastrointestinal digestion approach provides a straightforward approach to imitate peptide function by incubating the peptide with ACE before in vivo oral administration. Oral administration of ACE inhibitory peptides in hypertensive patients requires these peptides to pass through the digestive tract and be absorbed through the intestinal epithelium. Pepsin is widely used to represent gastrointestinal enzymes that function at acidic pH. Polypeptides are further truncated by pancreatic proteases, including trypsin, α-chymotrypsin, elastase, and carboxypeptidases A and B at alkaline pH. In vivo testing of peptides is frequently performed in spontaneously hypertensive rats as they mimic hypertension in humans. This animal model has been used to evaluate the effects of both short-and long-term administration of antihypertensive peptides. In human studies, food-derived peptides have been used to establish whether peptides exhibit an antihypertensive effect in humans with high-to-normal blood pressure. For example, the antihypertensive effect of the peptides IPP and VPP isolated from the commercial fermented milk show antihypertensive effects after long-term administration. The sour milk product Calpis from Japan has been examined in mildly hypertensive patients [112]. In some cases, ACE inhibitory peptides fail to show hypotensive activity after oral administration in vivo, possibly because of the hydrolysis of these peptides by ACE or gastrointestinal proteases [74,113]. It is difficult to evaluate a direct correlation between in vitro ACE inhibitory activity and in vivo antihypertensive activity because the bioavailability of these peptides after oral administration varies. ACE inhibitory peptides must remain active during gastrointestinal digestion and reach the specific organ. However, it is possible that ACE inhibitory peptides are degraded before reaching the specific organ. The antihypertensive mechanism of ACE inhibitory peptides, rather than the ACE inhibition mechanism, may be of greater interest [77,114].

In silico methods are used to predict the structure of ACE inhibitory peptides based on similarity between sequences available in databases. The molecular docking approach is widely used to predict and characterize the binding site of target proteins according to ligand conformation and binding affinity score [115]. The most convenient approach to elucidate the accuracy of molecular docking is to determine the distance of binding conformation using the scoring function in the docking program [116]. Several scoring functions are used to evaluate the docking procedure, such as CDocker Energy, CDocker Interaction Energy, LibDockScore, PLP1, PLP2, LigScore1, LigScore2, Jain, PMF, and PMFO4. Besides, BIOPEP-UWM and BLAST database is increasingly popular to be in silico approaches for investigating biological activities from tilapia and chickpea [117]. BIOPEP-UWM database is used to predict bioactive peptides composed in protein sequences. This method has benefits such as time and cost reduction, as well as being a rapid method to identify and characterize proteins. Briefly, the bioactivities, sequences, number, and location of the peptides were obtained from the sequences of the identified proteins analyzed using the "profiles of potential bioactivity" tool. Moreover, the sequences of the identified proteins were examined using the "enzyme action" tool to simulate enzymatic hydrolysis [118]. Knowing the position of the binding site before docking significantly increases the docking efficiency. Moreover, knowledge of the structure and activity relationship is important to explore potential ACE inhibitory peptides. The ACE structure contains a Zn site, which usually coordinates with oxygen, nitrogen, and sulphur donors of Asp, Cys, and His, respectively, wherein His is the most regularly encountered in the sphere of Zn^{2+} ion. The other Zn ligand in catalytic sites is water; it is activated for polarization, ionization, and arrangement of ligands in coordination with Zn [11]. The Zn^{2+} ion is also important for the binding strength between ACE and its inhibitors [119]. Generally, ACE inhibitors contain one or more molecular functionalities, such as Zn-binding ligand, a hydrogen bond donor, and a carboxyl-terminal group [120]. The ability of a protein to interact with small molecules plays a major role in the dynamics of that protein, which may enhance or inhibit its biological function. Studies on the catalytic mechanism of ACE have revealed that the 19 amino acid residues in the active site of ACE, including His353, Ala354, Ser355, Ala356, His383, Glu384, His387, Phe391, Pro407, His410, Glu411, Phe512, His513, Ser516, Ser517, Val518, Pro519, Arg522, and Tyr523, bind to small molecules or to protein (ligand).

5. Conclusions

Bioactive peptides derived from marine resources have potential ACE inhibitory activity and are considered as therapeutic agents to combat hypertension. The main characteristic of ACE inhibitory peptides is the position of the hydrophobic residue, usually Pro, at the C-terminus. In vitro and in vivo testing are the most challenging tasks in antihypertensive research as their results do not always show direct correlation, although gastrointestinal digestion is suggested to mimic peptide release in human body. Marine organisms represent sustainable sources of ACE inhibitory peptides for the production of pharmaceuticals and nutraceuticals at an industrial scale. Due to the importance of pure peptide inhibiting ACE for future pharmaceutical and nutraceutical industry, the purification techniques of identified peptide is highly crucial. Therefore, upscaling research on bioactive peptide purification should trigger biotechnologists to perform the research.

Highlights:

- Angiotensin I-converting enzyme (ACE) is a key target for treating hypertension.
- Food-derived bioactive peptides inhibit ACE activity, decreasing blood pressure.
- These peptides improve bodily functions and human health, without adverse effects.
- Marine organisms are sustainable sources of ACE inhibitory peptides.
- Various methods for their industrial production and testing are available.

Author Contributions: Conceptualization, writing original draft preparation, D.Y.P.; English editing, M.N.G.A. and J.-L.H.; project administration, M.A.A.; supervision J.-L.H., review, editing, read and approve the final manuscript, ALL.

Acknowledgments: We gratefully acknowledge to Scientific Publication and Journal Development Center (PPJPI) Universitas Airlangga for English proofreading and Department of Biological Science and Technology, NPUST, Taiwan for supporting this work.

References

1. World Health Organization. World Health Day 2013. *Glob. Brief Hypertens.* **2013**, 9–11.
2. Ferreira-Santos, P.; Carrón, R.; Recio, I.; Sevilla, M.Á.; Montero, M.J. Effects of milk casein hydrolyzate supplemented with phytosterols on hypertension and lipid profile in hypercholesterolemic hypertensive rats. *J. Funct. Foods* **2017**, *28*, 168–176. [CrossRef]
3. Volpe, M.; Battistoni, A.; Chin, D.; Rubattu, S.D.; Tocci, G. Renin as a biomarker of cardiovascular disease in clinical practice. *Nutr. Metab. Cardiovasc. Dis.* **2012**, *22*, 312–317. [CrossRef]
4. Meng, Q.C.; Oparil, S. Purification and assay methods for angiotensin-converting enzyme. *J. Chromatogr. A* **1996**, *743*, 105–122. [CrossRef]
5. Bhullar, K.S.; Lassalle-Claux, G.; Touaibia, M.; Rupasinghe, H.V. Antihypertensive effect of caffeic acid and its analogs through dual renin–angiotensin–aldosterone system inhibition. *Eur. J. Pharmacol.* **2014**, *730*, 125–132. [CrossRef]
6. Guang, C.; Phillips, R.D.; Jiang, B.; Milani, F. Three key proteases–angiotensin-I-converting enzyme (ACE), ACE2 and renin–within and beyond the renin-angiotensin system. *Arch. Cardiovasc. Dis.* **2012**, *105*, 373–385. [CrossRef]

7. Lee, S.-H.; Qian, Z.-J.; Kim, S.-K. A novel angiotensin I converting enzyme inhibitory peptide from tuna frame protein hydrolysate and its antihypertensive effect in spontaneously hypertensive rats. *Food Chem.* **2010**, *118*, 96–102. [CrossRef]
8. Shahidi, F.; Zhong, Y. Bioactive Peptides. *J. AOAC Int.* **2008**, *91*, 914–931.
9. Bougatef, A.; Nedjar-Arroume, N.; Ravallec-Plé, R.; Leroy, Y.; Guillochon, D.; Barkia, A.; Nasri, M. Angiotensin I-converting enzyme (ACE) inhibitory activities of sardinelle (Sardinella aurita) by-products protein hydrolysates obtained by treatment with microbial and visceral fish serine proteases. *Food Chem.* **2008**, *111*, 350–356. [CrossRef]
10. Chen, J.; Wang, Y.; Zhong, Q.; Wu, Y.; Xia, W. Purification and characterization of a novel angiotensin-I converting enzyme (ACE) inhibitory peptide derived from enzymatic hydrolysate of grass carp protein. *Peptides* **2012**, *33*, 52–58. [CrossRef]
11. Spyroulias, G.; Galanis, A.; Pairas, G.; Manessi-Zoupa, E.; Cordopatis, P. Structural Features of Angiotensin-I Converting Enzyme Catalytic Sites: Conformational Studies in Solution, Homology Models and Comparison with Other Zinc Metallopeptidases. *Curr. Top. Med. Chem.* **2004**, *4*, 403–429. [CrossRef]
12. Lee, J.K.; Hong, S.; Jeon, J.-K.; Kim, S.-K.; Byun, H.-G. Purification and characterization of angiotensin I converting enzyme inhibitory peptides from the rotifer, Brachionus rotundiformis. *Bioresour. Technol.* **2009**, *100*, 5255–5259. [CrossRef]
13. Udenigwe, C.C. Bioinformatics approaches, prospects and challenges of food bioactive peptide research. *Trends Food Sci. Technol.* **2014**, *36*, 137–143. [CrossRef]
14. Möller, N.P.; Scholz-Ahrens, K.E.; Roos, N.; Schrezenmeir, J. Bioactive peptides and proteins from foods: Indication for health effects. *Eur. J. Nutr.* **2008**, *47*, 171–182. [CrossRef]
15. Li, G.-H.; Le, G.-W.; Shi, Y.-H.; Shrestha, S. Angiotensin I–converting enzyme inhibitory peptides derived from food proteins and their physiological and pharmacological effects. *Nutr. Res.* **2004**, *24*, 469–486. [CrossRef]
16. Wilson, J.; Hayes, M.; Carney, B. Angiotensin-I-converting enzyme and prolyl endopeptidase inhibitory peptides from natural sources with a focus on marine processing by-products. *Food Chem.* **2011**, *129*, 235–244. [CrossRef]
17. Li, Y.; Sadiq, F.A.; Liu, T.; Chen, J.; He, G. Purification and identification of novel peptides with inhibitory effect against angiotensin I-converting enzyme and optimization of process conditions in milk fermented with the yeast Kluyveromyces marxianus. *J. Funct. Foods* **2015**, *16*, 278–288. [CrossRef]
18. Yu, Y.; Hu, J.; Miyaguchi, Y.; Bai, X.; Du, Y.; Lin, B. Isolation and characterization of angiotensin I-converting enzyme inhibitory peptides derived from porcine hemoglobin. *Peptides* **2006**, *27*, 2950–2956. [CrossRef]
19. Chen, Y.; Wang, Z.; Chen, X.; Liu, Y.; Zhang, H.; Sun, T. Identification of angiotensin I-converting enzyme inhibitory peptides from koumiss, a traditional fermented mare's milk. *J. Dairy Sci.* **2010**, *93*, 884–892. [CrossRef]
20. Yang, Y.; Tao, G.; Liu, P.; Liu, J. Peptide with Angiotensin I-Converting Enzyme Inhibitory Activity from Hydrolyzed Corn Gluten Meal. *J. Agric. Food Chem.* **2007**, *55*, 7891–7895. [CrossRef]
21. Suh, H.J.; Whang, J.H.; Kim, Y.S.; Bae, S.H.; Noh, D.O. Preparation od angiotensin I converting enzyme inhibitor from corn gluten. *Process Biochem.* **2003**, *38*, 1239–1244. [CrossRef]
22. Huang, Q.; Li, S.-G.; Teng, H.; Jin, Y.-G.; Ma, M.-H.; Song, H.-B. Optimizing preparation conditions for Angiotensin-I-converting enzyme inhibitory peptides derived from enzymatic hydrolysates of ovalbumin. *Food Sci. Biotechnol.* **2015**, *24*, 2193–2198. [CrossRef]
23. Zhang, Y.; Pechan, T.; Chang, S.K. Antioxidant and angiotensin-I converting enzyme inhibitory activities of phenolic extracts and fractions derived from three phenolic-rich legume varieties. *J. Funct. Foods* **2018**, *42*, 289–297. [CrossRef]
24. Boschin, G.; Scigliuolo, G.M.; Resta, D.; Arnoldi, A. ACE-inhibitory activity of enzymatic protein hydrolysates from lupin and other legumes. *Food Chem.* **2014**, *145*, 34–40. [CrossRef]
25. Pujiastuti, D.Y.; Shih, Y.-H.; Chen, W.-L.; Hsu, J.-L. Screening of angiotensin-I converting enzyme inhibitory peptides derived from soft-shelled turtle yolk using two orthogonal bioassay-guided fractionations. *J. Funct. Foods* **2017**, *28*, 36–47. [CrossRef]
26. Rawendra, R.D.; Chang, C.-I.; Chen, H.-H.; Huang, T.-C.; Hsu, J.-L. A novel angiotensin converting enzyme inhibitory peptide derived from proteolytic digest of Chinese soft-shelled turtle egg white proteins. *J. Proteom.* **2013**, *94*, 359–369. [CrossRef]

27. Priyanto, A.D.; Doerksen, R.J.; Chang, C.-I.; Sung, W.-C.; Widjanarko, S.B.; Kusnadi, J.; Lin, Y.-C.; Wang, T.-C.; Hsu, J.-L. Screening, discovery, and characterization of angiotensin-I converting enzyme inhibitory peptides derived from proteolytic hydrolysate of bitter melon seed proteins. *J. Proteom.* **2015**, *128*, 424–435. [CrossRef]
28. Lu, Y.; Govindasamy-Lucey, S.; Lucey, J.A. Angiotensin-I-converting enzyme-inhibitory peptides in commercial Wisconsin Cheddar cheeses of different ages. *J. Dairy Sci.* **2016**, *99*, 41–52. [CrossRef]
29. Sieber, R.; Bütikofer, U.; Egger, C.; Portmann, R.; Walther, B.; Wechsler, D. ACE-inhibitory activity and ACE-inhibiting peptides in different cheese varieties. *Dairy Sci. Technol.* **2010**, *90*, 47–73. [CrossRef]
30. Majumder, K.; Chakrabarti, S.; Morton, J.S.; Panahi, S.; Kaufman, S.; Davidge, S.T.; Wu, J. Egg-derived ACE-inhibitory peptides IQW and LKP reduce blood pressure in spontaneously hypertensive rats. *J. Funct. Foods* **2015**, *13*, 50–60. [CrossRef]
31. Miguel, M.; Alonso, M.J.; Salaices, M.; Aleixandre, A.; López-Fandiño, R. Antihypertensive, ACE-inhibitory and vasodilator properties of an egg white hydrolysate: Effect of a simulated intestinal digestion. *Food Chem.* **2007**, *104*, 163–168. [CrossRef]
32. Yoshii, H.; Tachi, N.; Ohba, R.; Sakamura, O.; Takeyama, H.; Itani, T. Antihypertensive effect of ACE inhibitory oligopeptides from chicken egg yolks. *Comp. Biochem. Physiol. Part C Toxicol. Pharmacol.* **2001**, *128*, 27–33. [CrossRef]
33. Yu, Z.; Liu, B.; Zhao, W.; Yin, Y.; Liu, J.; Chen, F. Primary and secondary structure of novel ACE-inhibitory peptides from egg white protein. *Food Chem.* **2012**, *133*, 315–322. [CrossRef] [PubMed]
34. Jiang, Z.; Wang, L.; Che, H.; Tian, B. Effects of temperature and pH on angiotensin-I-converting enzyme inhibitory activity and physicochemical properties of bovine casein peptide in aqueous Maillard reaction system. *LWT* **2014**, *59*, 35–42. [CrossRef]
35. Lin, K.; Zhang, L.-W.; Han, X.; Cheng, D.-Y. Novel angiotensin I-converting enzyme inhibitory peptides from protease hydrolysates of Qula casein: Quantitative structure-activity relationship modeling and molecular docking study. *J. Funct. Foods* **2017**, *32*, 266–277. [CrossRef]
36. Yamada, A.; Sakurai, T.; Ochi, D.; Mitsuyama, E.; Yamauchi, K.; Abe, F. Novel angiotensin I-converting enzyme inhibitory peptide derived from bovine casein. *Food Chem.* **2013**, *141*, 3781–3789. [CrossRef] [PubMed]
37. Hayes, M.; Mora, L.; Hussey, K.; Aluko, R.E.; Soler, L.M. Boarfish protein recovery using the pH-shift process and generation of protein hydrolysates with ACE-I and antihypertensive bioactivities in spontaneously hypertensive rats. *Innov. Food Sci. Emerg. Technol.* **2016**, *37*, 253–260. [CrossRef]
38. Itou, K.; Akahane, Y. Antihypertensive effect of heshiko, a fermented mackerel product, on spontaneously hypertensive rats. *Fish. Sci.* **2004**, *70*, 1121–1129. [CrossRef]
39. Neves, A.C.; Harnedy, P.A.; O'Keeffe, M.B.; Fitzgerald, R.J. Bioactive peptides from Atlantic salmon (Salmo salar) with angiotensin converting enzyme and dipeptidyl peptidase IV inhibitory, and antioxidant activities. *Food Chem.* **2017**, *218*, 396–405. [CrossRef] [PubMed]
40. Suetsuna, K.; Chen, J.-R. Identification of Antihypertensive Peptides from Peptic Digest of Two Microalgae, Chlorella vulgaris and Spirulina platensis. *Mar. Biotechnol.* **2001**, *3*, 305–309. [CrossRef] [PubMed]
41. Suetsuna, K.; Maekawa, K.; Chen, J.-R. Antihypertensive effects of Undaria pinnatifida (wakame) peptide on blood pressure in spontaneously hypertensive rats. *J. Nutr. Biochem.* **2004**, *15*, 267–272. [CrossRef] [PubMed]
42. Aneiros, A.; Garateix, A. Bioactive peptides from marine sources: Pharmacological properties and isolation procedures. *J. Chromatogr. B* **2004**, *803*, 41–53. [CrossRef] [PubMed]
43. Suleria, H.A.R.; Gobe, G.; Masci, P.; Osborne, S.A. Marine bioactive compounds and health promoting perspectives; innovation pathways for drug discovery. *Trends Food Sci. Technol.* **2016**, *50*, 44–55. [CrossRef]
44. Yasuhara-Bell, J.; Lu, Y. Marine compounds and their antiviral activities. *Antivir. Res.* **2010**, *86*, 231–240. [CrossRef] [PubMed]
45. Harnedy, P.A.; Fitzgerald, R.J. Bioactive peptides from marine processing waste and shellfish: A review. *J. Funct. Foods* **2012**, *4*, 6–24. [CrossRef]
46. Ryan, J.T.; Ross, R.P.; Bolton, D.; Fitzgerald, G.F.; Stanton, C. Bioactive Peptides from Muscle Sources: Meat and Fish. *Nutrients* **2011**, *3*, 765–791. [CrossRef]
47. Ngo, D.-H.; Ryu, B.; Kim, S.-K. Active peptides from skate (Okamejei kenojei) skin gelatin diminish angiotensin-I converting enzyme activity and intracellular free radical-mediated oxidation. *Food Chem.* **2014**, *143*, 246–255. [CrossRef]

48. Martins, A.; Vieira, H.M.; Gaspar, H.; Santos, S. Marketed Marine Natural Products in the Pharmaceutical and Cosmeceutical Industries: Tips for Success. *Mar. Drugs* **2014**, *12*, 1066–1101. [CrossRef]
49. Ni, H.; Li, L.; Liu, G.; Hu, S.-Q. Inhibition Mechanism and Model of an Angiotensin I-Converting Enzyme (ACE)-Inhibitory Hexapeptide from Yeast (Saccharomyces cerevisiae). *PLoS ONE* **2012**, *7*, e37077. [CrossRef]
50. Shi, L.; Mao, C.; Xu, Z.; Zhang, L. Angiotensin-converting enzymes and drug discovery in cardiovascular diseases. *Drug Discov. Today* **2010**, *15*, 332–341. [CrossRef]
51. Gavras, H. Angiotensin converting enzyme inhibition and its impact on cardiovascular disease. *Circulation* **1990**, *81*, 381–388. [CrossRef] [PubMed]
52. Wijesekara, I.; Kim, S.-K. Angiotensin-I-Converting Enzyme (ACE) Inhibitors from Marine Resources: Prospects in the Pharmaceutical Industry. *Mar. Drugs* **2010**, *8*, 1080–1093. [CrossRef] [PubMed]
53. Wijesinghe, W.A.J.P.; Ko, S.C.; Jeon, Y.J. Effect of phlorotannins isolated from Ecklonia cava on angiotensin I-converting enzyme (ACE) inhibitory activity. *Nutr. Res. Pract.* **2011**, *5*, 93–100. [CrossRef] [PubMed]
54. Wu, H.; He, H.-L.; Chen, X.-L.; Sun, C.-Y.; Zhang, Y.-Z.; Zhou, B.-C. Purification and identification of novel angiotensin-I-converting enzyme inhibitory peptides from shark meat hydrolysate. *Process Biochem.* **2008**, *43*, 457–461. [CrossRef]
55. Byun, H.-G.; Kim, S.-K. Purification and characterization of angiotensin I converting enzyme (ACE) inhibitory peptides from Alaska pollack (Theragra chalcogramma) skin. *Process Biochem.* **2001**, *36*, 1155–1162. [CrossRef]
56. Wang, Y.-K.; He, H.-L.; Chen, X.-L.; Sun, C.-Y.; Zhang, Y.-Z.; Zhou, B.-C. Production of novel angiotensin I-converting enzyme inhibitory peptides by fermentation of marine shrimp Acetes chinensis with Lactobacillus fermentum SM 605. *Appl. Microbiol. Biotechnol.* **2008**, *79*, 785–791. [CrossRef]
57. Ono, S.; Hosokawa, M.; Miyashita, K.; Takahashi, K. Inhibition properties of dipeptides from salmon muscle hydrolysate on angiotensin I-converting enzyme. *Int. J. Food Sci. Technol.* **2006**, *41*, 383–386. [CrossRef]
58. Liu, J.; Yu, Z.; Zhao, W.; Lin, S.; Wang, E.; Zhang, Y.; Hao, H.; Wang, Z.; Chen, F. Isolation and identification of angiotensin-converting enzyme inhibitory peptides from egg white protein hydrolysates. *Food Chem.* **2010**, *122*, 1159–1163. [CrossRef]
59. Wu, J.; Aluko, R.E.; Nakai, S. Structural Requirements of Angiotensin I-Converting Enzyme Inhibitory Peptides: Quantitative Structure–Activity Relationship Study of Di- and Tripeptides. *J. Agric. Food Chem.* **2006**, *54*, 732–738. [CrossRef]
60. Robert, M.-C.; Razaname, A.; Mutter, M.; Juillerat, M.A. Identification of Angiotensin-I-Converting Enzyme Inhibitory Peptides Derived from Sodium Caseinate Hydrolysates Produced byLactobacillus helveticusNCC 2765. *J. Agric. Food Chem.* **2004**, *52*, 6923–6931. [CrossRef]
61. Saito, T.; Nakamura, T.; Kitazawa, H.; Kawai, Y.; Itoh, T. Isolation and Structural Analysis of Antihypertensive Peptides That Exist Naturally in Gouda Cheese. *J. Dairy Sci.* **2000**, *83*, 1434–1440. [CrossRef]
62. Fahmi, A.; Morimura, S.; Guo, H.; Shigematsu, T.; Kida, K.; Uemura, Y. Production of angiotensin I converting enzyme inhibitory peptides from sea bream scales. *Process Biochem.* **2004**, *39*, 1195–1200. [CrossRef]
63. Lan, X.; Liao, D.; Wu, S.; Wang, F.; Sun, J.; Tong, Z.; Wu, S. Rapid purification and characterization of angiotensin converting enzyme inhibitory peptides from lizard fish protein hydrolysates with magnetic affinity separation. *Food Chem.* **2015**, *182*, 136–142. [CrossRef] [PubMed]
64. Wu, S.; Feng, X.; Lan, X.; Xu, Y.; Liao, D. Purification and identification of Angiotensin-I Converting Enzyme (ACE) inhibitory peptide from lizard fish (Saurida elongata) hydrolysate. *J. Funct. Foods* **2015**, *13*, 295–299. [CrossRef]
65. Gu, R.-Z.; Li, C.-Y.; Liu, W.-Y.; Yi, W.-X.; Cai, M.-Y. Angiotensin I-converting enzyme inhibitory activity of low-molecular-weight peptides from Atlantic salmon (*Salmo salar* L.) skin. *Food Res. Int.* **2011**, *44*, 1536–1540. [CrossRef]
66. Intarasirisawat, R.; Benjakul, S.; Wu, J.; Visessanguan, W. Isolation of antioxidative and ACE inhibitory peptides from protein hydrolysate of skipjack (Katsuwana pelamis) roe. *J. Funct. Foods* **2013**, *5*, 1854–1862. [CrossRef]
67. Jung, W.-K.; Mendis, E.; Je, J.-Y.; Park, P.-J.; Son, B.W.; Kim, H.C.; Choi, Y.K.; Kim, S.-K. Angiotensin I-converting enzyme inhibitory peptide from yellowfin sole (Limanda aspera) frame protein and its antihypertensive effect in spontaneously hypertensive rats. *Food Chem.* **2006**, *94*, 26–32. [CrossRef]
68. Ngo, D.-H.; Vo, T.-S.; Ryu, B.; Kim, S.-K. Angiotensin-I-converting enzyme (ACE) inhibitory peptides from Pacific cod skin gelatin using ultrafiltration membranes. *Process Biochem.* **2016**, *51*, 1622–1628. [CrossRef]

69. Ko, J.-Y.; Kang, N.; Lee, J.-H.; Kim, J.-S.; Kim, W.-S.; Park, S.-J.; Kim, Y.-T.; Jeon, Y.-J. Angiotensin I-converting enzyme inhibitory peptides from an enzymatic hydrolysate of flounder fish (Paralichthys olivaceus) muscle as a potent anti-hypertensive agent. *Process Biochem.* **2016**, *51*, 535–541. [CrossRef]
70. Ghassem, M.; Arihara, K.; Babji, A.S.; Said, M.; Ibrahim, S. Purification and identification of ACE inhibitory peptides from Haruan (Channa striatus) myofibrillar protein hydrolysate using HPLC–ESI-TOF MS/MS. *Food Chem.* **2011**, *129*, 1770–1777. [CrossRef]
71. Ko, S.-C.; Kang, N.; Kim, E.-A.; Kang, M.C.; Lee, S.-H.; Kang, S.-M.; Lee, J.-B.; Jeon, B.-T.; Kim, S.-K.; Park, S.-J.; et al. A novel angiotensin I-converting enzyme (ACE) inhibitory peptide from a marine Chlorella ellipsoidea and its antihypertensive effect in spontaneously hypertensive rats. *Process Biochem.* **2012**, *47*, 2005–2011. [CrossRef]
72. Zhao, Y.; Li, B.; Dong, S.; Liu, Z.; Zhao, X.; Wang, J.; Zeng, M. A novel ACE inhibitory peptide isolated from Acaudina molpadioidea hydrolysate. *Peptides* **2009**, *30*, 1028–1033. [CrossRef] [PubMed]
73. Balti, R.; Nedjar-Arroume, N.; Bougatef, A.; Guillochon, D.; Nasri, M. Three novel angiotensin I-converting enzyme (ACE) inhibitory peptides from cuttlefish (Sepia officinalis) using digestive proteases. *Food Res. Int.* **2010**, *43*, 1136–1143. [CrossRef]
74. Balti, R.; Bougatef, A.; Sila, A.; Guillochon, D.; Dhulster, P.; Nedjar-Arroume, N. Nine novel angiotensin I-converting enzyme (ACE) inhibitory peptides from cuttlefish (Sepia officinalis) muscle protein hydrolysates and antihypertensive effect of the potent active peptide in spontaneously hypertensive rats. *Food Chem.* **2015**, *170*, 519–525. [CrossRef]
75. Alemán, A.; Gómez-Guillén, M.C.; Montero, P. Identification of ace-inhibitory peptides from squid skin collagen after in vitro gastrointestinal digestion. *Food Res. Int.* **2013**, *54*, 790–795. [CrossRef]
76. Tsai, J.; Lin, T.; Chen, J.; Pan, B. The inhibitory effects of freshwater clam (Corbicula fluminea, Muller) muscle protein hydrolysates on angiotensin I converting enzyme. *Process Biochem.* **2006**, *41*, 2276–2281. [CrossRef]
77. Jao, C.-L.; Huang, S.-L.; Hsu, K.-C. Angiotensin I-converting enzyme inhibitory peptides: Inhibition mode, bioavailability, and antihypertensive effects. *BioMedicine* **2012**, *2*, 130–136. [CrossRef]
78. Ko, S.-C.; Jang, J.; Ye, B.-R.; Kim, M.-S.; Choi, I.-W.; Park, W.-S.; Jung, W.-K. Purification and molecular docking study of angiotensin I-converting enzyme (ACE) inhibitory peptides from hydrolysates of marine sponge Stylotella aurantium. *Process Biochem.* **2016**, *54*, 180–187. [CrossRef]
79. Wu, Q.; Jia, J.; Yan, H.; Du, J.; Gui, Z. A novel angiotensin-I converting enzyme (ACE) inhibitory peptide from gastrointestinal protease hydrolysate of silkworm pupa (Bombyx mori) protein: Biochemical characterization and molecular docking study. *Peptides* **2015**, *68*, 17–24. [CrossRef]
80. Jemil, I.; Mora, L.; Nasri, R.; Abdelhedi, O.; Aristoy, M.-C.; Hajji, M.; Nasri, M.; Toldrá, F.; Soler, L.M. A peptidomic approach for the identification of antioxidant and ACE-inhibitory peptides in sardinelle protein hydrolysates fermented by Bacillus subtilis A26 and Bacillus amyloliquefaciens An6. *Food Res. Int.* **2016**, *89*, 347–358. [CrossRef]
81. Lin, H.-C.; Alashi, A.M.; Aluko, R.E.; Pan, B.S.; Chang, Y.-W. Antihypertensive properties of tilapia (Oreochromis spp.) frame and skin enzymatic protein hydrolysates. *Food Nutr. Res.* **2017**, *61*, 1391666. [CrossRef] [PubMed]
82. Ondetti, M.A.; Cushman, D.W. Enzymes of the renin-angiotensin system and their inhibitors. *Annu. Rev. Biochem.* **1982**, *51*, 283–308. [CrossRef] [PubMed]
83. López-Fandiño, R.; Otte, J.; Van Camp, J. Physiological, chemical and technological aspects of milk-protein-derived peptides with antihypertensive and ACE-inhibitory activity. *Int. Dairy J.* **2006**, *16*, 1277–1293. [CrossRef]
84. Lassoued, I.; Mora, L.; Barkia, A.; Aristoy, M.C.; Nasri, M.; Toldrá, F. Bioactive peptides identified in thornback ray skin's gelatin hydrolysates by proteases from Bacillus subtilis and Bacillus amyloliquefaciens. *J. Proteom.* **2015**, *128*, 8–17. [CrossRef]
85. So, P.B.T.; Rubio, P.; Lirio, S.; Macabeo, A.P.; Huang, H.-Y.; Corpuz, M.J.-A.T.; Villaflores, O.B. In vitro angiotensin I converting enzyme inhibition by a peptide isolated from Chiropsalmus quadrigatus Haeckel (box jellyfish) venom hydrolysate. *Toxicon* **2016**, *119*, 77–83. [CrossRef] [PubMed]
86. Sato, M.; Hosokawa, T.; Yamaguchi, T.; Nakano, T.; Muramoto, K.; Kahara, T.; Funayama, K.; Kobayashi, A.; Nakano, T. Angiotensin I-Converting Enzyme Inhibitory Peptides Derived from Wakame (Undaria pinnatifida) and Their Antihypertensive Effect in Spontaneously Hypertensive Rats. *J. Agric. Food Chem.* **2002**, *50*, 6245–6252. [CrossRef] [PubMed]

87. Nakagomi, K.; Fujimura, A.; Ebisu, H.; Sakai, T.; Sadakane, Y.; Fujii, N.; Tanimura, T. Acein-1, a novel angiotensin-I-converting enzyme inhibitory peptide isolated from tryptic hydrolysate of human plasma. *FEBS Lett.* **1998**, *438*, 255–257. [CrossRef]
88. Fujita, H.; Yoshikawa, M. LKPNM: A prodrug-type ACE-inhibitory peptide derived from fish protein. *Immunopharmacol.* **1999**, *44*, 123–127. [CrossRef]
89. Vercruysse, L.; Van Camp, J.; Morel, N.; Rougé, P.; Herregods, G.; Smagghe, G. Ala-Val-Phe and Val-Phe: ACE inhibitory peptides derived from insect protein with antihypertensive activity in spontaneously hypertensive rats. *Peptides* **2010**, *31*, 482–488. [CrossRef]
90. Shahidi, F.; Ambigaipalan, P. Novel functional food ingredients from marine sources. *Curr. Opin. Food Sci.* **2015**, *2*, 123–129. [CrossRef]
91. Agyei, D.; Ongkudon, C.M.; Wei, C.Y.; Chan, A.S.; Danquah, M.K. Bioprocess challenges to the isolation and purification of bioactive peptides. *Food Bioprod. Process.* **2016**, *98*, 244–256. [CrossRef]
92. Sánchez-Rivera, L.; Martínez-Maqueda, D.; Cruz-Huerta, E.; Miralles, B.; Recio, I. Peptidomics for discovery, bioavailability and monitoring of dairy bioactive peptides. *Food Res. Int.* **2014**, *63*, 170–181. [CrossRef]
93. Jemil, I.; Abdelhedi, O.; Mora, L.; Nasri, R.; Aristoy, M.-C.; Jridi, M.; Hajji, M.; Toldrá, F.; Nasri, M.; Soler, L.M. Peptidomic analysis of bioactive peptides in zebra blenny (Salaria basilisca) muscle protein hydrolysate exhibiting antimicrobial activity obtained by fermentation with Bacillus mojavensis A21. *Process Biochem.* **2016**, *51*, 2186–2197. [CrossRef]
94. Sheih, I.-C.; Wu, T.-K.; Fang, T.J. Antioxidant properties of a new antioxidative peptide from algae protein waste hydrolysate in different oxidation systems. *Bioresour. Technol.* **2009**, *100*, 3419–3425. [CrossRef] [PubMed]
95. Ustyuzhanina, N.E.; Ushakova, N.A.; Zyuzina, K.A.; Bilan, M.I.; Elizarova, A.L.; Somonova, O.V.; Madzhuga, A.V.; Krylov, V.B.; Preobrazhenskaya, M.E.; Usov, A.I.; et al. Influence of Fucoidans on Hemostatic System. *Mar. Drugs* **2013**, *11*, 2444–2458. [CrossRef]
96. Korhonen, H.; Pihlanto, A. Bioactive peptides: Production and functionality. *Int. Dairy J.* **2006**, *16*, 945–960. [CrossRef]
97. Rizzello, C.G.; Tagliazucchi, D.; Babini, E.; Rutella, G.S.; Saa, D.L.T.; Gianotti, A. Bioactive peptides from vegetable food matrices: Research trends and novel biotechnologies for synthesis and recovery. *J. Funct. Foods* **2016**, *27*, 549–569. [CrossRef]
98. Sanjukta, S.; Rai, A.K. Production of bioactive peptides during soybean fermentation and their potential health benefits. *Trends Food Sci. Technol.* **2016**, *50*, 1–10. [CrossRef]
99. Kleekayai, T.; Harnedy, P.A.; O'Keeffe, M.B.; Poyarkov, A.A.; CunhaNeves, A.; Suntornsuk, W.; Fitzgerald, R.J. Extraction of antioxidant and ACE inhibitory peptides from Thai traditional fermented shrimp pastes. *Food Chem.* **2015**, *176*, 441–447. [CrossRef]
100. Cushman, D.; Cheung, H. Spectrophotometric assay and properties of the angiotensin-converting enzyme of rabbit lung. *Biochem. Pharmacol.* **1971**, *20*, 1637–1648. [CrossRef]
101. Li, G.-H.; Liu, H.; Shi, Y.-H.; Le, G.-W. Direct spectrophotometric measurement of angiotensin I-converting enzyme inhibitory activity for screening bioactive peptides. *J. Pharm. Biomed. Anal.* **2005**, *37*, 219–224. [CrossRef] [PubMed]
102. Belović, M.M.; Ilić, N.M.; Tepić, A.N.; Šumić, Z. Selection of conditions for angiotensin-converting enzyme inhibition assay: Influence of sample preparation and buffer. *Food Feed Res.* **2013**, *40*, 11–16.
103. Shalaby, S.M.; Zakora, M.; Otte, J. Performance of two commonly used angiotensin-converting enzyme inhibition assays using FA-PGG and HHL as substrates. *J. Dairy Res.* **2006**, *73*, 178–186. [CrossRef] [PubMed]
104. Murray, B.; Walsh, D.; Fitzgerald, R. Modification of the furanacryloyl-l-phenylalanylglycylglycine assay for determination of angiotensin-I-converting enzyme inhibitory activity. *J. Biochem. Biophys. Methods* **2004**, *59*, 127–137. [CrossRef] [PubMed]
105. Sentandreu, M.Á.; Toldrá, F. A rapid, simple and sensitive fluorescence method for the assay of angiotensin-I converting enzyme. *Food Chem.* **2006**, *97*, 546–554. [CrossRef]
106. Van Der Ven, C.; Gruppen, H.; De Bont, D.B.; Voragen, A.G. Optimisation of the angiotensin converting enzyme inhibition by whey protein hydrolysates using response surface methodology. *Int. Dairy J.* **2002**, *12*, 813–820. [CrossRef]

107. Vermeirssen, V.; Van Camp, J.; Verstraete, W. Optimisation and validation of an angiotensin-converting enzyme inhibition assay for the screening of bioactive peptides. *J. Biochem. Biophys. Methods* **2002**, *51*, 75–87. [CrossRef]
108. Anzenbacherová, E.; Anzenbacher, P.; Macek, K.; Květina, J. Determination of enzyme (angiotensin convertase) inhibitors based on enzymatic reaction followed by HPLC. *J. Pharm. Biomed. Anal.* **2001**, *24*, 1151–1156. [CrossRef]
109. Sentandreu, M.A.; Toldrá, F. A fluorescence-based protocol for quantifying angiotensin-converting enzyme activity. *Nat. Protoc.* **2006**, *1*, 2423–2427. [CrossRef]
110. Betancourt, L.H.; De Bock, P.-J.; Staes, A.; Timmerman, E.; Perez-Riverol, Y.; Sánchez, A.; Besada, V.; González, L.J.; Vandekerckhove, J.; Gevaert, K. SCX charge state selective separation of tryptic peptides combined with 2D-RP-HPLC allows for detailed proteome mapping. *J. Proteom.* **2013**, *91*, 164–171. [CrossRef]
111. Geng, F.; He, Y.; Yang, L.; Wang, Z. A rapid assay for angiotensin-converting enzyme activity using ultra-performance liquid chromatography-mass spectrometry. *Biomed. Chromatogr. BMC* **2010**, *24*, 312–317. [CrossRef] [PubMed]
112. Hernández-Ledesma, B.; Contreras, M.D.M.; Recio, I. Antihypertensive peptides: Production, bioavailability and incorporation into foods. *Adv. Colloid Interface Sci.* **2011**, *165*, 23–35. [CrossRef] [PubMed]
113. Wu, J.; Ding, X. Characterization of inhibition and stability of soy-protein-derived angiotensin I-converting enzyme inhibitory peptides. *Food Res. Int.* **2002**, *35*, 367–375. [CrossRef]
114. Vermeirssen, V.; Van Camp, J.; Verstraete, W. Bioavailability of angiotensin I converting enzyme inhibitory peptides. *Br. J. Nutr.* **2004**, *92*, 357–366. [CrossRef] [PubMed]
115. Meng, X.-Y.; Zhang, H.-X.; Mezei, M.; Cui, M. Molecular Docking: A Powerful Approach for Structure-Based Drug Discovery. *Curr. Comput. Drug Des.* **2011**, *7*, 146–157. [CrossRef]
116. Politi, A.; Durdagi, S.; Moutevelis-Minakakis, P.; Kokotos, G.; Mavromoustakos, T. Development of accurate binding affinity predictions of novel renin inhibitors through molecular docking studies. *J. Mol. Graph. Model.* **2010**, *29*, 425–435. [CrossRef]
117. Panjaitan, F.C.A.; Gomez, H.L.R.; Chang, Y.-W. In Silico Analysis of Bioactive Peptides Released from Giant Grouper (Epinephelus lanceolatus) Roe Proteins Identified by Proteomics Approach. *Molecules* **2018**, *23*, 2910. [CrossRef]
118. Tejano, L.A.; Peralta, J.P.; Yap, E.E.S.; Panjaitan, F.C.A.; Chang, Y.-W. Prediction of Bioactive Peptides from Chlorella sorokiniana Proteins Using Proteomic Techniques in Combination with Bioinformatics Analyses. *Int. J. Mol. Sci.* **2019**, *20*, 1786. [CrossRef]
119. Pan, D.; Guo, H.; Zhao, B.; Cao, J. The molecular mechanisms of interactions between bioactive peptides and angiotensin-converting enzyme. *Bioorganic Med. Chem. Lett.* **2011**, *21*, 3898–3904. [CrossRef]
120. Andrews, P.R.; Carson, J.M.; Caselli, A.; Spark, M.J.; Woods, R. Conformational analysis and active site modeling of angiotensin-converting enzyme inhibitors. *J. Med. Chem.* **1985**, *28*, 393–399. [CrossRef]

13

Antinociceptive Effects of Cardamonin in Mice: Possible Involvement of $TRPV_1$, Glutamate and Opioid Receptors

Chung Pui Ping [1], Tengku Azam Shah Tengku Mohamad [1], Muhammad Nadeem Akhtar [2], Enoch Kumar Perimal [1], Ahmad Akira [1], Daud Ahmad Israf Ali [1,3] and Mohd Roslan Sulaiman [1,3,*]

1 Department of Biomedical Sciences, Faculty of Medicine and Health Sciences, Universiti Putra Malaysia Selangor, Serdang 43400, Malaysia; puiping.chung@gmail.com (C.P.P.); azamshah@upm.edu.my (T.A.S.T.M.); enoch@upm.edu.my (E.K.P.); ahmadakira@upm.edu.my (A.A.); daudaia@upm.edu.my (D.A.I.A.)

2 Laboratory of Natural Products, Institute of Bioscience, Universiti Putra Malaysia, Selangor, Serdang 43400, Malaysia; nadeemupm@gmail.com

3 Faculty of Industrial Sciences & Technology, University Malaysia Pahang, Pahang, Gambang 26300, Malaysia

* Correspondence: mrs@upm.edu.my;

Abstract: Pain is one of the most common cause for hospital visits. It plays an important role in inflammation and serves as a warning sign to avoid further injury. Analgesics are used to manage pain and provide comfort to patients. However, prolonged usage of pain treatments like opioids and NSAIDs are accompanied with undesirable side effects. Therefore, research to identify novel compounds that produce analgesia with lesser side effects are necessary. The present study investigated the antinociceptive potentials of a natural compound, cardamonin, isolated from *Boesenbergia rotunda* (L) Mansf. using chemical and thermal models of nociception. Our findings showed that intraperitoneal and oral administration of cardamonin (0.3, 1, 3, and 10 mg/kg) produced significant and dose-dependent inhibition of pain in abdominal writhing responses induced by acetic acid. The present study also demonstrated that cardamonin produced significant analgesia in formalin-, capsaicin-, and glutamate-induced paw licking tests. In the thermal-induced nociception model, cardamonin exhibited significant increase in response latency time of animals subjected to hot-plate thermal stimuli. The rota-rod assessment confirmed that the antinociceptive activities elicited by cardamonin was not related to muscle relaxant or sedative effects of the compound. In conclusion, the present findings showed that cardamonin exerted significant peripheral and central antinociception through chemical- and thermal-induced nociception in mice through the involvement of $TRPV_1$, glutamate, and opioid receptors.

Keywords: cardamonin; antinociceptive; $TRPV_1$; glutamate; opioid

---

1. Introduction

Cardamonin or 2′,4′-dihydroxy-6′-methoxychalcone ($C_{16}H_{14}O_4$) is a naturally occurring chalcone. Cardamonin was firstly isolated from the seeds of *Amomum subulatum* [1] and later from other plant species, such as *Boesenbergia pandurata*, *Alpinia rafflesiana*, *Alpinia katsumadai*, *Alpinia henryi*, and *Campomanesia adamantium*. Previous report showed that cardamonin exerted antiproliferative activity and induced apoptosis in PC-3 [2], myeloma [3], and A549 cell lines [4]. In addition, cardamonin was capable to protect lipopolysaccharide (LPS)-induced septic mice against acute lung injury [5] and showed nephroprotective effect against cisplatin-induced renal injury [6]. Furthermore, cardamonin could exert inhibition of platelet aggregation [7], vasorelaxant effect [8], improvement in insulin resistance and vascular complication in a high fructose-fed rat model [9], suppression of lipid accumulation in vitro [10], inhibition of pigmentation in human normal melanocytes [11], and anti-pruritic activity [12].

In vitro study showed that cardamonin inhibits the release of pro-inflammatory mediators [13] and it was supported by the findings on inhibitory action of cardamonin upon the expression of NO and PGE_2 via interruption of the NF-κB pathway [14,15]. This mechanism of action is common to phenolic compounds showing protective effects [16,17]. In vivo study also presented the capability of cardamonin in suppressing NO generation in LPS-challenged ICR mice [18]. NO has been reported to be involved in generation of pain perception through a series of pathway [19]. Since cardamonin reduces generation of NO, we believe that cardamonin may show antinociceptive activityies.

Recently, the antinociceptive profile of cardamonin has been reported through PBQ-induced writhing and carrageenan-induced hyperalgesia test [20], but there is still no report on the possible mechanism of antinociceptive action of cardamonin. Thus, the present study was aimed to examine the antinociceptive effect of cardamonin in chemical- and thermal-induced nociception using mice models.

2. Results

2.1. Evaluation of the Antinociceptive Activity

2.1.1. Acetic Acid–Induced Abdominal Writhing Test

The effect of cardamonin in acetic acid-induced abdominal writhing response in mice is depicted in Figure 1. Cardamonin produced significant reduction in the number of writhing in both routes of administration, intraperitoneally (Panel a) and orally (Panel b) at $p < 0.001$. Cardamonin administered intraperitoneally (i.p.) showed 45, 56, 80, and 100% of inhibition against acetic acid-induced pain as compared to control at doses of 0.3, 1, 3, and 10 mg/kg respectively, with calculated ED_{50} (and its respective confidence interval) of 2.1 (1.9–2.5) mg/kg. Oral administration (p.o.) of cardamonin exhibited 39%, 40%, 63% and 77% of inhibition as compared to control at doses of 0.3, 1, 3, and 10 mg/kg, respectively, with calculated ED_{50} (and its respective confidence interval) of 2.5 (2.0–3.3) mg/kg. Indomethacin, produced significant inhibition in acetic acid-induced abdominal pain with 80% (i.p.) and 60% (p.o.) of inhibition respectively, as compared to control at $p < 0.001$.

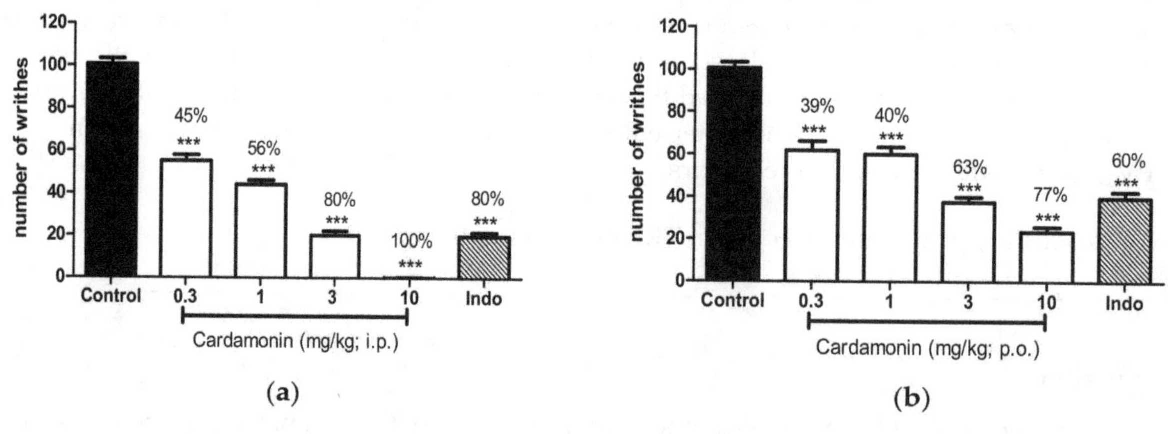

Figure 1. (**a**) Effect of cardamonin (0.3, 1, 3, 10 mg/kg, i.p.) administered intraperitoneally against acetic acid-induced nociception. (**b**) Effect of cardamonin (0.3, 1, 3, 10 mg/kg, i.p.) administered orally against acetic acid-induced nociception. Each column represents the mean ± S.E.M. of 6 mice. Control group received only the vehicle (ethanol: Tween 20: distilled water in 5:5:90, *v/v/v*) used to dilute the compound. Indomethacin (Indo, 10 mg/kg) was used as positive control. The asterisks denote the significance levels compared with the control group (one-way ANOVA, followed by Dunnett's post hoc test); *** $p < 0.001$. Values in parentheses were percentage of inhibition.

2.1.2. Formalin-Induced Paw Licking Test

Cardamonin treated animals showed significant analgesic effect on both early neurogenic phase (0–5 min) and late inflammatory phase (15–35 min) in the formalin-induced paw licking test as shown in Figure 2 (Panel a and b respectively). Cardamonin inhibited the inflammatory pain better in comparison with the neurogenic pain at all dosage use, especially at 1 mg/kg (98%) and 3 mg/kg (99%) against inflammatory pain. Morphine (5 mg/kg; s.c.) produced significant inhibition ($p < 0.001$) against formalin-induced pain at both the early neurogenic phase (96%) and late inflammatory phase (99%). In contrast, indomethacin significantly inhibits formalin-induced pain better at the late inflammatory phase (70% of inhibition) than the early neurogenic phase (31% of inhibition).

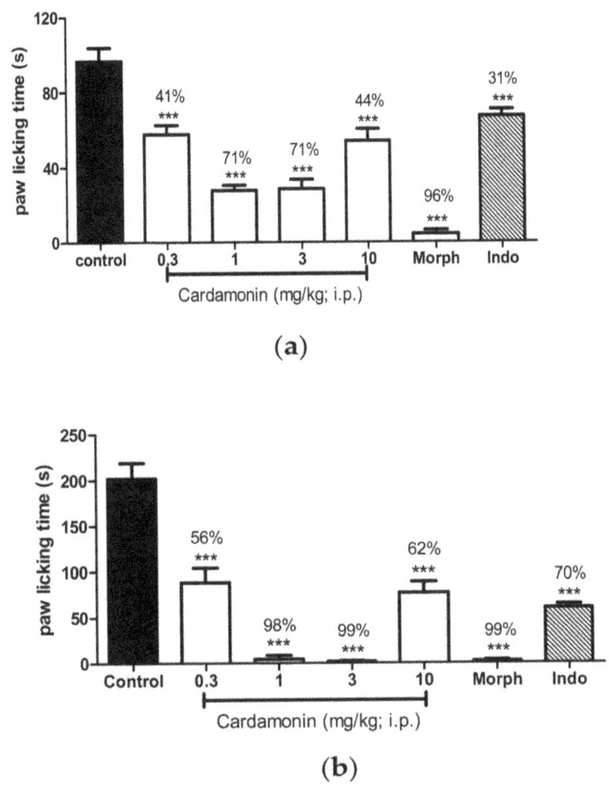

Figure 2. (**a**) Effect of cardamonin (0.3, 1, 3, 10 mg/kg, i.p.) in formalin-induced paw licking test (early phase) in mice. (**b**) Effect of cardamonin (0.3, 1, 3, 10 mg/kg, i.p.) in formalin-induced paw licking test (late phase) in mice. Each column represents the mean ± S.E.M. of 6 mice. Control group received only the vehicle used to dilute the compound. Morphine (Morph, 5 mg/kg, s.c.) and indomethacin (Indo, 10 mg/kg, i.p.) were used as positive control. The asterisks denote the significance levels compared with the control group (one-way ANOVA, followed by Dunnett's post hoc test); *** $p < 0.001$. Values in parentheses were percentage of inhibition.

2.1.3. Hot Plate Test

i.p. administration of cardamonin and morphine significantly increased the latency time of nociceptive responses in the hot plate test at the temperature of 52 ± 0.2 °C compared with vehicle-treated animals (Table 1).

Table 1. Effect of cardamonin on the hot plate test in mice. Results were expressed in mean ± S.E.M of latency time (s) of 6 mice. Statistical significance was determined by two-way ANOVA followed by Bonferroni post hoc test.

Treatment	Dose	Latency Time (s)							
	(mg/kg)	0 min	30 min	60 min	90 min	120 min	150 min	180 min	210 min
Control		6.17 ± 0.17	6.83 ± 0.31	6.67 ± 0.33	6.67 ± 0.21	6.83 ± 0.31	6.67 ± 0.21	6.83 ± 0.31	6.33 ± 0.21
Cardamonin (i.p.)	0.3	6.34 ± 0.16	6.99 ± 0.52	7.01 ± 0.27	8.26 ± 0.33	8.28 ± 0.56	9.08 ± 1.09 *	8.36 ± 0.59	6.83 ± 0.55
	1	7.05 ± 0.22	6.84 ± 0.56	7.03 ± 0.16	7.11 ± 0.28	8.04 ± 0.67	8.97 ± 0.44 *	8.50 ± 0.37	7.22 ± 0.26
	3	6.95 ± 0.25	6.83 ± 0.25	7.59 ± 0.25	7.65 ± 0.16	8.37 ± 0.41	8.92 ± 0.24 *	7.52 ± 0.51	6.71 ± 0.36
	10	6.63 ± 0.20	7.45 ± 0.46	8.08 ± 0.46	9.14 ± 0.72 *	10.09 ± 0.89 ***	9.21 ± 0.83 **	8.07 ± 0.33	7.48 ± 0.15
Naloxone (i.p.) + Cardamonin (i.p.)	1 + 5	7.30 ± 0.24	8.70 ± 0.28	8.54 ± 0.32	8.60 ± 0.25	11.33 ± 0.59 ###	11.62 ± 0.50 ##	9.40 ± 0.58	8.45 ± 0.66
Morphine (s.c.)	5	7.50 ± 0.34	18.33 ± 0.67 ***	17.00 ± 0.82 ***	16.33 ± 0.42 ***	16.33 ± 0.99 ***	15.33 ± 0.62 ***	15.17 ± 0.40 ***	14.83 ± 0.40 ***
Naloxone (i.p.) + Morphine (s.c.)	5 + 5	7.30 ± 0.29	8.93 ± 0.82 ###	11.18 ± 0.74 ###	10.76 ± 0.61 ###	10.10 ± 0.84 ###	9.01 ± 0.83 ###	7.64 ± 0.30 ###	6.92 ± 0.30 ###

* $p < 0.05$ as compared to control; ** $p < 0.01$ as compared to control; *** $p < 0.001$ as compared to control; ## $p < 0.01$ as compared to the group receiving appropriate drug/compound at the same dose without naloxone; ### $p < 0.001$ as compared to the group receiving appropriate drug/compound at the same dose without naloxone.

2.2. *Investigation of the Mechanisms of Action*

2.2.1. Involvement of the $TRPV_1$ Receptor

Cardamonin showed significant inhibition against capsaicin-induced nociception at 1, 3 and 10 mg/kg with $p < 0.001$ in Figure 3. The maximum inhibition was produced by cardamonin at the dose of 3 mg/kg with 66% inhibition compared to control. Likewise, capsazepine and indomethacin significantly exhibited 89% and 74% inhibition, respectively.

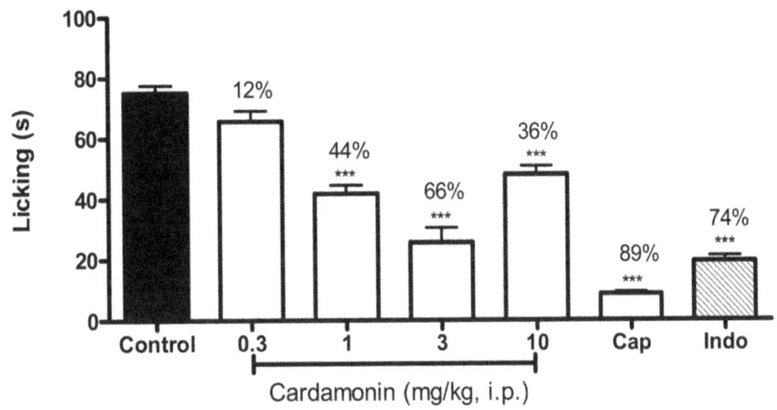

Figure 3. Effect of cardamonin (0.3, 1, 3, 10 mg/kg, i.p.) against capsaicin-induced nociception. Each column represents the mean ± S.E.M. of 6 mice. Control group receives only the vehicle used to dilute the compound. Capsazepine (Cap, 0.17 mmol/kg, i.p.) was used as the positive control for capsaicin-induced nociception. Indomethacin (Indo, 10 mg/kg, i.p.) was used as positive control. The asterisks denote the significance levels compared with the control group (one-way ANOVA, followed by Dunnett's post hoc test); *** $p < 0.001$. Values in parentheses are percentage of inhibition.

2.2.2. Involvement of the Glutamate Receptor

Using the glutamate-induced nociception study, it was observed that cardamonin produced significant antinociceptive activities at all dosage (Figure 4). The percentage of inhibition for were 46%, 44%, 66%, and 84% for 0.3, 1, 3, and 10 mg/kg of cardamonin, respectively, as in comparison with control. Indomethacin showed 69% of significant inhibition against glutamate-induced nociception at $p < 0.001$.

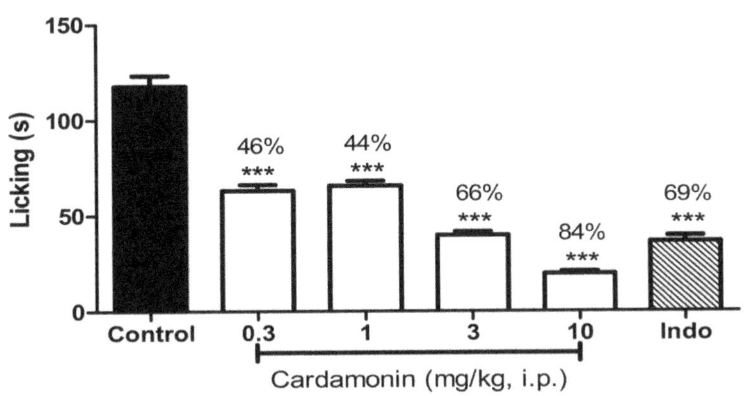

Figure 4. Effect of cardamonin (0.3, 1, 3, 10 mg/kg, i.p.) against glutamate-induced nociception. Each column represents the mean ± S.E.M. of 6 mice. Control group receives only the vehicle used to dilute the compound. Indomethacin (Indo, 10 mg/kg, i.p.) was used as positive control. The asterisks denote the significance levels compared with the control group (one-way ANOVA, followed by Dunnett's post hoc test), *** $p < 0.001$. Values in parentheses are percentage of inhibition.

2.2.3. Involvement of the Opioid Receptors

Pre-treatment of mice with the non-specific opioid receptor antagonist, naloxone (5 mg/kg; i.p.) significantly reversed the antinociceptive effect of cardamonin (1 mg/kg; i.p.) at $p < 0.001$ only in the early neurogenic phase, but not the late inflammatory phase (Figure 5). The effect of morphine (5 mg/kg; s.c.) was significantly reversed by naloxone in both the early neurogenic phase as well as late inflammatory phase. This suggested that opioid system might be involved in the centrally activated antinociceptive activity by cardamonin.

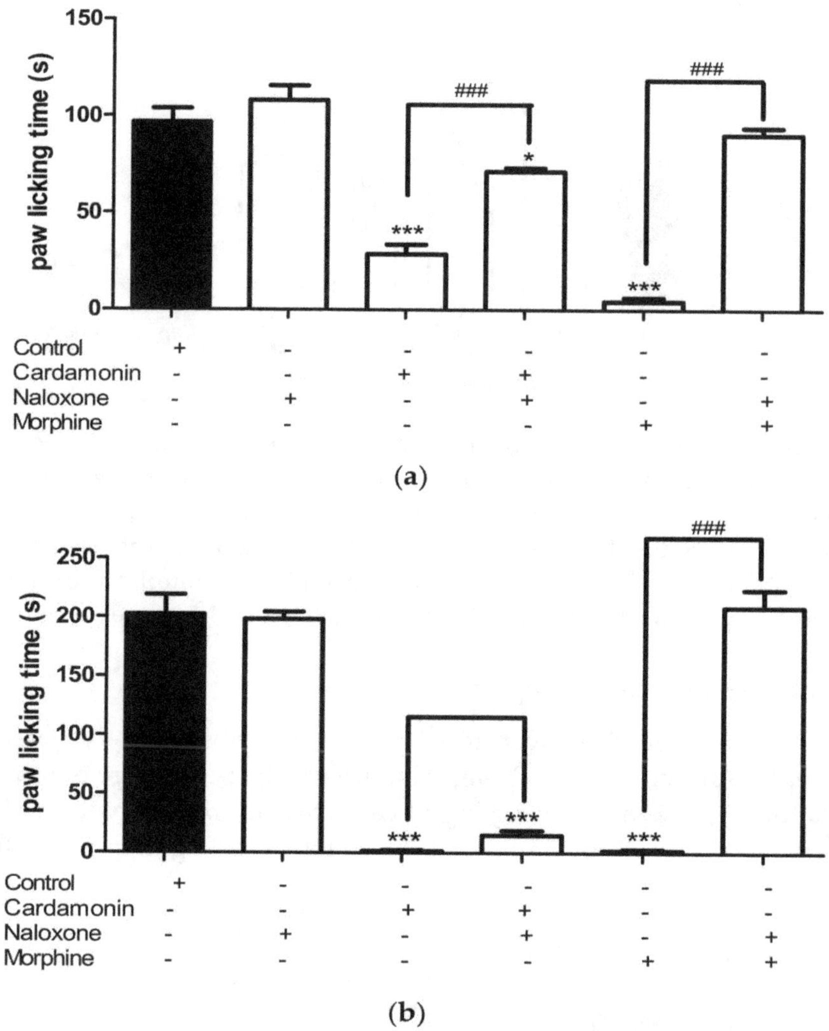

Figure 5. (**a**) Effect of naloxone (5 mg/kg, i.p.) on antinociception caused by cardamonin (1 mg/kg, i.p.) in the early phase in formalin-induced paw licking test. (**b**) Effect of naloxone (5 mg/kg, i.p.) on antinociception caused by cardamonin (1 mg/kg, i.p.) in the and the late phase in formalin-induced paw licking test. The asterisks and hash denote the significance levels (one-way ANOVA, followed by Tukey's post hoc test), * $p < 0.05$, *** $p < 0.001$, ### $p < 0.001$.

2.3. Toxicity Assessment

After seven days of observation, no mortality was reported at all doses of cardamonin used. During the observation period, the animals did not show any signs of abnormal behavior and locomotor activity. The observations were done qualitatively.

2.4. Motor Coordination Evaluation

Animals subjected to rota rod task after administration of cardamonin (10 mg/kg; i.p.) did not show any disturbance in motor coordination. The mean $\pm$ S.E.M. in the rota rod test for control, cardamonin (10 mg/kg) and diazepam (4 mg/kg) were 114.7 $\pm$ 5.33 s, 120.0 $\pm$ 0.00 s, and 38.83 $\pm$ 4.38 s, respectively.

3. Discussion

According to the Third National Health and Morbidity Survey 2006, 7% of the Malaysian population were suffering from chronic persistent pain [21]. Chronic pain has become a prevalent health problem among the older generation in Malaysia [22]. This has led to higher hospitalization rates among the elderly and severely interferes with the quality of life.

Non-steroidal anti-inflammatory drugs (NSAIDs), opioids, and analgesic adjuvants are the major classes of pharmacological therapies for pain relief currently available in modern medicine [23]. In spite of pain relieving effects, prolonged usage of these drugs leads to undesirable side effects such as gastrointestinal bleeding, renal toxicity, hypotension and respiratory depression [24,25]. These adverse effects have limited the usage of well-known effective pain relieving medicines. Research has been continuously carried out to seek for alternative pharmacologically potent analgesic treatment with fewer or milder side effects.

Previous studies have demonstrated an increase in NOS and TNF-α gene expression in the injected paw of animals after intraplantar administration of CFA [26]. It was postulated that NO capable of inducing peripheral hyperalgesia by regulating the expression of cyclooxygenase (COX) which then results in an increase of prostaglandin release [27]. Thus, with the reports of the inhibitory effect of cardamonin upon the release of pro-inflammatory mediators and also inhibition of both the NO and PGE_2 [13–15], we suggest that cardamonin possess antinociceptive effect in both chemical- and thermal-induced nociception models in mice.

The present study demonstrated the antinociceptive effects of cardamonin, either through intraperitoneal or oral administration, at doses that did not produce impairment of motor coordination. It showed a dose-dependent inhibition in acetic acid-induced abdominal writhing test in mice. This result support the finding on antinociceptive activity of cardamonin in PBQ-induced writhing test [20]. The acetic acid–induced abdominal writhing model has been utilized as a screening tool for the assessment of antinociceptive and also anti-inflammatory properties of potential analgesic agents [28]. Following acetic acid administration into the peritoneal cavity of the animals, chemical mediators released directly or indirectly at the free nerve endings of sensory polymodal neurons. They also reported on the increase level of prostaglandins, especially PGE_2 in the peritoneal fluid following acetic acid injection [29]. In line with the in vitro finding where cardamonin exerted inhibitory action of PGE_2 secretion and down regulation of COX-2 gene expression, we suggest that the antinociceptive mechanism of cardamonin may be linked partly to the disruption of the LOX and/or COX in the peripheral tissues, leading to decrease in PGE_2 synthesis, which then interferes with the mechanism of signal transduction in primary afferent nociceptors. It has also been previously reported that cardamonin inhibits inflammatory cytokines like TNF-α, IL-1β and IL-6 and interferes with the NF-κB signaling pathway [15] that may additionally explain the antinociceptive effects of cardamonin.

The commonly used analgesic agent NSAIDs inhibits the synthesis of prostaglandin, and in the present study, indomethacin exerted a significant inhibition in the acetic acid–induced pain model. As shown in Figure 2, cardamonin at the dose of 3 mg/kg has similar analgesic effect as indomethacin at dose 10 mg/kg. However, acetic acid–induced nociceptive model has good sensitivity but poor specificity. This is due to the suppressing effect of abdominal writhes by muscle relaxants or other types of drugs to misinterpretation of the results [30,31]. Thus, formalin-induced paw licking and hot plate test were carried out in the present study to avoid this problem.

The responses of formalin-induced paw licking is biphasic [32]. The first phase reflects the neurogenic pain whereby formalin-injected into the paw directly sensitize the C-fiber primary afferent nociceptors. The second phase is the result of inflammatory response caused by the action of inflammatory mediators, or to some extent, the central sensitization of the dorsal horn neurons [32,33]. Substance P and bradykinin was reported release during the neurogenic phase, whereas histamine, serotonin, prostaglandins and also bradykinin were involved in the inflammatory phase [34]. Centrally acting analgesics such as morphine inhibit nociception in both phases equally; in contrast, peripherally acting analgesics such as indomethacin only inhibit the second phase [33,34]. The present study indicates that cardamonin at all doses reduce paw lickings induced by formalin in both phases. Thus it was suggested that cardamonin works both centrally and peripherally, which also implies that cardamonin not only possess antinociceptive response but also anti-inflammatory activity.

In line with its centrally acting properties, cardamonin exert significant prolongation in response latency time to thermal stimuli as in the hot plate assessment. Hot plate test is a sensitive and specific thermal model for the evaluation of the involvement of central analgesic activity, or in other words supra-spinal activity [35,36]. Thus, the present study provides strong evidence that cardamonin exert centrally mediated antinociceptive activity as it decreases nociception in the first phase of formalin test and increased nociceptive threshold in the hot plate test. In addition, pre-treatment with non-selective opioid antagonist, naloxone has significantly antagonized the antinociceptive effect of cardamonin and morphine in both the formalin-induced paw licking and hot plate test. These finding suggest that the central antinociceptive mechanism of cardamonin could involve the activation of opioid receptors or modulation of the effect of endogeneous opioid peptides.

In order to further understand the antinociceptive action of cardamonin, capsaicin-induced neurogenic paw licking test was carried out. Capsaicin, the pungent ingredient of hot chili peppers, upon administered, it directly stimulates the transient receptor potential cation channel V1 ($TRPV_1$) which found on the sensory C-fibers. Capsaicin also mediates the release of excitatory amino acids (glutamate and aspartate), nitric oxide and pro-inflammatory mediators and thus transmitting the nociceptive impulses to the central spinal system [37]. In this study, cardamonin also exhibit significant reduction in nociceptive responses in capsaicin-induced paw licking assessment.

Another interesting finding of this study reveals that cardamonin exhibit significant inhibitory nociceptive response against intraplantar injection of glutamate into mouse hind paw. Glutamate-induced nociceptive responses appears to involve peripheral, spinal and supra-spinal sites of action and is mediated by both of the activation of *N*-methyl-*D*-aspartate (NMDA) and α-amino-3-hydroxyl-5-methyl-isoxazolepropionate (non-NMDA) receptors, as well as by nitric oxide release or by some NO-derived substances. The release of nitric oxide eventually increased the synthesis or release of pro-inflammatory mediators such as cytokine, reactive oxygen species (ROS) as well as prostanoids followed by enhanced inflammatory reaction [38]. The present study strongly suggests that antinociceptive activity induced by cardamonin in the glutamate test, at least in part, could be due to its interaction with the glutamatergic system or its ability to inhibit NO production.

Finally, the present study provides convincing evidence that systemic administration of cardamonin was largely devoid of significant effect on motor coordination of animals in the rota rod assessment. Therefore, the possibility of non-specific muscle relaxation and sedative effects of cardamonin-induced antinociception could be eliminated. The result of preliminary acute toxicity investigation showed that no occurrence of animal mortality over the period of observation. The study conducted qualitatively by observing signs of toxicity indicated that cardamonin have a reasonably low toxicity profile and should be regarded as safe while detailed quantitative assessments to be carried out in the future.

4. Materials and Methods

4.1. Plant Material

Five kilograms of *Boesenbergia rotunda* were purchased from the local market in Serdang, Malaysia and was authenticated by a resident botanist at the Institute of Bioscience, Universiti Putra Malaysia (IBS, UPM), Malaysia. A voucher specimen (SK1780/10) was deposited at the Herbarium,

Laboratory of Natural Products, IBS, UPM and small part of the rhizomes were cultivated at the Medicinal Plant Garden, IBS, UPM for future reference.

4.2. Extraction and Isolation

The fresh rhizomes of *B. rotunda* were sliced into small flat pieces and dried under shadow for one weak. The dried rhizomes were ground into fine powder by using domestic food processor. The dried powder 2.5 kg was dissolved in distilled methanol for two-three days. The methanolic extract was filtrate and concentrate on rotary evaporator to obtained 255 gm crude extract. The methanolic extract was subjected to solvent extraction. The crude methanolic extract was dissolved in 250 mL distilled water and transferred into separating funnel. About 150 mL hexane was added into aqueous layer and subsequently extracted with chloroform, ethyl acetate, and butanol. The chloroform layer finally passed over sodium sulfate anhydrous to remove the moisture. The chloroform extract was subjected to flash column chromatography by using ethyl acetate and hexane as eluents. Finally, the compound (Figure 6) was purified from chloroform extract and identify as cardamonin (CARD) after performing the detailed NMR spectroscopic and chromatographic methods, respectively. The purity of the compound was 98.0%.

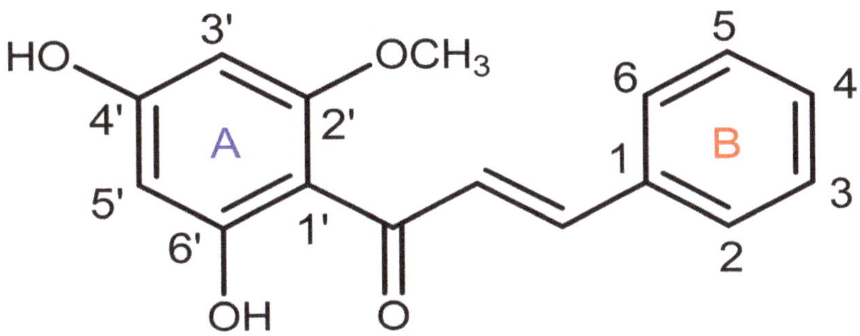

Figure 6. The chemical Structure of cardamonin.

(Cardamonin): (E)-1-(4′,6′dihydroxy-2′-methoxyphenyl)-3-phenylprop-2-en-1-one. (E)-1-(4′,6′-dihydroxy-2′-methoxyphenyl)-3-phenylprop-2-en-1-one: yellow needles crystals: m.p. 192–194 °C, EI-MS *m/z* 270.23, (molecular formula $C_{16}H_{16}O_4$). IR max (cm^{-1}, KBr disc): 3256 (OH), 1632 (C=O), 1544, 1490, 1288, 1326, 1228 cm^{-1}. ^{1}HNMR ($CDCl_3$, 500 MHz): δ 7.92 (d, 1H, J = 15.5 Hz, Hβ), 7.80 (d, 1H, J = 15.5 Hz, Hα), 7.62 (br, d, 2H, H-2,6), 7.46 (m, 3H, H-3,4,5), 6.12 (br, s, 1H, H-3′), 5.98 (br, s, 1H, H-5′), 3.85 (s, 3H, OMe, C-2′). int.): *m/z* 270 ([M^+], 269 (54), 253 (5), 193 (100), 131 (35, 103 (39), 77 (32).

4.3. Experimental Animals

All animal care and the antinociceptive experimental procedures performed were in accordance with the ethical guidelines for investigations of experimental pain in conscious animals (Zimmermann, 1983) and approved by the Animal Care Unit Committee (ACUC), Faculty of Medicine and Health Sciences, Universiti Putra Malaysia (UPM/FPSK/PADS/BR-UUH/00425). The antinociceptive experiments were carried out using male ICR mice (20–30 g). They were housed in groups of 10 per cage and maintained on a 12/12-h light/dark cycle (lights were switched on at 06:00 h), at the animal house facility, Faculty of Medicine and Health Sciences, Universiti Putra Malaysia. Food and water were available ad libitum, except during the experimental procedure. The animals were habituated to the condition of the laboratory at least 2 h before testing and were used only once throughout the experiments. The number of animals and intensities of noxious stimuli used were the minimum necessary to demonstrate consistent effects of drug treatments. All efforts were made to minimize animal suffering. At the end of the experiments, the animals were anesthetized and euthanized by cervical dislocation. In all experiments, data were collected by a blinded, randomized, and controlled design.

4.4. Drugs and Chemicals

Tween 20, absolute ethanol, acetic acid, formalin, morphine hydrochloride, naloxone, indomethacin, diazepam, capsaicin, capsazepine, and glutamate were purchased from Sigma Chemical Co. (St. Louis, MO, USA). All drugs used were dissolved in physiological saline (0.9% NaCl). Cardamonin and indomethacin were dissolved in ethanol, Tween 20 and distilled water in 5:5:90 (*v*/*v*/*v*) fractions. Respective controls received only solvent vehicle, whereby it had no effect per se on nociceptive responses. All drugs, chemicals, and CARD solutions were freshly prepared and administered intraperitoneally (i.p.) in a volume of 10 mL/kg, unless otherwise stated in the method.

4.5. Evaluation of the Antinociceptive Activity

4.5.1. Acetic Acid–Induced Abdominal Writhing Test

The acetic acid–induced abdominal writhing test was conducted as previously described [39]. Mice were pre-treated with CARD (0.3, 1, 3 and 10 mg/kg; i.p.), 30 min prior to injection of 0.6% acetic acid (10 mL/kg; i.p.). Indomethacin (10 mg/kg) was used as reference drug and was administered by i.p. route, 30 min before the nociceptive agent. Following the injection of acetic acid, the animals were immediately placed into a perspex chamber, and the number of writhing was recorded for 30 min, starting from 5 min post-injection. Antinociceptive activity of CARD was expressed as a reduction in the mean number of abdominal writhes in the group pre-treated with CARD compared with the control group.

4.5.2. Formalin-Induced Paw Licking Test

The formalin-induced paw licking test was carried out as previously described [40]. Mice used were individually adapted in an observation chamber made of transparent acrylic. CARD (0.3, 1, 3, and 10 mg/kg; i.p.) or vehicle (10 mL/kg; i.p.) was administered 30 min before the formalin injection. Indomethacin (10 mg/kg; i.p.) and morphine (5 mg/kg; s.c.) were used as positive control drug and were administered 30 min and 1 h before the test. After 30 min, 20 μL of 2.5% of formalin solution (*v*/*v* in distilled water) was injected subcutaneously into the ventral surface of the right hind paw of the mice. The amount of time (in seconds) spent on licking and biting the injected paw was recorded up to 35 min after formalin injection as an indicator of nociceptive behavior. The initial nociceptive scores normally peaked at 0–5 min (early phase) and 15–35 min (late phase) after formalin injection, representing the neurogenic and inflammatory pain responses, respectively.

4.5.3. Hot Plate Test

The antinociceptive property of cardamonin for thermal noxious stimuli was evaluated according to the method described previously [41]. The metal surface of the hot plate (Model 7280, Ugo Basile, VA, Italy) was set and maintained at temperature of 52 ± 0.2 °C. Mice were then placed into the Plexiglas cylinder on the heated metal surface individually and the time elapsed between placement and licking the forepaws, or jumping were recorded as response latency time. The reaction time was recorded before and at 30, 60, 90, 120, 180 and 210 min after administration of cardamonin (0.3, 1, 3, and 10 mg/kg; i.p.) or vehicle (10 mL/kg; i.p.). Morphine (5 mg/kg; s.c.) was used as a reference drug. A cut-off time of 20 s was defined as complete analgesia and to avoid tissue damage.

4.6. Investigation of the Mechanisms of Action

4.6.1. Involvement of the $TRPV_1$ Receptor

The involvement of $TRPV_1$ in antinociceptive activity by CARD was investigated by using capsaicin-induced paw licking model. The procedure implemented was similar to that described previously [42]. Mice were pre-treated with CARD (0.3, 1, 3, and 10 mg/kg; i.p.), capsazepine (0.17 mmol/kg; i.p.), indomethacin (10 mg/kg; i.p.) or vehicle (10 mL/kg; i.p.) prior to injection of

20 μL of capsaicin (1.6 μg/paw) intraplantarly (i.pl) into the ventral surface of the right hind paw of the mice. The animals were observed individually for 5 min after capsaicin injection. The amount of time spent licking the injected paw was recorded and was considered as an indication of pain behavior.

4.6.2. Involvement of the Glutamate Receptor

The participation of glutamate receptor in antinociceptive activity by cardamonin was investigated through glutamate-induced paw licking model. The experiment was carried out as previously described [38]. Mice were pre-treated with CARD (0.3, 1, 3, and 10 mg/kg; i.p.), indomethacin (10 mg/kg; i.p.) or vehicle (10 mL/kg; i.p.). After 30 min, 20 μL of glutamate (10 μmol/paw; i.pl.) was injected into the ventral surface of right hind paw of the mice. The mice were then observed individually for 15 min after glutamate injection. The amount of time spent licking the glutamate-injected paw was recorded and was considered as an indication of pain behavior.

4.6.3. Involvement of the Opioid Receptors

To investigate the possible involvement of the opioid system in the antinociceptive activity of cardamonin, separate groups of mice were pre-treated with the non-selective opioid receptor antagonist, naloxone (5 mg/kg; i.p.) 15 min prior to the administration of cardamonin (1 mg/kg; i.p.), morphine (5 mg/kg; s.c.) or vehicle (10 mL/kg; i.p.). After 30 min (for i.p. administration) and 60 min (for s.c. administration), the mice were subjected to the formalin-induced paw licking test and hot plate test [42].

4.7. Toxicity Assessment

The acute toxicity study was conducted to assess the toxicity of cardamonin as described previously [41]. Animals were fasted overnight prior to the test with free access to water ad libitum. Mice were divided into groups and were administered with experimental doses of cardamonin (0.3, 1, 3 and 10 mg/kg) orally (p.o.) and intraperitoneally (i.p.). The control group received the vehicle (10 mL/kg). After administration of cardamonin, the animals were observed for 4 h for any abnormal behaviors, respiratory distress, motor impairment, sedation, and hyper-excitability qualitatively. In addition, any incidence of mortality was recorded up to 24 h after administration of cardamonin. Animals were given free access to standard pellet and water throughout the study.

4.8. Motor Coordination Test

Rota-rod test was conducted to investigate the possible sedative and motor-coordination effect of cardamonin. The method employed was similar to that described previously with slight modification [43]. Mice that successfully remain on the revolving bar of the rota rod apparatus (Model 7600, Ugo Basile) revolving at a speed of 20 rounds per min for two consecutive periods of 60 s were selected 24 h prior to the test. The selected mice were administered with cardamonin (10 mg/kg; i.p.), vehicle (10 mL/kg; i.p.) or diazepam (4 mg/kg; i.p.) 30 min prior to the experiment. Motor performance was evaluated as the latency of permanence(s) on the revolving bar up to 120 s at the time of 30, 60, and 90 s after the treatment. The average time of the animals remain on the revolving bar was recorded.

4.9. Statistical Analysis

The data collected was expressed as mean ± S.E.M. obtained from 6 animals per group and analyzed using one-way ANOVA followed by Dunnett's post hoc test, unless otherwise stated. The differences between means were considered as statistically significant at $p < 0.05$. The experimental ED_{50} (effective dose producing a 50% reduction in abdominal writhes) and its 95% confidence intervals (CI) were determined by linear regression using GraphPad Prism (Version 5, GraphPad Software,

La Jolla, CA, USA). The percentages of inhibition were calculated by comparing the results of treatment group with control group.

5. Conclusions

In conclusion, the present study demonstrated that systemic administration of cardamonin at a dose which does not cause any toxic effects and interference of motor co-ordination exerted significant peripheral and central antinociception when assessed in the chemical- and thermal-induced nociception test models in mice through the involvement of $TRPV_1$, glutamate, and opioid receptors. The precise mechanism underlying the antinociceptive activity of cardamonin remains to be investigated. Currently, a study to determine the possible mechanism(s) of action responsible for cardamonin-induced antinociceptive activity is in progress.

Author Contributions: Conceptualization, M.R.S., E.K.P., A.A., D.A.I.A. and C.P.P.; Methodology, C.P.P.; Software, C.P.P.; Validation, T.A.S.T.M., M.N.A., E.K.P., and A.A.; Formal Analysis, C.P.P.; Investigation, C.P.P.; Resources, T.A.S.T.M., M.N.A., E.K.P., A.A., D.A.I.A. and M.R.S.; Data Curation, All authors; Writing-Original Draft Preparation, All authors; Writing-Review & Editing, All authors; Visualization, All authors; Supervision, T.A.S.T.M., M.N.A., E.K.P., A.A., D.A.I.A. and M.R.S.; Project Administration, M.R.S.; Funding Acquisition, M.R.S.

Acknowledgments: The authors would like to thank the Faculty of Medicine and Health Sciences and Institute of Bioscience, Universiti Putra Malaysia, for providing the necessary support for this study.

References

1. Bheemasankara, R.C.; Namosiva, R.T.; Suryaprakasam, S. Cardamonin and alpinetin from the seeds of *Amomum subulatum*. *Planta Medica* **1976**, *29*, 391–392.
2. Pascoal, A.C.; Ehrenfried, C.A.; Lopez, B.G.; de Araujo, T.M.; Pascoal, V.D.; Gilioli, R.; Anhe, G.F.; Ruiz, A.L.; Carvalho, J.E.; Stefanello, M.E. Antiproliferative Activity and Induction of Apoptosis in PC-3 Cells by the Chalcone Cardamonin from *Campomanesia adamantium* (Myrtaceae) in a Bioactivity-Guided Study. *Molecules* **2014**, *19*, 1843. [CrossRef] [PubMed]
3. Qin, Y.; Sun, C.-Y.; Lu, F.-R.; Shu, X.-R.; Yang, D.; Chen, L.; She, X.-M.; Gregg, N.M.; Guo, T.; Hu, Y. Cardamonin exerts potent activity against multiple myeloma through blockade of NF-κB pathway in vitro. *Leuk. Res.* **2012**, *36*, 514–520. [CrossRef] [PubMed]
4. Tang, Y.; Fang, Q.; Shi, D.; Niu, P.; Chen, Y.; Deng, J. mTOR inhibition of cardamonin on antiproliferation of A549 cells is involved in a FKBP12 independent fashion. *Life Sci.* **2014**, *99*, 44–51. [CrossRef] [PubMed]
5. Wei, Z.; Yang, J.; Xia, Y.F.; Huang, W.Z.; Wang, Z.T.; Dai, Y. Cardamonin protects septic mice from acute lung injury by preventing endothelial barrier dysfunction. *J. Biochem. Mol. Toxicol.* **2012**, *26*, 282–290. [CrossRef] [PubMed]
6. El-Naga, R.N. Pre-treatment with cardamonin protects against cisplatin-induced nephrotoxicity in rats: Impact on NOX-1, inflammation and apoptosis. *Toxicol. Appl. Pharmacol.* **2014**, *274*, 87–95. [CrossRef] [PubMed]
7. Jantan, I.; Raweh, S.M.; Sirat, H.M.; Jamil, S.; Mohd Yasin, Y.H.; Jalil, J.; Jamal, J.A. Inhibitory effect of compounds from Zingiberaceae species on human platelet aggregation. *Phytomedicine* **2008**, *15*, 306–309. [CrossRef] [PubMed]
8. Wang, Z.-T.; Lau, C.-W.; Chan, F.L.; Yao, X.; Chen, Z.-Y.; He, Z.-D.; Huang, Y. Vasorelaxant effects of cardamonin and alpinetin from *Alpinia henryi* K. Schum. *J. Cardiovasc. Pharmacol.* **2001**, *37*, 596–606. [CrossRef] [PubMed]
9. Liao, Q.; Shi, D.-H.; Zheng, W.; Xu, X.-J.; Yu, Y.-H. Antiproliferation of cardamonin is involved in mTOR on aortic smooth muscle cells in high fructose-induced insulin resistance rats. *Eur. J. Pharmacol.* **2010**, *641*, 179–186. [CrossRef] [PubMed]
10. Zhang, T.; Yamamoto, N.; Yamashita, Y.; Ashida, H. The chalcones cardamonin and flavokawain B inhibit the differentiation of preadipocytes to adipocytes by activating ERK. *Arch. Biochem. Biophys.* **2014**, *554*, 44–54. [CrossRef] [PubMed]

11. Cho, M.; Ryu, M.; Jeong, Y.; Chung, Y.-H.; Kim, D.-E.; Cho, H.-S.; Kang, S.; Han, J.-S.; Chang, M.-Y.; Lee, C.-K.; et al. Cardamonin suppresses melanogenesis by inhibition of Wnt/β-catenin signaling. *Biochem. Biophys. Res. Commun.* **2009**, *390*, 500–505. [CrossRef] [PubMed]
12. Park, M.K.; Choi, J.K.; Kim, H.J.; Nakahata, N.; Lim, K.M.; Kim, S.Y.; Lee, C.H. Novel inhibitory effects of cardamonin on thromboxane A_2-induced scratching response: Blocking of Gh/transglutaminase-2 binding to thromboxane A_2 receptor. *Pharmacol. Biochem. Behav.* **2014**, *126*, 131–135. [CrossRef] [PubMed]
13. Ahmad, S.; Israf, D.A.; Lajis, N.H.; Shaari, K.; Mohamed, H.; Wahab, A.A.; Ariffin, K.T.; Hoo, W.Y.; Aziz, N.A.; Kadir, A.A.; et al. Cardamonin, inhibits pro-inflammatory mediators in activated RAW 264.7 cells and whole blood. *Eur. J. Pharmacol.* **2006**, *538*, 188–194. [CrossRef] [PubMed]
14. Israf, D.A.; Khaizurin, T.A.; Syahida, A.; Lajis, N.H.; Khozirah, S. Cardamonin inhibits COX and iNOS expression via inhibition of p65NF-κB nuclear translocation and κ-B phosphorylation in RAW 264.7 macrophage cells. *Mol. Immunol.* **2007**, *44*, 673–679. [CrossRef] [PubMed]
15. Chow, Y.-L.; Lee, K.-H.; Vidyadaran, S.; Lajis, N.H.; Akhtar, M.N.; Israf, D.A.; Syahida, A. Cardamonin from *Alpinia rafflesiana* inhibits inflammatory responses in IFN-γ/LPS-stimulated BV2 microglia via NF-κB signalling pathway. *Int. Immunopharmacol.* **2012**, *12*, 657–665. [CrossRef] [PubMed]
16. Menghini, L.; Ferrante, C.; Leporini, L.; Recinella, L.; Chiavaroli, A.; Leone, S.; Pintore, G.; Vacca, M.; Orlando, G.; Brunetti, L. An hydroalcoholic chamomile extract modulates inflammatory and immune response in HT29 cells and isolated rat colon. *Phytother. Res.* **2016**, *30*, 1513–1518. [CrossRef] [PubMed]
17. Locatelli, M.; Macchione, N.; Ferrante, C.; Chiavaroli, A.; Recinella, L.; Carradori, S.; Zengin, G.; Cesa, S.; Leporini, L.; Leone, S. Graminex Pollen: Phenolic Pattern, Colorimetric Analysis and Protective Effects in Immortalized Prostate Cells (PC3) and Rat Prostate Challenged with LPS. *Molecules* **2018**, *23*, e1145. [CrossRef] [PubMed]
18. Takahashi, A.; Yamamoto, N.; Murakami, A. Cardamonin suppresses nitric oxide production via blocking the IFN-γ/STAT pathway in endotoxin-challenged peritoneal macrophages of ICR mice. *Life Sci.* **2011**, *89*, 337–342. [CrossRef] [PubMed]
19. Schmidtko, A.; Tegeder, I.; Geisslinger, G. No NO, no pain? The role of nitric oxide and cGMP in spinal pain processing. *Trends Neurosci.* **2009**, *32*, 339–346. [CrossRef] [PubMed]
20. Park, M.K.; Lee, H.J.; Choi, J.K.; Kim, H.J.; Kang, J.H.; Lee, E.J.; Kim, Y.R.; Kang, J.H.; Yoo, J.K.; Cho, H.Y.; et al. Novel anti-nociceptive effects of cardamonin via blocking expression of cyclooxygenase-2 and transglutaminase-2. *Pharmacol. Biochem. Behav.* **2014**, *118*, 10–15. [CrossRef] [PubMed]
21. Cardosa, M.; Osman, Z.J.; Nicholas, M.; Tonkin, L.; Williams, A.; Aziz, K.A.; Ali, R.M.; Dahari, N.M. Self-management of chronic pain in Malaysian patients: Effectiveness trial with 1-year follow-up. *Transl. Behav. Med.* **2012**, *2*, 30–37. [CrossRef] [PubMed]
22. Zaki, L.R.M.; Hairi, N.N. Chronic pain and pattern of health care utilization among Malaysian elderly population: National Health and Morbidity Survey III (NHMS III, 2006). *Maturitas* **2014**, *79*, 435–441. [CrossRef] [PubMed]
23. Williams, M.; Kowaluk, E.A.; Arneric, S.P. Emerging molecular approaches to pain therapy. *J. Med. Chem.* **1999**, *42*, 1481. [CrossRef] [PubMed]
24. Smith, M.D.; Wang, Y.; Cudnik, M.; Smith, D.A.; Pakiela, J.; Emerman, C.L. The Effectiveness and Adverse Events of Morphine versus Fentanyl on a Physician-staffed Helicopter. *J. Emerg. Med.* **2012**, *43*, 69–75. [CrossRef] [PubMed]
25. Sostres, C.; Gargallo, C.J.; Arroyo, M.T.; Lanas, A. Adverse effects of non-steroidal anti-inflammatory drugs (NSAIDs, aspirin and coxibs) on upper gastrointestinal tract. *Best Pract. Res. Clin. Gastroenterol.* **2010**, *24*, 121–132. [CrossRef] [PubMed]
26. Chen, Y.; Boettger, M.K.; Reif, A.; Schmitt, A.; Uceyler, N.; Sommer, C. Nitric oxide synthase modulates CFA-induced thermal hyperalgesia through cytokine regulation in mice. *Mol. Pain* **2010**, *6*, 1–11. [CrossRef] [PubMed]
27. Cury, Y.; Picolo, G.; Gutierrez, V.P.; Ferreira, S.H. Pain and analgesia: The dual effect of nitric oxide in the nociceptive system. *Nitric Oxide* **2011**, *25*, 243–254. [CrossRef] [PubMed]
28. De Souza, M.M.; Pereira, M.A.; Ardenghi, J.V.; Mora, T.C.; Bresciani, L.F.; Yunes, R.A.; Monache, F.D.; Cechinel Filho, V. Filicene obtained from *Adiantumcuneatum* interacts with the cholinergic, dopaminergic, glutamatergic, GABAergic, and tachykinergic systems to exert antinociceptive effect in mice. *Pharmacol. Biochem. Behav.* **2009**, *93*, 40–46. [CrossRef] [PubMed]

29. Deraedt, R.; Jouquey, S.; Delevallee, F.; Flahaut, M. Release of prostaglandins E and F in an algogenic reaction and its inhibition. *Eur. J. Pharmacol.* **1980**, *61*, 17–24. [CrossRef]
30. Ikeda, Y.; Ueno, A.; Naraba, H.; Oh-ishi, S. Involvement of vanilloid receptor VR1 and prostanoids in the acid-induced writhing responses of mice. *Life Sci.* **2001**, *69*, 2911–2919. [CrossRef]
31. Le Bars, D.; Gozariu, M.; Cadden, S.W. Animal models of nociception. *Pharmacol. Rev.* **2001**, *53*, 597–652. [PubMed]
32. Omote, K.; Kawamata, T.; Kawamata, M.; Namiki, A. Formalin-induced release of excitatory amino acids in the skin of the rat hindpaw. *Brain Res.* **1998**, *787*, 161–164. [CrossRef]
33. Hunskaar, S.; Hole, K. The formalin test in mice: Dissociation between inflammatory and non-inflammatory pain. *Pain* **1987**, *30*, 103–114. [CrossRef]
34. Shibata, M.; Ohkubo, T.; Takahashi, H.; Inoki, R. Modified formalin test: Characteristic biphasic pain response. *Pain* **1989**, *38*, 347–352. [CrossRef]
35. Abbott, F.V.; Melzack, R. Brainstem lesions dissociate neural mechanisms of morphine analgesia in different kinds of pain. *Brain Res.* **1982**, *251*, 149–155. [CrossRef]
36. Nemirovsky, A.; Chen, L.; Zelman, V.; Jurna, I. The antinociceptive effect of the combination of spinal morphine with systemic morphine or buprenorphine. *Anesthesia Analg.* **2001**, *93*, 197–203. [CrossRef]
37. Sakurada, T.; Matsumura, T.; Moriyama, T.; Sakurada, C.; Ueno, S.; Sakurada, S. Differential effects of intraplantar capsazepine and ruthenium red on capsaicin-induced desensitization in mice. *Pharmacol. Biochem. Behav.* **2003**, *75*, 115–121. [CrossRef]
38. Beirith, A.; Santos, A.R.S.; Calixto, J.B. Mechanisms underlying the nociception and paw oedema caused by injection of glutamate into the mouse paw. *Brain Res.* **2002**, *924*, 219–228. [CrossRef]
39. Sulaiman, M.R.; Tengku Mohamad, T.A.; Shaik Mossadeq, W.M.; Moin, S.; Yusof, M.; Mokhtar, A.F.; Zakaria, Z.A.; Israf, D.A.; Lajis, N. Antinociceptive activity of the essential oil of *Zingiber zerumbet*. *Planta Medica* **2010**, *76*, 107. [CrossRef] [PubMed]
40. Mohamad, A.S.; Akhtar, M.N.; Zakaria, Z.A.; Perimal, E.K.; Khalid, S.; Mohd, P.A.; Khalid, M.H.; Israf, D.A.; Lajis, N.H.; Sulaiman, M.R. Antinociceptive activity of a synthetic chalcone, flavokawin B on chemical and thermal models of nociception in mice. *Eur. J. Pharmacol.* **2010**, *647*, 103–109. [CrossRef] [PubMed]
41. Ong, H.M.; Mohamad, A.S.; Makhtar, N.; Khalid, M.H.; Khalid, S.; Perimal, E.K.; Mastuki, S.N.; Zakaria, Z.A.; Lajis, N.; Israf, D.A. Antinociceptive activity of methanolic extract of *Acmella uliginosa* (Sw.) Cass. *J. Ethnopharmacol.* **2011**, *133*, 227–233. [CrossRef] [PubMed]
42. Ming-Tatt, L.; Khalivulla, S.I.; Akhtar, M.N.; Mohamad, A.S.; Perimal, E.K.; Khalid, M.H.; Akira, A.; Lajis, N.; Israf, D.A.; Sulaiman, M.R. Antinociceptive activity of a synthetic curcuminoid analogue, 2, 6-bis-(4-hydroxy-3-methoxybenzylidene) cyclohexanone, on nociception-induced models in mice. *Basic Clin. Pharmacol. Toxicol.* **2012**, *110*, 275–282. [CrossRef] [PubMed]
43. Perimal, E.K.; Akhtar, M.N.; Mohamad, A.S.; Khalid, M.H.; Ming, O.H.; Khalid, S.; Tatt, L.M.; Kamaldin, M.N.; Zakaria, Z.A.; Israf, D.A. Zerumbone-induced antinociception: Involvement of the L-arginine-nitric oxide-cGMP-PKC-K^+ ATP channel pathways. *Basic Clin. Pharmacol. Toxicol.* **2011**, *108*, 155–162. [CrossRef] [PubMed]

Permissions

All chapters in this book were first published by MDPI; hereby published with permission under the Creative Commons Attribution License or equivalent. Every chapter published in this book has been scrutinized by our experts. Their significance has been extensively debated. The topics covered herein carry significant findings which will fuel the growth of the discipline. They may even be implemented as practical applications or may be referred to as a beginning point for another development.

The contributors of this book come from diverse backgrounds, making this book a truly international effort. This book will bring forth new frontiers with its revolutionizing research information and detailed analysis of the nascent developments around the world.

We would like to thank all the contributing authors for lending their expertise to make the book truly unique. They have played a crucial role in the development of this book. Without their invaluable contributions this book wouldn't have been possible. They have made vital efforts to compile up to date information on the varied aspects of this subject to make this book a valuable addition to the collection of many professionals and students.

This book was conceptualized with the vision of imparting up-to-date information and advanced data in this field. To ensure the same, a matchless editorial board was set up. Every individual on the board went through rigorous rounds of assessment to prove their worth. After which they invested a large part of their time researching and compiling the most relevant data for our readers.

The editorial board has been involved in producing this book since its inception. They have spent rigorous hours researching and exploring the diverse topics which have resulted in the successful publishing of this book. They have passed on their knowledge of decades through this book. To expedite this challenging task, the publisher supported the team at every step. A small team of assistant editors was also appointed to further simplify the editing procedure and attain best results for the readers.

Apart from the editorial board, the designing team has also invested a significant amount of their time in understanding the subject and creating the most relevant covers. They scrutinized every image to scout for the most suitable representation of the subject and create an appropriate cover for the book.

The publishing team has been an ardent support to the editorial, designing and production team. Their endless efforts to recruit the best for this project, has resulted in the accomplishment of this book. They are a veteran in the field of academics and their pool of knowledge is as vast as their experience in printing. Their expertise and guidance has proved useful at every step. Their uncompromising quality standards have made this book an exceptional effort. Their encouragement from time to time has been an inspiration for everyone.

The publisher and the editorial board hope that this book will prove to be a valuable piece of knowledge for researchers, students, practitioners and scholars across the globe.

List of Contributors

B. Angélica Pilón-Jiménez, Fernanda I. Saldívar-González, Bárbara I. Díaz-Eufracio and José L. Medina-Franco
Department of Pharmacy, National Autonomous University of Mexico, Mexico City 04510, Mexico

Elena Lucarini, Laura Micheli, Carmen Parisio, Lorenzo Di Cesare Mannelli and Carla Ghelardini
Department of Neuroscience, Psychology, Drug Research and Child Health—NEUROFARBA—Pharmacology and Toxicology Section, University of Florence, 50139 Florence, Italy

Eleonora Pagnotta, Roberto Matteo and Luca Lazzeri
CREA-Council for Agricultural Research and Economics, Research Centre for Cereal and Industrial Crops, 40128 Bologna, Italy

Lara Testai, Alma Martelli and Vincenzo Calderone
Department of Pharmacy, University of Pisa, 56126 Pisa, Italy
Interdepartmental Research Centre "Nutraceuticals and Food for Health (NUTRAFOOD)", University of Pisa, 56126 Pisa, Italy
Interdepartmental Research Centre of Ageing Biology and Pathology, University of Pisa, 56126 Pisa, Italy

Aldo Tava and Luciano Pecetti
CREA Research Centre for Animal Production and Aquaculture, viale Piacenza 29, 26900 Lodi, Italy

Łukasz Pecio and Anna Stochmal
Department of Biochemistry and Crop Quality, Institute of Soil Science and Plant Cultivation, State Research Institute, ul. Czartoryskich 8, 24-100 Pulawy, Poland

Roberto Lo Scalzo
CREA Research Centre for Engineering and Agro-Food Processing, via G. Venezian 26, 20133 Milano, Italy

María L. Del Prado-Audelo
Laboratorio de Posgrado en Tecnología Farmacéutica, FES-Cuautitlán, Universidad Nacional Autónoma de México, Cuautitlán Izcalli 54740, Mexico

Isaac H. Caballero-Florán
Departamento de Fisiología, Biofísica & Neurociencias, Centro de Investigación y de Estudios Avanzados del Instituto Politécnico Nacional, Ciudad de México 07360, Mexico
Departamento de Farmacia, Facultad de Química, Universidad Nacional Autónoma de México, Ciudad Universitaria, Circuito Exterior S/N, Del. Coyoacán, C.P. Ciudad de México 04510, Mexico

Jorge A. Meza-Toledo
Departamento de Farmacia, Facultad de Química, Universidad Nacional Autónoma de México, Ciudad Universitaria, Circuito Exterior S/N, Del. Coyoacán, C.P. Ciudad de México 04510, Mexico
Escuela de Ciencias de la Salud, Universidad del Valle de México, Campus Coyoacán, Ciudad de México, 04910, Mexico

Néstor Mendoza-Muñoz
Facultad de Ciencias Químicas, Universidad de Colima, C.P. Colima 28400, México

Maykel González-Torres
CONACyT-Laboratorio de Biotecnología, Instituto Nacional de Rehabilitación Luis Guillermo Ibarra Ibarra, Ciudad de México 14389, Mexico
Instituto Tecnológico y de Estudios Superiores de Monterrey, Campus Ciudad de México 14380, Mexico

Benjamín Florán
Departamento de Fisiología, Biofísica & Neurociencias, Centro de Investigación y de Estudios Avanzados del Instituto Politécnico Nacional, Ciudad de México 07360, Mexico

Hernán Cortés
Laboratorio de Medicina Genómica, Departamento de Genética, Instituto Nacional de Rehabilitación Luis Guillermo Ibarra Ibarra, Ciudad de México 14389, Mexico

Gerardo Leyva-Gómez
Departamento de Farmacia, Facultad de Química, Universidad Nacional Autónoma de México, Ciudad Universitaria, Circuito Exterior S/N, Del. Coyoacán, C.P. Ciudad de México 04510, Mexico

Ping Zhao
Institute for Medical Biology & Hubei Provincial Key Laboratory for Protection and Application of Special Plants in the Wuling Area of China, College of Life Sciences, South-Central University for Nationalities, Wuhan 430074, China
National Demonstration Center for Experimental Ethnopharmacology Education, South-Central University for Nationalities, Wuhan 430074, China

Qian Ming, Junying Qiu, Di Tian, Jia Liu, Jinhua Shen and Qing-Hua Liu
Institute for Medical Biology & Hubei Provincial Key Laboratory for Protection and Application of Special Plants in the Wuling Area of China, College of Life Sciences, South-Central University for Nationalities, Wuhan 430074, China

Xinzhou Yang
National Demonstration Center for Experimental Ethnopharmacology Education, South-Central University for Nationalities, Wuhan 430074, China
School of Pharmaceutical Sciences, South-Central University for Nationalities, 182 Min-Zu Road, Wuhan 430074, China

Tong Zhang, De-Hua Duan, Yi-Hao Zhang and Ying Chang
College of Life Science, Northeast Agricultural University, Harbin 150030, China

Li Wang and Sheng-Xiong Huang
State Key Laboratory of Phytochemistry and Plant Resources in West China, Kunming Institute of Botany, Chinese Academy of Sciences, Kunming 650201, China

Laetitia Bocquet, Sevser Sahpaz, Natacha Bonneau, Jennifer Samaillie, Vincent Roumy, Justine Jacquin, Simon Bordage, Thierry Hennebelle and Céline Rivière
EA 7394—ICV, Charles Viollette Research Institute, SFR Condorcet FR CNRS 3417, Univ. Lille, INRA, ISA-Yncréa, Univ. Artois, Univ. Littoral Côte d'Opale, 3 rue du Professeur Laguesse, 59000 Lille, France

Claire Beaufay and Joëlle Quetin-Leclercq
Pharmacognosy Research group, Louvain Drug Research Institute, Université Catholique de Louvain, 1200 Brussels, Belgium

Séverine Mahieux and Christel Neut
U995—LIRIC, Lille Inflammation Research International Center, Univ. Lille, Inserm, CHU Lille, 59000 Lille, France

Feng Chai
U1008—Controlled Drug Delivery Systems and Biomaterials, Univ. Lille, Inserm, CHU Lille, 59000 Lille, France

Juan Carlos Sánchez-Salgado
Instituto de Medicina Molecular y Ciencias Avanzadas, Mexico City 01900, Mexico
Facultad de Farmacia, Universidad Autónoma del Estado de Morelos, Cuernavaca, MOR 62209, Mexico

Samuel Estrada-Soto and Sara García-Jiménez
Facultad de Farmacia, Universidad Autónoma del Estado de Morelos, Cuernavaca, MOR 62209, Mexico

Sergio Montes
Instituto Nacional de Neurología y Neurocirugía, Mexico City 14269, Mexico

Jaime Gómez-Zamudio
Unidad de Investigación Médica en Bioquímica, Hospital de Especialidades, Centro Médico Nacional Siglo XXI, IMSS, México City 06720, Mexico

Rafael Villalobos-Molina
Unidad de Biomedicina, Facultad de Estudios Superiores-Iztacala, Universidad Nacional Autónoma de México, Tlalnepantla 54090, Mexico
Departamento de Bioquímica, Facultad de Medicina, Universidad Nacional Autónoma de México, Ciudad de México 04510, México

Antonio Francioso
Department of Bioorganic Chemistry, Leibniz Institute of Plant Biochemistry, 06120 Halle (Saale), Germany
Department of Biochemical Sciences "A. Rossi Fanelli", Sapienza University of Rome, 00185 Roma, Italy
Department of Plant Biology, Faculty of Biology, University of Havana, 10 200 La Habana, Cuba

Katrin Franke, Wolfgang Brandt and Ludger Wessjohann
Department of Bioorganic Chemistry, Leibniz Institute of Plant Biochemistry, 06120 Halle (Saale), Germany

Luciana Mosca and Maria D'Erme
Department of Biochemical Sciences "A. Rossi Fanelli", Sapienza University of Rome, 00185 Roma, Italy

Angel Sanchez-Lamar
Department of Plant Biology, Faculty of Biology, University of Havana, 10 200 La Habana, Cuba

Claudio Villani
Department of Chemistry and Technology of Drugs, Sapienza University of Rome, 00185 Roma, Italy

Stefan Frischbutter
Department of Dermatology and Allergy, Charité, Universitätsmedizin Berlin, 10117 Berlin, Germany
German Rheumatism Research Centre, a Leibniz Institute, 10117 Berlin, Germany

Pinarosa Avato and Maria Pia Argentieri
Dipartimento di Farmacia-Scienze del Farmaco, Università degli Studi di Bari Aldo Moro, via Orabona 4, 70125 Bari, Italy

Fernando D. Prieto-Martínez and José L. Medina-Franco
Facultad de Química, Departamento de Farmacia, Universidad Nacional Autónoma de México, Avenida Universidad 3000, Mexico City 04510, Mexico

Dwi Yuli Pujiastuti, Muhamad Nur Ghoyatul Amin and Mochammad Amin Alamsjah
Department of Marine, Faculty of Fisheries and Marine, Universitas Airlangga, Surabaya 60115, Indonesia

Jue-Liang Hsu
Department of Biological Science and Technology, National Pingtung University of Science and Technology, Pingtung 91201, Taiwan
Research Center for Austronesian Medicine and Agriculture, National Pingtung University of Science and Technology, Pingtung 91201, Taiwan

Chung Pui Ping, Tengku Azam Shah Tengku Mohamad, Enoch Kumar Perimal and Ahmad Akira
Department of Biomedical Sciences, Faculty of Medicine and Health Sciences, Universiti Putra Malaysia Selangor, Serdang 43400, Malaysia

Muhammad Nadeem Akhtar
Laboratory of Natural Products, Institute of Bioscience, Universiti Putra Malaysia, Selangor, Serdang 43400, Malaysia

Daud Ahmad Israf Ali and Mohd Roslan Sulaiman
Department of Biomedical Sciences, Faculty of Medicine and Health Sciences, Universiti Putra Malaysia Selangor, Serdang 43400, Malaysia
Faculty of Industrial Sciences & Technology, University Malaysia Pahang, Pahang, Gambang 26300, Malaysia

Index

www.ingramcontent.com/pod-product-compliance
Lightning Source LLC
LaVergne TN
LVHW060551210926
848485LV00005B/1295